Neuropsychological Explorations of Memory and Cognition

Essays in Honor of Nelson Butters

CRITICAL ISSUES IN NEUROPSYCHOLOGY

Series Editors

Antonio E. Puente
University of North Carolina, Wilmington

Cecil R. Reynolds
Texas A&M University

Current Volumes in this Series

BEHAVIORAL INTERVENTIONS WITH BRAIN-INJURED CHILDREN
A. MacNeil Horton, Jr.

CLINICAL NEUROPSYCHOLOGICAL ASSESSMENT
A Cognitive Approach
Edited by Robert L. Mapou and Jack Spector

NEUROPSYCHOLOGICAL EVALUATION OF THE
SPANISH SPEAKER
Alfredo Ardila, Monica Rosselli, and Antonio E. Puente

NEUROPSYCHOLOGICAL EXPLORATIONS OF
MEMORY AND COGNITION:
Essays in Honor of Nelson Butters
Edited by Laird S. Cermak

NEUROPSYCHOLOGICAL TOXICOLOGY
Identification and Assessment of Human Neurotoxic Syndromes,
Second Edition
David E. Hartman

THE NEUROPSYCHOLOGY OF ATTENTION
Ronald A. Cohen

A PRACTICAL GUIDE TO HEAD INJURY REHABILITATION:
A Focus on Postacute Residential Treatment
Michael D. Wesolowski and Arnie H. Zencius

PRACTITIONER'S GUIDE TO CLINICAL NEUROPSYCHOLOGY
Robert M. Anderson, Jr.

REHABILITATION AFTER TRAUMATIC BRAIN INJURY:
The Role of Family Support Programs
Louise Margaret Smith and Hamish P. D. Godfrey

A Continuation Order Plan is available for this series. A continuation order will bring delivery of each new volume immediately upon publication. Volumes are billed only upon actual shipment. For further information please contact the publisher.

Neuropsychological Explorations of Memory and Cognition

Essays in Honor of Nelson Butters

Edited by

Laird S. Cermak

Veterans Administration Medical Center
Boston, Massachusetts

Plenum Press • New York And London

Library of Congress Cataloging-in-Publication Data

On file

ISBN 0-306-44983-8

© 1994 Plenum Press, New York
A Division of Plenum Publishing Corporation
233 Spring Street, New York, N. Y. 10013

Printed in the United States of America

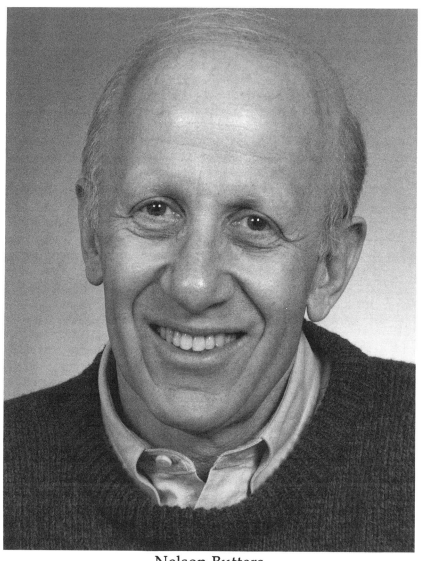

Nelson Butters

Contributors

Michael P. Alexander, M.D. • Braintree Hospital, Department of Neurology, Boston University

William W. Beatty, Ph.D. • Department of Psychiatry and Behavioral Sciences, University of Oklahoma Health Sciences Center

James T. Becker, Ph.D. • Alzheimer's Disease Research Center, Departments of Psychiatry and Neurology, University of Pittsburgh Medical Center

Marlene Oscar Berman, Ph.D. • Department of Veterans Affairs, Boston; Division of Psychiatry, and Department of Neurology, Boston University School of Medicine

Jason Brandt, Ph.D. • Department of Psychiatry, The John Hopkins University School of Medicine

Meryl A. Butters, Ph.D. • Department of Psychiatry, Western Psychiatric Institute and Clinic, University of Pittsburgh Medical Center

Laird S. Cermak, Ph.D. • Memory Disorders Research Center, Boston University School of Medicine and Department of Veterans Affairs Medical Center, Boston

Agnes S. Chan • Department of Psychiatry, School of Medicine, University of California, San Diego, and Department of Psychology, San Diego State University

Dean C. Delis, Ph.D. • Department of Veterans Affairs Medical Center, San Diego and Department of Psychiatry, University of California

Guila Glosser, Ph.D. • Department of Neurology, The Graduate Hospital, Philadelphia

Gerald Goldstein, Ph.D. • Department of Veterans Affairs Medical Center, Pittsburgh and Unversity of Pittsburgh

Eric Granholm, Ph.D. • Psychology Service, San Diego Department of Veterans Affairs Medical Center; Department of Psychiatry, University of California, San Diego

Murray Grossman, M.D. • Department of Neurology, University of Pennsylvania School of Medicine

William C. Heindel, Ph.D. • Department of Psychology, Brown University

John R. Hodges, M.D., FRCP • University Neurology Unit, Addenbrooke's Hospital, Cambridge

Felicia A. Huppert, PH.D. • Department of Psychiatry, University of Cambridge, and Addenbrooke's Hospital, Cambridge

Terry Jernigan, Ph.D. • Department of Veterans Affairs Medical Center, San Diego, CA

Barbara Pendleton Jones, Ph.D. • Laboratory of Psychology and Psychopathology, National Institute of Mental Health

Edith Kaplan, Ph.D. • Department of Neurology, Boston University School of Medicine

Narinder Kapur, Ph.D. • Wessex Neurological Centre, Southampton General Hospital, England

Christopher M. Ryan, Ph.D. • Western Psychiatric Institute and Clinic, Department of Psychiatry, University of Pittsburgh School of Medicine

David P. Salmon, Ph.D. • Department of Neurosciences, School of Medicine, University of California, San Diego

Donald G. Stein, Ph.D. • Dean, The Graduate School, Associate Provost for Research, Rutgers, The State University of New Jersey

Donald T. Stuss, Ph.D. • Rotman Research Institute of Bayrest Centre, Departments of Psychology and Medicine (Neurology), University of Toronto

Morton Wiener, Ph.D. • Department of Psychology, Clark University

Jessica Wolfe, Ph.D. • Department of Veterans Affairs, Boston and Tufts University School of Medicine

Foreword

It has now been almost 17 months since I awoke one morning with what appeared to be laryngitis and my usual January flu. When my hypophonia did not subside and my speech became mildy dysarthric, I consulted several physicians, all of whom reassured me that my symptoms were due to "aging" and overuse of my vocal chords. It was not until March 11, 1993, three days before my father's death, that an internist at UCSD noticed that I had developed fasciculations in both arms and informed me that I probably had amyotropic lateral sclerosis (ALS). Subsequent visits to several eminent neurologists confirmed the diagnosis that I had the bulbar form of ALS, and I was advised to put my financial affairs in order and to decide how I wished to spend the remaining 5 to 18 months of my life. Since I am now confined to a wheelchair and my speech is no longer comprehensible, I feel some urgency to express my gratitude to you, all my friends and colleagues, to let you know my thoughts as I approach the final stages of the disease. After watching my brother die of a chronic neurological problem 22 years ago, I had already rid myself of all misconceptions about my own mortality. I decided years ago that if I ever developed a chronic fatal disease I would try to make the process of dying an opportunity for growth, closure and resolution.

On a professional level I have devoted myself to completing a number of research reports and book chapters with students and collaborators and to the editing of the APA's new journal *Neuropsychology*. I am most gratified by the journal's great success and view it as my legacy to the field. Without the extensive assistance of David Salmon, Dean Delis, Mark Bondi, Andreas Monsch, Agnes Chan, Deborah Cahn, Shannon Johnson, Christine Fennema, Eric Granholm and Angela Drake I would not have been able to finish any of the reports and chapters. Without the encouragement and hard work of my Editorial Assistant, Diana Snyder, and my three Associate Editors, Laird Cermak, Julia Hannay, and Robert Heaton, I would have resigned the editorship of the journal long ago. In addition to the extra work these individuals had to assume, they were forced to watch my progressive physical deterioration and to adapt to my worsening dysarthria and other bulbar problems on a daily basis. Their job descriptions did not require them to share the pain of my disease, but they all did so gladly and without complaint. There is no way I can ever adequately express my thanks to these individuals for making the past year a productive one.

Besides my research and editorial collaborators a number of other colleagues have aided me greatly during the past year. My two "bosses," Lewis Judd (UCSD) and Jacqueline Parthemore (VA), allowed me to relinquish the most burdensome administrative aspects of my position and to focus on those activities (teaching and research) that provided me with the most pleasure. I owe a special debt of gratitude to Sandra Brown who assumed the duties of Chief of Psychology at the VA with virtually no advance warning. Sandy knew that she would likely be my successor as Chief within a year or two, and I had planned to educate her gradually as to the explicit and implicit features of the job. Unfortunately, due to the acute onset and rapid progression of my illness this gradual transfer of power was not possible, and Sandy had to assume the position of Chief without ample opportunity to delegate some of her demanding clinical, teaching and research duties to others. As I had expected, Sandy has performed brilliantly as Chief despite having to deal with a number of unexpected personnel problems. It is a great relief to me to know that the course I set for the Psychology Service will be continued under Sandy's leadership.

Although I have remained professionally active during the past year, I have still had to accommodate to a progressively debilitating illness that would likely kill me within a year or two. Given the moodiness that has always characterized my personality, I feared that I would become severely depressed and bitter and would be unable to function at all. While I cannot offer you a cogent explanation for my current mental state, neither of these dire predictions has come to pass. In fact, the past 15 months have been marked by serenity and extensive introspection. I realize that I shall not enjoy a long retirement during which Arlene and I had planned to travel and watch our grandchildren grow up. Nor shall I have the opportunity to devote the final decades of my life to a number of photographic ventures I had planned. However, despite these disappointments I now have a sense of fulfillment and closure with regard to my family and professional lives that were missing prior to my illness.

For the past 37 years I have been most fortunate to have been married to Arlene who has always been my best friend and partner through life. I consider myself to have been most fortunate to have shared my life with such a compassionate and loving woman. I am most grateful that Arlene and I had the opportunity to watch our three children - Meryl, Paul and Lisa - mature into responsible adults. They, as well as our two granddaughters Alicia and Samantha and our daughter-in-law Jill, have been a source of great happiness and pride. During the past year members of my family have made great personal and career sacrifices in order to provide me with the excellent physical care needed to ensure my comfort and a good quality of life. No husband or father could have asked for more.

When I think about my professional career, I have a similar sense of contentment and completion. As a few of you may know, my career as a reseacher is a matter of serendipity. Throughout graduate school my intent was to teach psychology in a small New England college. Several of my elementary, high school, and college teachers had been instrumental in helping me through some troubled times, and I had decided to dedicate my career to doing the same for other students. My intentions now are not to detail the chance events that derailed my college teaching plans and landed me in a research career in medical school settings. Rather, I wish to thank all of the students (undergraduate, graduate and postdoctoral) I have had the opportunity to work with. I am proud of my research in memory disorders, but I view the positive influences I have had on the careers and lives of my students to be my greatest achievement. In truth, I never was sure how my students felt about me until I became ill last year. I had feared that my moodiness and my obsessive editing of all their manuscripts had left many of them with ambivalent or even negative feelings about the time they spent with me. However, the chapters in this festschrift and the numerous personal letters I have received from former students and colleagues during the past year have reassured me that my influence has been significant and beneficial. I have found your statements of gratitude and concerns for my health to be most comforting and more meaningful than any of the awards I have received for my research and contributions to the profession of neuropsychology. When I depart this world, I shall do so with the knowledge that I have had some lasting positive effects on your lives and perhaps on the field of neuropsychology. Despite the physical burdens imposed by my present illness, I am content and consider myself to be most fortunate with regard to the family, career and friends I have had.

Finally, I would like to express special thanks to two colleagues, Laird Cermak and Saul Levine. Without Laird's extensive efforts this festschrift would not have been published. Having edited a few books during my career, I am fully aware of the substantial amount of time that Laird invested in this project. My family and I also owe a great debt to Saul for helping us cope psychologically with my illness and for guiding my attempts to place my life in some perspective.

Nelson Butters, Ph.D.
June 5, 1994

Preface

This text is for and about the career of Nelson Butters. It is written by the colleagues with whom he has worked over the last three decades and it reflects the extent to which he has shaped and influenced their careers. The intent is to show how each investigator's current line of research was impacted by, or emanated from, their earlier experiences collaborating with Nelson Butters. As a consequence, the text serves additionally as an historical forum for the flow of research theory and paradigmatic shifts within the field of cognitive neuropsychology. This group of individuals, through their myriad interconnections with Nelson form, possibly more than any other single grouping, the fabric of the field of Neuropsychology as it exists today. This in no way negates the tremendous influence other individuals have had upon the direction the field has taken, nor upon the bodies of data and theory they introduced. But, it is meant to demonstrate the phenomenal positive effect the career and interpersonal contributions of Nelson Butters has provided to this large group of people who have formed the threads which Nelson has woven together to form a very large portion of the tapestry of our discipline.

I have had the good fortune to know Nelson throughout most of this period and have had the opportunity to experience firsthand his concern for the development of others' careers and lives. I have seen him prod and cajole students, fellows, and colleagues into producing to the very limits of their abilities and into becoming professionals in their own right. I have seen him do the same to the entire profession through his work in guiding the International Neuropsychological Society, Division 40 of APA and, most recently, the journal *Neuropsychology* through their birthing process and early formative years. Through these efforts he has done more than any other one individual to advance the field of Neuropsychology to the status within the Neurosciences that it enjoys today. This book is intended to serve as a testimony to these accomplishments.

From a very personal standpoint, my name and life have been inextricably linked with those of Nelson Butters. Our careers have been intertwined throughout three decades and our lives have been similarly interconnected. I would not have come into the field of the study of amnesia, nor would I have become an investigator of any form of cognitive neuropsychology were it not for Nelson. Realizing the road that experimental psychology has taken, the extent to which it has merged with the neurosciences, and the manner in which it has embraced the cognitive revolution, I am fully aware that my own career would probably now exist on a road rarely intersecting this major highway were it not for the fact that Nelson and I met at a crossroads in our professional lives. I shall miss the signposts he sets up, but most of all, I shall miss seeing him on the horizon.

Laird S. Cermak, Ph.D.
June 24, 1994

ACKNOWLEDGEMENT. I, and all the contributors to this volume, wish to acknowledge the remarkable contribution of Mary R. Fitzgerald to the production of this text. Mary processed, formatted, edited and proofed this entire work. For this effort we are all exceedingly grateful.

Contents

xv

Recovery of Function After Serial Lesions of Prefrontal Cortex in the Rhesus Monkey

A Retrospective

DONALD G. STEIN[1]

I first met Nelson Butters at a Clark University reception in the late 1960's where I had joined the faculty as a new assistant professor. Nelson had just returned to Boston from Kent State University in Ohio to take a position in neuropsychology at the Veteran's Administration hospital in Roxbury, Massachusetts. Nelson had taken his degree in clinical psychology from Clark University and followed this training with a post-doctoral research fellowship in the laboratory of Mortimer Mishkin and Enger Rosvold at the National Institutes of Health. At the time, the NIH laboratory was the leading place to be for primate research on the cortical mechanisms of learning and memory. Using selective damage to the monkey cortex as an investigative technique, the NIH investigators performed dozens of studies to examine the role of the frontal cortex in cognitive performance and spatial learning. The many papers coming from that laboratory set the standard for thinking about structure function relationships in the central nervous system.

---

[1] DONALD G. STEIN, Ph.D., • Dean, The Graduate School, Associate Provost for Research, Rutgers, The State University of New Jersey

Neuropsychological Explorations of Memory and Cognition: Essays in Honor of Nelson Butters, edited by Laird S. Cermak, Ph.D. Plenum Press, New York, 1994

Nelson and I were introduced to one another by Jeffrey Rosen, who was my first graduate student at Clark. He had come up from Washington, D.C. as a graduate of the George Washington University. It turned out that Jeff had been working as an assistant to Mortimer Mishkin and had helped Nelson to do the monkey studies at the NIH.

Where is all this leading? Bear with me a bit longer and it will all fall into place. Jeff and I had begun a series of studies designed to test the concept of localization in the central nervous system, which, as I mentioned, was a strongly established paradigm during the 1950's and 60's when the three of us were students. Why did we decide to move against a mainstream paradigm when we had been trained to accept localization as a bedrock principle of cerebral organization? In fact, I had done my dissertation research on the role of the hippocampus in mediating memory consolidation. I was creating bilateral aspiration lesions of the hippocampus and then, in the traditional lesion approach, I tested the animals on a variety of behavioral tasks to determine the extent of the lesion-induced deficits. As I tested the rats, I noticed that several of the animals with hippocampal injury were able to perform the tests almost as well as normal controls. This was disturbing because histological reconstructions of the lesions revealed that some of the rats had complete hippocampectomies, yet they were able to solve the tasks with no difficulty.

At the time I was doing my thesis, I had also read a few studies which had reported that, if brain damage was inflicted slowly, the subjects were able to perform as well as intact controls. In particular, one report by John Adametz (Adametz, 1959) really attracted my attention. He created either single or multistage lesions in the rostral reticular formation of adult cats. The multi-stage lesions were spaced three weeks apart while the one-stage coagulations destroyed the structure in a single sitting. At that time the reticular formation was conceived as a rather diffuse structure that was thought to be a center for consciousness and arousal--a view that was supported, among others, by the highly regarded electrophysiological and lesion experiments of Donald Lindsey and Horace Magoun at UCLA (Magoun, 1963 for review).

Briefly stated, Adametz found that the cats with single stage surgeries went into deep comas and could only be temporarily aroused by highly intense and noxious stimulation. These animals soon died without ever regaining normal sleep-wake cycles or basic consummatory behaviors. In contrast, Adametz reported that all of the cats with staged lesions survived the extensive damage of the reticular core and went on to slow sleep-wake cycles, consummatory responses and grooming behaviors that were very close to normal.

How then, could one talk about the role of a given structure in the brain, when in its absence, subjects were able to perform just as well as normals? The Adametz work plus my own casual observations began to make me feel uncomfortable about doing lesion experiments as a means to understand the localization of functions in the central nervous system. However, I needed to get my degree and didn't want to create additional complications in my life so I put the question aside until I got my first job at Clark University and that brings me to the work I did with Jeff Rosen and eventually with Nelson Butters.

To follow up on the Adametz experiments and several others who had reported serial lesion effects (see Finger, et al 1973, for review), Jeff and I and our students at Clark decided to create one- or two-stage bilateral lesions of the frontal cortex, the hippocampus or the amygdala in adult, male rats and then test the animals on a variety of learning tasks. In the case of the two stage injuries there was a 30 day interval between the first and second operations. However, to emphasize, none of the different lesion groups received any training or testing until all of the surgery was complete. To make a long story shorter, we were able to show that in the case of one-stage injury, the rats demonstrated very much the 'classical' symptoms attributed to damage of the area under study. In marked contrast, the animals with two stage lesions which destroyed the same amount of brain tissue, were virtually unimpaired on all of the behavioral tests we applied.

The implications for theories of cerebral organization, especially those strongly emphasizing strict association between intact structure and specific functions were not lost on us, but the fact is that, in the 1960's and early 70's most people in the field were not ready to accept either the idea of recovery of function after massive brain damage or the notion that there might be a need to reconsider the doctrine of cerebral localization. Now enter Nelson Butters.

The first paper on our serial lesion results was published in Science (Stein, et al, 1969) and it did create quite a bit of interest, most of it not very positive. However, when opponents granted that some degree of sparing after massive brain damage was possible, they attributed it to the fact that the lissencephalic rat brain was no match for the highly complex, primate central nervous system where structure function relationships were much more precise and determined. To some extent, our findings were being dismissed because rats didn't need much of a brain to learn. This was an important question to answer but the animal laboratory at Clark University was very small and I had no experience with monkeys. But Nelson Butters did have a primate colony at the Boston, Veterans Administration Hospital and thanks to his connection with Clark and with Jeff Rosen, he was willing to support a research collaboration to see whether we could get similar sparing of function(s) after serial lesions in the monkey. What started out to be a single experiment, led to about seven years of close collaboration and a long-standing friendship.

In the first study (Rosen, Stein & Butters, 1971), 10 adult, rhesus monkeys were initially trained on a delayed spatial alternation (DSA) task and then operated upon 10 weeks after they were able to perform a 5-sec DSA problem. Monkeys in the one-stage group then received bilateral, aspiration lesions of the banks and depths of sulcus principalis. In the multiple-stage group (MS), the sulcus principalis was removed in 4 operations spaced three weeks apart. Each stage consisted on removing one bank and depth of the sulcus (e.g. lower bank-left hemisphere; upper bank-right hemisphere, etc) until the structure had been removed. Two weeks after all surgery had been completed, the animals began testing first for post-operative retention of DSA and then for acquisition of delayed response learning DR and position reversal. These were all tasks which had been used previously to demonstrate severe and permanent deficits in cognitive performance after prefrontal cortex lesions.

The results nicely paralleled what we had previously found in our rats. On the DSA retention task, the multiple stage monkeys were initially impaired, but generally made less errors than their single-stage counterparts--especially during the later phases of retesting (i.e. after 500 trials). On the DR acquisition and position reversal tasks, the MS monkeys were significantly better in every regard.

The histological findings were also very interesting in that the MS monkeys had what appeared to be substantially larger total lesions than their one-stage counterparts. So, here was an unambiguous case where, in the adult monkey, more extensive prefrontal cortex damage, occurring slowly, led to significantly better sparing and recovery of function than smaller lesions inflicted all at once.

These findings were important because we were able to demonstrate that recovery of cognitive functions after massive, bilateral damage in the adult primate nervous system could be induced under the right circumstances. Remember, at the time this research was done, it was believed that only brain injuries occurring early in life would result in such sparing of function; especially with respect to cognitive tasks. Our work together actually replicated the earlier experiments of Ades & Raab (1946; 1949) who had obtained similar findings after cortical damage to the motor and striate cortex in monkeys.

At the time, we were unable to offer more than a phenomenological 'explanation' for what we thought might be occurring. We suggested that the serial lesions might somehow 'permit' more 'reorganization of function' in the face of extensive practice--a not very satisfying mechanism.

In a second study (Rosen, Butters, Soeldner & Stein, 1975) we thought we could focus in on what potential mechanisms might account for the function sparing we observed after serial lesions. While working with Jeffrey Rosen and myself, Nelson was also collaborating with Depak Pandya a neuroanatomist interested in behavior and in delineating the connections of the frontal cortex to other CNS structures (see for example Butters & Pandya, 1969; Butters, et al 1971). Butters, Pandya and their students had shown that severe behavioral impairments were produced by removal of SP when only the middle third of the upper and lower banks were damaged in a single, bilateral operation.

The hypothesis we would test was that full and complete behavioral recovery should occur, on DSA retention, when serial lesions were restricted to the middle third of SP. This was because we thought adjacent tissue would be available to compensate for the loss of the primary area mediating spatial learning. In contrast, we expected profound and permanent deficits in the one-stage lesion group. In brief, the results were fully in the predicted direction. There was no overlap in performance between the one-stage and serial lesion groups. We believed that the better sparing was due to the 'fact' that remaining SP tissue could mediate the functions restricted to the middle third that we removed.

Admittedly, these and several other studies that we did together, never provided a good explanation of why serial lesions produce better recovery than when the same lesions are created in a single setting. However, our findings did serve an important purpose. Even though we could not provide an adequate physiological substrate, we were able to demonstrate that, under the right circumstances, even the adult primate nervous system is capable of considerable plasticity in response to damage. I believe that the demonstration of extensive plasticity in the brain-damaged monkey made it possible for us to continue to examine what needed to be done to promote functional recovery independently of serial lesions. In other words, the 'monkey work' we did with Nelson gave more credibility to a phenomenon (recovery of function) that was essentially considered by many investigators of the time, to be only a curious anomaly not worthy of serious research.

In the twenty or so years since we performed those serial lesion studies much has been learned about the potential mechanisms underlying first, the injury cascade itself, and second, the endogenous repair mechanisms induced by traumatic brain damage (TBI). For example, in the early 1970's no one was thinking that (TBI) could unleash a storm of excitatory amino acids whose effects on already vulnerable neurons would be very cytotoxic (e.g. Faden, et al, 1989). We were unaware that TBI creates massive production of free radicals which then go on to destroy lipid membranes, produce severe edema and create further free radical cascades of tissue damage (e.g Hall & Braughler, 1993). We didn't know that TBI causes the release of massive amounts of calcium ions which, in their excess become neurotoxic (e.g. Choi, 1989). Neither did we know that brain injury itself stimulates neural tissue to produce trophic, repair factors, such as nerve growth factor, among others, which rescues injured nerve cells from further degeneration and promotes synaptic maintenance (e.g. Nieto-Sampedro, 1988). We didn't know that TBI can induce the production of neuron cell adhesion molecules (NCAMs) which help to guide growing nerve terminals to their postsynaptic targets. We didn't know that injury on one side of the brain induces neurotrophic and NCAM increases not only at the site of the injury itself, but even in the contralateral intact cortex and at sites far removed from the zone of injury (e.g. Jorgenson & Stein, 1992). All of these processes contribute to neuronal repair and functional recovery.

What we've since learned is that the brain's response to traumatic injury is far more systemic. When we were creating our serial lesions, in a sense we were 'prepping' the remaining brain tissue to respond to the cerebral emergency--not only in tissue adjacent to the damage, but at distant sites as well. When we then went back to create the second, third or fourth surgery, we were entering into an already vastly changed and dynamic system that had already began to respond to the initial damage.

Multiple stage injuries would, first of all, reduce the cascade of toxic injury by-products like free radicals and excess calcium simply because less tissue was disturbed at each operation. At the same time, the brain's ability to produce endogenous trophic factors at the injury site and in the contralateral hemisphere, would reduce the traumatic effects of the additional surgeries.

In retrospect, we could even explain why the multiple stage surgeries which led to bigger lesions, resulted in better behavioral recovery. At the time we did our initial histology, we believed that the excessive glial scarring we produced by multiple entries into the prefrontal cortex, was a detrimental event so it was paradoxical that the 4-stage animals should be better. We now know that glial cells helped to scavenge free radicals and excess excitatory amino acids from the injury zone. Glia are also among the primary sources of neurotrophic factors that are released by the brain in response to injury (e.g. Gage, et al, 1988). Thus, those glial 'scars' we observed in our monkeys may actually have been necessary for the better behavioral recovery we observed in the four stage groups.

Tremendous progress has been made in the field of recovery research--and it is now very much a sub-discipline of neuroscience with its own society (Neurotrauma Society) and several journals which emphasize recovery of function research (Restorative Neurology and Neuroscience, Experimental Neurology, Journal of Neurotransplantation, Brain Injury Rehabilitation, to name several). I very much believe that the early monkey work we did with Nelson Butters gave us the confidence to proceed at a time when it was very difficult to swim against the mainstream views of nervous system organization.

Nelson helped in other ways too. He was a loyal friend. There was a time when it was very difficult to get funding for this research and the one grant application I had was rejected for reasons that didn't seem to be completely objective. It turned out that Nelson was a reviewer for one of the government agencies and by chance, a copy of my proposal was given to him to review. The only problem was that it was not in my name. It was submitted by someone else who had been sitting on the review panel that turned down my application. Somehow the bulk of my proposal ended up being submitted to another agency, but with someone else's name as the principal investigator.

Nelson took a strong stand on this issue and "blew the whistle" even though this act could have created problems for him as well. He could have saved himself a lot of trouble, but he was there when he was needed. It was a tortuous and difficult process for everyone, but eventually the application was reconsidered and fully funded. Without Nelson's vigilance and help, my research on functional recovery might very well have been permanently blocked. I think that without the monkey experiments made possible by Nelson Butters, we probably would have had to turn to other, more traditional areas of research that I would have personally found much less fulfilling. Nelson made it possible to develop and pursue a career path that has kept me occupied for the last 25 years. We've been good friends for all of that time and that's the best note on which I can end this essay.

REFERENCES

Adametz, J.H. (1959) Rate of recovery of functioning in cats with rostral reticular lesions. *J. Neurosurg.* , *16*, 85-98.

Ades, H.W. & Raab, D.H. (1946) Recovery of motor function after two-stage extirpation of area 4 in monkeys. *J. Neurophysiol.* , *9*, 55-60.

Butters, N. & Pandya, D. (1969) Retention of delayed alternation: Effect of selective lesions of sulcus principalis. *Science, 165*, 1271-1273.

Butters, N. Pandya, D., Sanders, K. & Dye, P. (1971) Behavioral deficits in monkeys after selective lesions within the middle third of sulcus principalis. *J. Comp. physiol. Psychol. 76*, 8-14.

Choi, D. (1989) Calcium-mediated neurotoxicity: Relationship to specific channel types and its role in ischemic damage. *Trends. Neurosci. 11*, 21-26.

Finger, S., Walbran, B. & Stein, D.G. (1973) Brain damage and behavioral recovery: serial lesion phenomena. *Brain Res. 63*, 1-18.

Gage, F.H., Olejniczak, P. & Armstrong, D.M. (1988) Astrocytes are important for sprouting in the septohippocampal system. *Exp. Neurol. 102*, 2-13.

Hall, E.D. & Braughler, J.M. (1993) Free radicals in CNS injury. In: S.G. Waxman (Ed)., *Molecular and Cellular approaches to the treatment of neurological disease.* New York, Raven Press, 81-105.

Jorgenson, O.S. & Stein, D.G. (1992) Transplant and ganglioside Gm1- mediated recovery in rats with brain lesions. *Rest. Neurol. Neurosci. 3*, 311-320.

Lindsey, D.B., Schreiner, L.H., Knowles, W.B. & Magoun, H.W. (1949) Behavioral and EEG changes following chronic brain stem lesions in the cat. *Electroenceph. Clin. Neurol.* , *1*, 455-473.

Magoun, H.W. (1963) *The Waking Brain*, Springfield, Ill. Charles C. Thomas Publishers.

Nieto-Sampedro, M. (1988) Growth factor induction and order of events in CNS repair. In: Stein, D.G. & Sabel, B.A. (Eds) *Pharmacological approaches to the treatment of brain and spinal cord injury.* New York, Plenum Press, 309-332.

Rosen, J., Stein, D.G. & Butters, N. (1971) Recovery of function after serial ablation of prefrontal cortex in the rhesus monkey. *Science, 173*, 353-356.

Rosen, J., Butters, N., Soeldner, C. & Stein, D.G. (1975) Effects of one stage and serial ablations
    of the middle third of sulcus principalis on delayed alternation in monkeys. *J. Comp.
    physiol. Psychol., 89*, 1077-1082.

2

Comparative Neuropsychology

Brain Functions in Nonhuman Primates and Human Neurobehavioral Disorders

MARLENE OSCAR-BERMAN[1]

I am very pleased to be able to join in paying tribute to Professor Nelson Butters, a colleague and a friend for nearly 30 years. I get to extol not only his accomplishments during the early years in Boston, but also to mention his sense of humor. In fact, when remembering back to Nelson's years at the VA Medical Center in Boston, I first thought about his monkey work, and then, about his monkey *business*. I shall discuss the monkey work in the historical perspective of his career, and I'll mention his monkey business to provide hysterical perspective.

NONHUMAN PRIMATE RESEARCH

I first met Nelson in Los Angeles in 1964, at a convention of the American Psychological Association. I had reported the results of my Master's thesis on frontal lobe function in Rhesus monkeys (Oscar & Wilson, 1966), and

[1] MARLENE OSCAR BERMAN, Ph.D. • Department of Veterans Affairs, Boston; Division of Psychiatry, and Department of Neurology, Boston University School of Medicine

Neuropsychological Explorations of Memory and Cognition: Essays in Honor of Nelson Butters, edited by Laird S. Cermak, Ph.D. Plenum Press, New York, 1994

Nelson came up and introduced himself to me. Being considerably older than I was, he already had earned his Ph.D. degree from Clark University, and was working as a postdoctoral research fellow in the Neuropsychology Section of the National Institute of Mental Health. When he introduced himself to me, I remember thinking to myself that his name was familiar, but I actually had him confused with another colleague of ours who was doing research on monkey brain function around that time, Charles Butter from Michigan. Nelson told me that many people confused the two of them, not just because of the similarity in their names, but also because of their mutual interests in primate brain function (e.g., Butter, 1969).

A few years later, Nelson and Charlie collaborated together, with Donald Stein and Jeffrey Rosen, on the behavioral effects of sequential and one-stage surgical removals of prefrontal cortex in monkeys. The results of that collaboration were published in the journal, *Experimental Neurology* (Butters, Butter, Rosen & Stein, 1973) and summarized in a chapter of the book, *Plasticity and Recovery of Function in the Central Nervous System* (Stein, Rosen & Butters, 1974). The findings reported by Butter, Butters, and their colleagues were that while functional recovery occurred following serial removals of the dorsolateral prefrontal region (in particular the principal sulcus), serial ablation of orbital prefrontal cortex did not attenuate the deficits associated with single-stage lesions. These findings paralleled the discovery by Goldman and her colleagues around that time, that infant monkeys with lesions in dorsolateral prefrontal cortex were capable of recovering lost function over time, but that infant monkeys with orbitofrontal lesions were not (Goldman, 1971). In subsequent studies, Nelson and his collaborators looked for areas of the brain that might be responsible for the functional recovery that occurred after serial dorsolateral cortical lesions, and they showed that cortical tissue both proximal and distal to the principal sulcus played some role in taking over lost functions.

My next encounter with Nelson was in 1969, at Charles Gross's laboratory in William James Hall at Harvard University. I was finishing up a postdoctoral fellowship in Charley's laboratory, studying eye movement correlates of visual learning in normal people and in monkeys before and after lesions of inferotemporal cortex (Oscar-Berman & Bakoplus-Banos, 1971; Oscar-Berman, Heywood & Gross, 1971, 1974). By that time, Nelson already was settled into his job as a Research Psychologist at the Boston VA Hospital across town. He had come over to Harvard from the VA to visit Charley's lab. During the course of our conversation, Nelson mentioned that I should consider applying to be a Research Associate at the Boston VA. I would be able to learn about human neurological disorders through the preceptorship of Dr. Harold Goodglass, and I could collaborate with Nelson on studies of monkey cortical functions. I followed Nelson's advice, and it turned out that he had paved the way for many marvelous experiences I was to have at the Department of Veterans Affairs Medical Center in Boston (its current name), beginning in 1970.

Nelson had begun working at the Psychology Research Unit of the Boston VA Medical Center in 1967. The Psychology Research Unit had its origin about 10 years earlier, when Dr. Goodglass recruited Mrs. Edith Kaplan, then a graduate student in Psychology at Clark University, to work with him on problems of aphasia and related disorders, and on cerebral dominance (see Geschwind, 1974, and Oscar-Berman, 1989, for additional historical information). This beginning was enthusiastically supported by the Chief of Neurology at the VA, Fred A. Quadfasel, and subsequently, by Norman Geschwind, who succeeded Quadfasel. The aphasia-related aspect of the research program was bolstered by the addition of two psychologists, Edgar Zurif and Howard Gardner in 1972. Together with their neurological colleagues, D. Frank Benson and Martin L. Albert, a highly talented group was convened to work out their hunches about the nature of aphasia and related deficits of movement, perception, and cognitive functions (Albert, Goodglass, Helm, Rubens & Alexander, 1981; Geschwind, 1974; Goodglass, 1993).

The arrival of Nelson in 1967, added two new areas to the VA Psychology Unit's activity: First, the use of a monkey model for the study of recovery of brain function, and second, an organized program on the nature of memory functions in amnesic states — particularly alcoholic Korsakoff's disease. Thus, the interplay between nonhuman and human primate research at the Boston VA Hospital began at that time. In both approaches to the study of brain function, Nelson enjoyed collaborating with colleagues. This is exemplified in the Table of Contents of a book of readings that Nelson put together for his students (Butters, 1972). The book contains a set of articles reproduced from journals for easy access by students taking courses from Nelson. It reflects Nelson's continued interest in frontal and parietal lobe systems, especially functions of association cortex in human and nonhuman animal models, and it shows some of Nelson's many collaborators. Of the 24 papers that Nelson reproduced in the book, six of them were coauthored by Nelson and his colleagues. Three of the six came from his collaborative work on monkey brain function, and three were on human neurological patients.

The three collaborative papers based on nonhuman primate models included in the book centered around frontal system dysfunction after brain lesions. One paper dealt with lesions of the middle third sector of the *sulcus principalis* in monkeys (Butters, Pandya, Sanders & Dye, 1971). In the paper, Nelson and his colleagues reported that lesions of the middle third of the sulcus had to include both banks in order to be effective in producing retention deficits on prior learned tasks. Another of Nelson's monkey papers reproduced in the book (Butters & Rosvold, 1968b), explored the functional neuroanatomy of frontal systems, specifically the consequences of lesions of subcortical projection areas. Butters and Rosvold (1968a) reported earlier that lesions of two separate projection areas of orbitofrontal cortex, the ventrolateral sector of the head of the caudate nucleus, and medial septal nuclei, resulted in deficits similar to those

CONTENTS

Selected Readings in Neuropsychology, Edited by Nelson Butters, Ph.D.
      MSS Information Corporation
      655 Madison Ave, New York, NY 10021

following lesions of orbitofrontal cortex itself. The reproduced paper (Butters & Rosvold, 1968b) implicated a ventral septal contribution to the perseverative-like effects. The third of Nelson's monkey papers appearing in the book was a recovery-of-function paper published in *Science* (Rosen, Stein & Butters, 1971).

RESEARCH ON HUMAN NEUROBEHAVIORAL DISORDERS

In the edited book of readings (Butters, 1972), examples of Nelson's *human* research publications show his interest in the late 1960s and early 1970s, in parietal association cortex (Butters & Barton, 1970; Butters, Samuels, Goodglass & Brody, 1970; Cermak, Butters & Goodglass, 1971). Norman Geschwind had proposed that the posterior parietal cortex of the left hemisphere, receiving afferent inputs from all sensory association areas, is important in mediating cross-modal associations (Geschwind, 1965). According to this view, reading and object naming are psychological processes dependent upon the ability to perform tactual-visual and auditory-visual cross-modal associations. Nelson and his collaborators examined this hypothesis by testing the ability of brain-damaged patients to perform cross-modal matches using visual, tactual, and auditory sensory inputs (Butters, Barton & Brody, 1970). The results were consistent with Geschwind's hypothesis that the left parietal lobe plays a role in the completion of cross-modal connections. Patients with left parietal lobe damage were more severely impaired in their ability to perform cross-modal matches than patients with damage elsewhere in the left hemisphere, and patients with right parietal lesions showed an attenuated deficit on cross-modal matching. In addition, Nelson and his colleagues found an interesting relationship between dyslexia and the performance of auditory-visual matches: Deficits in reading ability were related to impairments in making auditory-visual associations (Butters, Samuels, Goodglass & Brody, 1971).

Nelson's research on human neurological patients in the 1970s also looked at the visual-spatial constructional deficits that followed parietal lobe damage. From the original descriptions of visual-spatial constructional deficits, it seemed that damage to either the right or the left parietal lobe resulted in visual-spatial deficits, with damage to the right having more severe consequences. However, the identification of the basic processes underlying these visual-spatial deficits had been elusive. Some of the proposed underlying causes were visual-sensory defects, restriction of visual attention, central vestibular pathology, and general apraxia, but these were found insufficient to account for all the visual-spatial constructional deficits associated with lesions of either hemisphere. Cautioned, then, by the probability that no single factor would explain all cases of constructional apraxia, Nelson and his collaborators examined the role of one cognitive factor, the ability to perform reversible operations in space, in the constructional deficits of right and left parietal lobe patients (Butters & Barton, 1970). They found that patients with right or left parietal damage were unable to rotate objects spatially through imagery, suggesting that loss of such capacity does play a role in constructional disorders after parietal lobe damage.

An early example of Nelson's collaboration with Laird Cermak on amnesia also appeared in the book of readings he assembled in 1972: A paper on Korsakoff's syndrome that appeared in *Neuropsychologia* (Cermak et al., 1971, listed in the Table of Contents with the names, Laird Cermack and Howard Goodglass). As we know now, the early work on amnesia was to launch an avalanche of knowledge about memory disorders, and about the consequences of alcoholism on brain function (e.g., Butters & Cermak, 1980; Butters, Granholm, Salmon & Grant, 1987; Butters, Heindel & Salmon, 1989; Butters & Ryan, 1986; Butters & Salmon, 1987).

Although the book clearly reflects Nelson's interests in functions of association cortex, it does not scratch the surface of the long list of Nelson's collaborators during his Boston years. They included, in addition to those mentioned earlier, Marilyn Albert, Jim Becker, Francois Boller, Jason Brandt, Sue Carey, Morris Freedman, Edith Kaplan, Nari Kapur, Walter Pohl, Marcel Mesulam, Howard Gardner, Mort Mishkin, Chris Ryan, Gary VanHoesen, Mort Weiner, and myself. Nelson and I conducted a study together on recovery from serial inferotemporal cortical lesions in monkeys (Oscar-Berman & Butters, 1976), and we also produced a film together called, "Techniques of Primate Brain Surgery," that we presented at the annual convention of the Eastern Psychological Association in 1972 (Butters & Oscar-Berman, 1972).

COMPARATIVE NEUROPSYCHOLOGY

The mix of interests in nonhuman and human brain function in the 1960s and 1970s, reflected the influence of Comparative Psychology to which students such as Nelson and I were heavily exposed in our graduate school training (e.g., see Bitterman, 1962, 1975; Bitterman, LoLordo, Overmier & Rashotte, 1979; Harlow, 1958; Hilgard & Bower, 1975; Jarrard, 1971; Masterton, Bitterman, Campbell & Hotton, 1976; Meador, Rumbaugh, Pate & Bard, 1987; and Pribram, 1955). It grew out of an interest in animal behaviors as models of human behaviors that could be controlled and manipulated in the laboratory. From it evolved the Comparative Neuropsychological approach as we know it today. It has come to be used as a framework for comparing and contrasting the performances of disparate neurobehavioral populations on similar tasks.

Comparative Neuropsychology as applied in our research, involves the adaptation of experimental paradigms originally developed in animal laboratories, for use with human clinical populations (e.g., Freedman & Oscar-Berman, 1986a,b,c; Oscar-Berman, 1980, 1984, 1991, 1994; Oscar-Berman, Zola-Morgan, Oberg & Bonner, 1982; Weiskrantz, 1978). We employ simple tasks that can be mastered without relying upon language skills or high levels of preserved cognitive abilities. Historically, over many decades of animal research, the paradigms were perfected to study the effects of well-defined brain lesions on specific behaviors. Many of the paradigms still are used widely to link specific deficits with focalized areas of neuropathology, and to aid researchers in understanding brain mechanisms underlying neurobehavioral functions (e.g., see Arnold, 1984, Fuster, 1989, Harlow, 1958, Luria, 1966, and Warren & Akert, 1964). In the next section, we review research findings from our use of two such simple tasks, classical delayed response (DR) and delayed alternation (DA), as applied to a variety of human neurobehavioral disorders in which prefrontal system damage is known or highly suspect. Both tasks have a proven record of sensitivity to the effects of lesions in prefrontal cortical tissue of monkeys. Likewise, performance on such tasks follows a uniform pattern across the phylogenetic scale (see Harlow, 1958, and Jarrard, 1971).

NEUROANATOMICAL SYSTEMS IN DR AND DA PERFORMANCE

Nonhuman primates. Two large subdivisions of prefrontal cortex have been recognized to be important in normal DR and DA performance: The dorsolateral surface of prefrontal cortex (especially area 46 in the principal sulcus), and the ventral prefrontal region including the orbitofrontal surface and inferior convexity. The dorsolateral and ventral subdivisions of prefrontal cortex have correspondingly different cytoarchitectonics, neurochemical sensitivities, and connections with the rest of the brain. In any case, whatever the important distinguishing features between DR and DA tasks, accurate performance on them relies upon two parallel but overlapping prefrontal subsystems: Dorsolateral and ventral. A summary description of the two systems is provided in Table 1.

Brain regions having connections with each of these two systems run through different areas in many of the same structures. The dorsolateral system maintains more intimate connections with other neocortical sites than the ventral system. However, the dorsolateral system's connections with limbic sites are less striking than the orbitofrontal system's. Also, although the dorsolateral system is important for successful performance on both DR and DA, it is especially important in DR. Visuospatial memory, and attentional functions are thought to be compromised with dorsolateral lesions. By contrast, functions involved in response inhibition have been linked to orbitofrontal cortex. The ventral frontal system, of which the orbitofrontal cortex is a part, is intimately connected with basal forebrain and limbic structures, but its connections with other neocortical regions are not as extensive as the dorsolateral system's. And, like the dorsolateral system, the ventral system supports successful performance on both DA and DR, but it is especially important for DA performance.

DORSOLATERAL PREFRONTAL SYSTEM	VENTRAL PREFRONTAL SYSTEM
1. Maintains intimate connections with other neocortical sites.	1. Maintains intimate connections with limbic and basal forebrain sites.
2. Connections with limbic and basal .forebrain sites are less striking than with cortex.	2. Connections with other neocortical sites are less striking than with limbic and basal forebrain sites.
3. Closely linked with catecholaminergic neurotransmitter system.	3. Closely linked with cholinergic neurotransmitter system.
4. Important for DR and DA performance (especially DR).	4. Important for DA performance (and some DR).
5. Visuospatial mnemonic and attentional functions.	5. Functions involved (somehow) in response inhibition.

Table 1. A simplified list of major differences between the dorsolateral and ventral (orbitofrontal) prefrontal systems. This information is based mainly on data obtained from work with nonhuman primates (e.g., see Arnold, 1984, Fuster, 1989, and Oscar-Berman et al., 1991).

Human prefrontal systems. The original work on behavioral and neuroanatomical systems involved in DR and DA performance was based upon nonhuman models. In humans, evidence regarding a prefrontal functional separation along dorsolateral and ventral dimensions is not quite as clear as with monkeys. One important reason for this is that many different and complex procedures have been used to assess the deficits. In our own attempts to clarify the functional significance of human prefrontal cortex, we have supplemented standard neuropsychological evaluations with DR and DA tasks. We chose DR and DA specifically because of their special sensitivity to frontal dysfunction in nonhuman primates.

HUMAN NEUROLOGICAL PATIENTS WITH PREFRONTAL PATHOLOGY

Table 2 lists the groups we have studied using DR and DA paradigms. In our studies, we tested all of the groups under similar laboratory conditions,

		++	=	**Impairment**
		---	=	**No Impairment**
		+/-	=	**Impairment in Some Patients**

TASKS

DR	DA	NEUROBEHAVIORAL DISORDERS
++	++	Bilateral frontal lobe lesions.
++	++	Alzheimer's disease.
+/-	++	Alcoholic Korsakoff's syndrome.
++	---	Parkinson's disease with dementia.
---	---	Parkinson's disease without dementia.
---	++	Closed head injury.
---	++	Olivopontocerebellar atrophy.
---	++	Huntington's disease.
---	++	Schizophrenia.
---	+/-	Anterior communicating artery disease.
---	---	Broca's aphasia.
---	---	Non-Korsakoff alcoholism.

Table 2. Performance by patients with known or suspected prefrontal pathology. Although DR and DA tasks overlap considerably in degree of sensitivity to impaired prefrontal functions, they overlap least on neuropsychological functions as follows: DR — Visuospatial, memory, and attentional functions; DA — Abnormal perseverative responding. Additional tests borrowed from Physiological Psychology (e.g., Object Alternation, DRL, Successive Reversals, etc.) are sensitive to abnormal perseveration. Likewise, there are other prefrontal functions that are not assessed directly by DR and DA (e.g., stimulus significance, affect, etc.).

and with pennies for reward. These results are described in detail in a recent chapter on frontal lobe function and dysfunction (Oscar-Berman et al., 1991), and in newer papers (Gansler, Covall, McGrath & Oscar-Berman, 1994; Seidman, Oscar-Berman, Kalinowski, Pai, Ajilor & Tsuang, 1994). Prefrontal dysfunction has been associated with the patient groups we tested. Except for the alcoholics and Broca's aphasics (who performed like normal controls), we observed that some of the groups had difficulty with DA, some had difficulty with DR, and some had deficits on both tasks. From our knowledge of the animal literature, it seemed that the groups were divided along lines that respected the subdivision of prefrontal cortex into dorsolateral and ventral systems.

Although most of the disorders we studied involve overlapping pathology of the dorsolateral and the ventral prefrontal systems, some groups seemed to be more heavily influenced by dorsolateral than by ventral prefrontal dysfunction, other groups appeared to be more heavily influenced by ventral than by dorsolateral dysfunction. However, it is important to stress the following caveat: This dichotomy is one of emphasis, and relies upon quantitatively different degrees of dysfunction and damage. Relative to other groups, two groups of patients performed poorly on DR: those with Parkinson's disease and dementia, and a subgroup of patients with Korsakoff's syndrome. Because of what we know about DR tasks, we think the frontal damage in these groups may be predominantly (but not exclusively) in the dorsolateral system. Six groups performed poorly on DA: those with olivopontocerebellar atrophy, closed head injury, anterior communicating artery disease, late stage Huntington's disease, schizophrenia, and a different subgroup of Korsakoff patients. Here, because of what we know about DA tasks, we think ventral system pathology may be prominent. Some patients performed poorly on both the DR and the DA tasks (i.e., Alzheimer patients and patients with bilateral prefrontal damage from trauma or tumors mainly); in these patients, there is extensive damage to both systems.

In summary, there is considerable evidence that the Comparative Neuropsychological approach can be used in trying to understand brain mechanisms of complex neurobehavioral functions. Experimental paradigms known to be reliable and valid tests of behavioral deficits in brain damaged nonhuman animals, can be adapted successfully for use with people. The tasks can supplement traditional neuropsychological assessment procedures. Research employing DR and DA tasks has been especially helpful because of the sensitivity of the paradigms to frontal lobe lesions, and the potential for giving a different perspective on human neurological syndromes with suspected prefrontal pathology. Results of our studies support the idea — highlighted as a result of research with nonhuman primates — that prefrontal cortex in humans contains at least two parallel systems: One on the dorsolateral surface, and one located ventrally. The disorders we sampled showed deficits compatible with this view. Remarkably, so do the neuropathology and neurochemistry of the disorders.

THE PSYCHOLOGY RESEARCH UNIT, DVA BOSTON, 1970s

Throughout his years in Boston, Nelson expanded his research interests, as well as his network of collaborators, many of whom had been his students. His research came to include comparative studies of memory patterns in a full range of dementing diseases, the development of differential diagnostic memory batteries, and the investigation of subclinical memory changes in chronic alcoholics (e.g., Butters & Salmon, 1987, Butters et al., 1987, 1989).

In the early 1970s, the Psychology Research Unit functioned as an integral part of the Psychology Service, under Dr. Ralph Fingar, Chief of the Service, and as a clinical and research adjunct of the Neurology Service, under

Dr. Robert Feldman. All of the members of the Unit with Ph.D. degrees, held (and continue to hold) faculty appointments at Boston University School of Medicine. Figure 1 is a group photograph of the Neurology Service in 1973, although only five psychologists showed up that day from our Unit, Nelson Butters, Laird Cermak, Edgar Zurif, Davis Howes, and myself (clustered together toward the left).

The next photograph is of the Psychology Research Unit itself, in 1976. In addition to the five people seen in the previous photograph, many of the faces in this photograph may be familiar (Do you recognize Murray Grossman, Howard Gardner, Don Stuss, Nari Kapur, Edith Kaplan, Esther Strauss, and David Rosenfield?)

Nelson worked at the Boston VA for 16 years, and it is there that he wrote about 150 of his over 200 publications. Much of his work during that time focused on alcoholic Korsakoff's syndrome, but he also studied patients with varieties of dementia. During his Boston years, he made important contributions to research and practice related to memory disorders, and he won the DVA's Career Scientist Award for Excellence in Research. It is important to emphasize that Nelson has always been an astute administrator, and he loves and is very good at teaching. His work for the International Neuropsychology Society began early in the history of the society, and he was Program Specialist for the Veterans Administration in the 1980s. He began teaching psychology in the early 1960s, first at George Washington University, then at Ohio State, and at Antioch College. While in Boston, he taught at Wellesley College, the University of Massachusetts, Northeastern University, Clark University, and Boston University.

In 1983, Nelson moved to California to become Chief of the Psychology Service at the San Diego VAMC, and Professor of Psychiatry at UCSD School of Medicine, to apply his teaching, mentoring, and administrative skills there. Many people wonder why he and his wife Arlene left Boston, and probably at least as many wonder why he shaved off his beard when he got to California. The following photographs tell the story. These photographs were taken in 1972, without Nelson's knowledge, at an annual Psychology Research and Neurology Service picnic at the home of Harold Goodglass.

Nelson had a suspicion that day, that Edith was up to something. He said to two of the research assistants, David Loiselle, and Ted Peck, "Hey, David and Ted, I think I heard Edith saying that she's going to cut off my beard."

Beards were in fashion at the VA in the early 1970s. Even Howard Gardner had one. "See, Norman, I grew a beard to look more like you and Nelson."

Norman replied, "Howard, I think beards are great, but there's a rumor that Edith will cut Nelson's off — his *beard* that is."

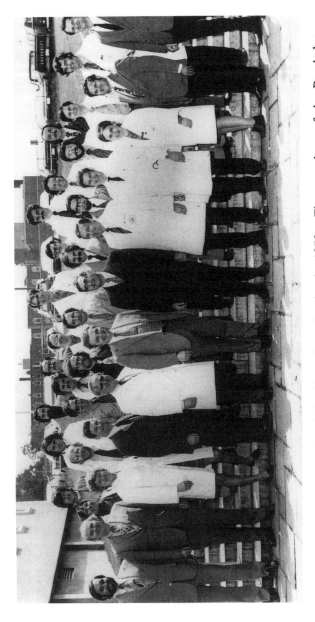

Figure 1. Group photograph of the Neurology Service in 1973. Five members of the Psychology Research Unit are Nelson Butters, Laird Cermak, Edgar Zurif, Davis Howes, and myself (left portion of the photograph).

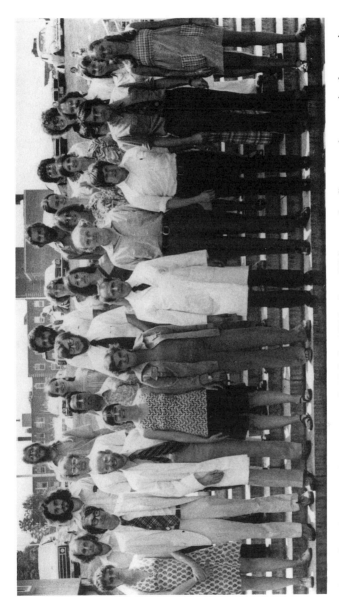

Figure 2. The Psychology Research Unit in 1976. In addition to the five people seen in the previous photograph, many of the faces in this photograph may be familiar. (Do you recognize Murray Grossman, Howard Gardner, Don Stuss, Nari Kapur, Edith Kaplan, Esther Strauss, and David Rosenfield?)

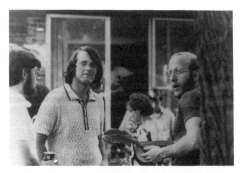

"Hey, David and Ted, I think I heard Edith
saying that she's going to cut off my beard."

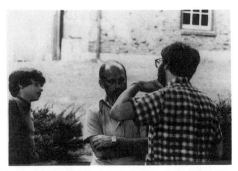

"See, Norman, I grew a beard to look more like
you and Nelson."

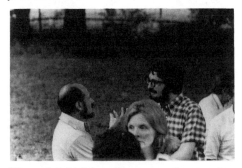

"Howard, I think beards are great, but there's a
rumor that Edith will cut Nelson's off-- his
beard that is."

Figure 3. Photographs taken in 1972, at an annual Psychology Research and
Neurology Service picnic at the home of Harold Goodglass.

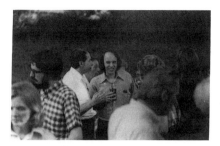

"Marty, do you think we should warn Nelson about the rumor?"

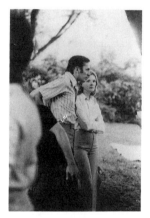

"Hon, do you think Nelson would continue to be
productive if he lost his beard?"

"Sure, Frank. But maybe Nelson and Arlene would use
it as an excuse to leave Boston and move to California."

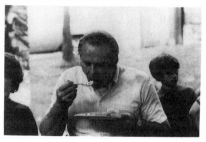

"No! Nelson would never be seen in public
without his beard. And there's no way he will
ever move to California."

Figure 4. Photographs taken in 1972, at an annual Psychology Research and
Neurology Service picnic at the home of Harold Goodglass.

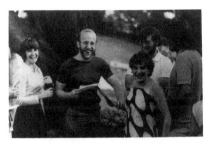

"Arlene, Ted, and David: Grab his arms! I'm gonna do it."

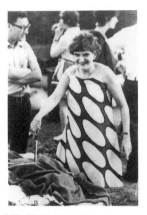

"I DID IT! I think it looks great."

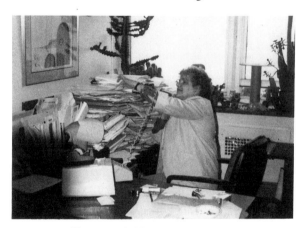

"Look at all this protest mail!
And the phone doesn't stop ringing."

Figure 5. Photographs taken in 1972, at an annual Psychology Research and Neurology Service picnic at the home of Harold Goodglass.

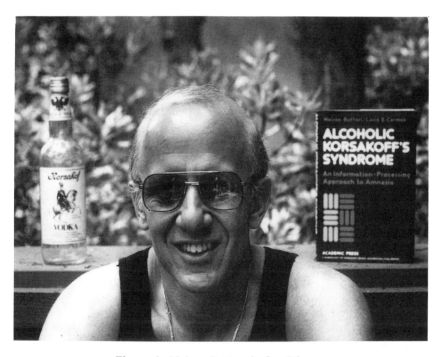

Figure 6. Nelson Butters in San Diego.

Harold also had heard the rumor, and was concerned; he said to Marty Albert, "Marty, do you think we should warn Nelson about the rumor?"

At the same time, Frank Benson and his wife Donna were discussing the same thing. Frank expressed his concerns to Donna: "Hon, do you think Nelson would continue to be productive if he lost his beard?"

Using her intuition, Donna replied, "Sure, Frank. But maybe Nelson and Arlene would use it as an excuse to leave Boston and move to California."

Using *his* intuition, Ralph Fingar said emphatically, "No! Nelson would never be seen in public without his beard. And there's no way he will ever move to California."

At this point, Edith move in swiftly, shouting, "Arlene! Ted! David! Grab his arms! I'm gonna do it."

Triumphantly, Edith then said, "I DID IT!"

Of course, after Edith cut off Nelson's beard, she had to deal with the consequences: "Look at all this protest mail! And the phone doesn't stop ringing."

The beautiful result is obvious in the photograph of Nelson in California.

So, Donna Benson was right, and Ralph Fingar was wrong. Nelson did go to California, and he remained clean-shaven for many years. He also remained very productive. The Psychology Service at the San Diego VA Medical Center has thrived under Nelson's leadership. In San Diego, as in Boston, Nelson continued to attract talented young scientists, to publish prolifically, to plan workshops for presentation all over the world, to mentor and train clinical neuropsychologists, and to receive honors for his contributions to the field. His many honors include his election to the office of President of the Division of Clinical Neuropsychology of the American Psychological Association in 1982, his election as President of the International Neuropsychology Society in 1984, his being chosen in 1980 for a three-year term as VA Program Specialist for Behavioral Sciences nationally, and his membership in numerous societies and editorial boards of professional organizations and journals. In his recently acquired job as Editor-in-Chief of APA's publication, *Neuropsychology*. Nelson is crafting his journal with the same skill and devotion that he gives to his students, and inspires in his colleagues. And finally, in the summer of 1993, Professor Nelson Butters was informed by the Department of Veterans Affairs Central Office that he was the recipient of the VA's highly prestigious Career Contribution Award for his decades of loyal service.

It's no wonder: Professor Nelson Butters is a Wonder.

ACKNOWLEDGEMENTS. The writing of this chapter was supported by funds from the Medical Research Service of the US Department of Veterans Affairs, and by a grant from the US Department of Health and Human Services, NIAAA (AA07112) to Boston University.

REFERENCES

Albert, M.L., Goodglass, H., Helm, N.A., Rubens, A.B., & Alexander, M.P. (1981). Clinical aspects of dysphasia. In G.E. Arnold, F. Winckel, & B.D. Wyke (Eds.), *Disorders of human communication 2*. (Whole volume). NY: Springer-Verlag.

Arnold, M.B. (1984). *Memory and the brain*. London: Lawrence Erlbaum.

Bitterman, M.E. (1962). Techniques for the study of learning in animals: analysis and classification. *Psychological Bulletin, 59*, 81-93.

Bitterman, M.E. (1975). The comparative analysis of learning. *Science, 188*, 699-709.

Bitterman, M.E., LoLordo, V.M., Overmier, J.B. & Rashotte, M.E. (Eds.) (1979). *Animal learning. Survey and analysis*. NY: Plenum.

Butter, C.M. (1969). Perseveration in extinction and in discrimination reversal tasks following selective frontal ablations in Macaca Mulatta. *Physiology and Behavior, 4*, 163-171.

Butters, N. (Ed.) (1972) *Selected readings in neuropsychology*. NY: MSS Information Corp.

Butters, N. & Barton, M. (1970). Effect of parietal lobe damage on the performance of reversible operations in space. *Neuropsychologia, 8*, 205-214.

Butters, N., Barton, M., & Brody, B.A. (1970). Role of the right parietal lobe in the mediation of cross-modal associations and reversible operations in space. *Cortex, 6(2)*, 174-190.

Butters, N., Butter, C., Rosen, J., & Stein, D. (1973). Behavioral effects of sequential and one-stage ablations of orbital prefrontal cortex in the monkey. *Experimental Neurology, 39(2)*, 204-214.

Butters, N. & Cermak, L.S. (1980). *Korsakoff's syndrome: An information-processing approach to amnesia*. NY: Academic Press.

Butters, N., Granholm, E., Salmon, D.P., & Grant, I. (1987). Episodic and semantic memory: A comparison of amnesic and demented patients. *Journal of Clinical and Experimental Neuropsychology, 9(5)*, 479-497.

Butters, N., Heindel, W., & Salmon, D. (1989). Neuropsychological differentiation of memory impairments in dementia. In G. Gilmore, P. Whitehouse, & M. Wykle (Eds.), *Memory, aging and dementia*. NY: Springer, pp. 112-139.

Butters, N. & Oscar-Berman, M. (1972). "Techniques of Primate Brain Surgery: Cortical Aspiration and Subcortical Stereotaxic Lesions." Presented at the Eastern Psychological Association Convention, Boston, MA.

Butters, N., Pandya, D., Sanders, K., & Dye, P. (1971). Behavioral deficits in monkeys after selective lesions within the middle third of sulcus principalis. *Journal of Comparative and Physiological Psychology, 76*, 8-14.

Butters, N., & Rosvold, H.E. (1968a). Effect of caudate and septal nuclei lesions on resistance to extinction and delayed-alternation. *Journal of Comparative and Physiological Psychology, 65(*3), 397-403.

Butters, N., & Rosvold, H.E. (1968b). Effect of septal lesions on resistance to extinction and delayed alternation in monkeys. *Journal of Comparative and Physiological Psychology, 66,* 389-395.

Butters, N. & Ryan, C. (1986). The neuropsychology of alcoholism. In D. Wedding, A.M. Horton, & J. Webster (Eds.), *The Neuropsychology Handbook: Behavioral and Clinical Perspectives.* NY: Springer, pp. 376-409.

Butters, N. & Salmon, D. (1987). The etiology and neuropathology of alcoholic Korsakofff's syndrome: Some evidence for the role of the basal forebrain. In M. Galanter (Ed.), *Recent developments in alcoholism, Vol. 5.* NY: Plenum, pp. 27-58.

Butters, N., Samuels, I., Goodglass, H., & Brody, B. (1970). Short-term and auditory memory disorders after parietal and frontal lobe damage. *Cortex, 6,* 440-459.

Butters, N., Samuels, I., Goodglass, H., & Brody, B. (1971). A comparison of subcortical and cortical damage on short-term visual and auditory memory. *Neuropsychologia, 9,* 307-315.

Cermak, L.S., Butters, N., & Goodglass, H. (1971). The extent of memory loss in Korsakoff patients. *Neuropsychologia, 9,* 307-315.

Freedman, M. & Oscar-Berman, M. (1986a). Bilateral frontal lobe disease and selective delayed-response deficits in humans. *Behavioral Neuroscience, 100,* 337-342.

Freedman, M. & Oscar-Berman, M. (1986b). Selective delayed response deficits in Parkinson's and Alzheimer's disease. *Archives of Neurology, 43,* 886-890.

Freedman M, & Oscar-Berman M. (1986c). Comparative neuropsychology of cortical and subcortical dementia. *Canadian Journal of Neurological Science, 13,* 410-414.

Fuster, J.M. (1989). *The prefrontal cortex.* NY: Raven Press.

Gansler, D.A., Covall, S., McGrath, N. & Oscar-Berman, M. (1994). Measures of prefrontal dysfunction after closed head injury. (Manuscript submitted for publication in *Brain and Cognition.*)

Geschwind, N. (1965). Disconnexion syndromes in animals and man. Part I. *Brain, 88,* 237-294.

Geschwind, N. (1974). Selected papers on language and the brain. In R.S. Cohen & M.W. Wartofsky (Eds.), *Boston studies in the philosophy of science, Vol. XVI.* Boston: D. Reidel.

Goldman, P.S. (1971). Functional development of the prefrontal cortex in early life and the problem of neuronal plasticity. *Experimental Neurology, 32,* 366-387.

Goodglass, H. (1993). *Understanding aphasia.* NY: Academic Press.

Harlow, H.F. (1958). The evolution of learning. In A. Roe & G.G. Simpson (Eds.), *Behavior and evolution.* New Haven: Yale University Press.

Hilgard, E.R. & Bower, G.H. (1975). *Theories of learning.* Englewood Cliffs, NJ: Prentice Hall.

Jarrard, L.E. (Ed.) (1971). *Cognitive processes of nonhuman primates.* NY: Academic Press.

Luria, A.R. (1966). *Higher cortical functions in man.* NY: Basic Books.

Masterton, R.B., Bitterman, M.E., Campbell, C.B.G., & Hotton, N. (Eds.). (1976). *Evolution of brain and behavior.* Hillsdale, NJ: Erlbaum.

Meador, D.M., Rumbaugh, D.M., Pate J.L., & Bard, K.A. (1987). Learning, problem solving, cognition, and intelligence. In G. Mitchell & J. Erwin (Eds.), *Comparative primate biology. Vol. 2, Part B. Behavior, cognition, and motivation.* NY: Alan R. Liss, pp. 17-83.

Oscar, M. and Wilson, M. Tactual and visual discrimination learning in monkeys with frontal lesions. (1966). *Journal of Comparative and Physiological Psychology, 62*(1), 108-114.

Oscar-Berman, M. (1980). Neuropsychology of long-term chronic alcoholism. *American Scientist, 68,* 410-419.

Oscar-Berman, M. (1984). Comparative neuropsychology and alcoholic Korsakoff's disease. In Squire, L. & Butters, N. (Eds.), *Neuropsychology of memory.* NY: Guilford Press, pp. 194-202.

Oscar-Berman, M. (1989). Links between clinical and experimental neuropsychology. *Journal of Clinical and Experimental Neuropsychology, 11*(4), 571-588.

Oscar-Berman, M. (1991). Clinical and experimental approaches to varieties of memory. *International Journal of Neuroscience, 58,* 135-150.

Oscar-Berman, M. (1992). Alcoholism and the frontal lobes. Invited lecture, Massachusetts Neuropsychological Society, Boston, MA.

Oscar-Berman, M. (1994). A comparative neuropsychological approach to alcoholism and the brain. Paper presented at the Seventh Congress of the International Society for Biomedical Research on Alcoholism. Gold Coast, Queensland, Australia.

Oscar-Berman, M. & Bakoplus-Banos, J. (1971). Eye orientation during visual discrimination learning by humans. *Perceptual and Motor Skills, 33* (3), 1311-1316.

Oscar-Berman, M. & Butters, N. (1976). Sequential and single-stage lesions of posterior association cortex in Rhesus monkeys. *Physiology and Behavior, 17* (2), 287-295.

Oscar-Berman, M., Heywood, S.P. & Gross, C.G. (1971). Eye orientation during visual discrimination learning by monkeys. *Neuropsychologia, 9* (3), 351-358.

Oscar-Berman, M., Heywood, S.P. & Gross, C.G. (1974). The effects of posterior cortical lesions on eye orientation during visual discrimination by monkeys. *Neuropsychologia, 12*(2), 175-183.

Oscar-Berman, M., McNamara, P. & Freedman, M. (1991). Delayed response tasks: Parallels between experimental ablation studies and findings in patients with frontal lesions. In Levin, H.S., Eisenberg, H.M. & Benton, A.L. (Eds.), *Frontal lobe function and injury.* NY: Oxford University Press, pp. 120-138.

Oscar-Berman, M., Zola-Morgan, S.M., Oberg, R.G.E. & Bonner, R.T. (1982). Comparative neuropsychology and Korsakoff's syndrome III: Delayed response, delayed alternation and DRL performance. *Neuropsychologia, 20,* 187-202.

Pribram, K.H. (1955). Toward a science of neuropsychology (method and data). In *Current trends in psychology and the behavioral sciences.* Pittsburgh, PA: University of Pittsburgh Press, pp. 115-142.

Rosen, J., Stein, D. & Butters, N. (1971) Recovery of function after serial ablation of prefrontal cortex in the rhesus monkey. *Science, 173,* 353-356.

Seidman, L.J., Oscar-Berman, M., Kalinowski, A.G., Pai, T., Ajilor, O. & Tsuang, M.T. (1994). Experimental and clinical neuropsychological measures of prefrontal dysfunction in schizophrenia. Submitted to *Neuropsychology*.

Stein, D., Rosen, J., & Butters, N., Eds. (1974). *Plasticity and recovery of function in the central nervous system.* NY: Academic Press.

Warren, J.M. & Akert, K. (Eds.) (1964). *The frontal granular cortex and behavior.* NY: McGraw-Hill.

Weiskrantz, L.A. (1978). A comparison of hippocampal pathology in man and other animals. In K. Elliott & J. Whelan (Eds.), *Functions of the septo-hippocampal system: Ciba Foundation symposium 58.* NY: Elsevier Science, pp. 373-406.

3

Processing Deficits of Amnesic Patients

Nearly Full Cycle?

LAIRD S. CERMAK[1]

The topic of "Encoding Deficits in Amnesia" was the first thing that Nelson and I talked about upon initially meeting back in 1970. At the time, I was an Assistant Professor in the Psychology Department at Tufts University and he had been at the Boston VA for approximately five years after having spent the first few years of his career at the NIH. We met at a meeting of the Boston area cognition interest group that convened once a month at Bolt, Beranek and Neuman, or at MIT. Founded by Drs. Norman and Waugh, and attended by notables such Nickerson, Wickelgren, Collins, Potter and Wingfield, we were clearly in over our heads. This particular meeting was one of the first I had attended and Nelson was the invited speaker, so I assumed that he was a regular member. It turned out that he was not a member and that the members were not all that interested in the results of testing brain-injured patients, feeling, as I was soon to learn was not an isolated reaction to this data, that little to nothing about normal memory could be learned from studying the injured brain. But, I thought otherwise and was fascinated by the possibilities of studying information processing by testing amnesics. Nelson was, of course, magnetic in his presentation, both entertaining and informative and, for a young investigator who was still feeling around for a niche in the field, compelling in his presentation. I remember telling my wife that night that I thought I had met

[1] LAIRD S. CERMAK, Ph.D.. • Memory Disorders Research Center, Boston University School of Medicine and Department of Veterans Affairs Medical Center, Boston

Neuropsychological Explorations of Memory and Cognition: Essays in Honor of Nelson Butters, edited by Laird S. Cermak, Ph.D. Plenum Press, New York, 1994

someone with whom I could collaborate on a project or two. I probably never had a better prediction in my life.

At any rate, we talked about Korsakoff patients and information processing and continued to do so for several weeks, during which time we designed a dozen or so experiments and began to write a grant together. Left to my own devices, I doubt that I would have begun thinking "Grant" so early in the game, but this turned out to be Nelson's way of doing research. So before our first study was completed, NIAAA had received our grant for the next three years and I was working on a position description for me to leave Tufts and join the small, in numbers only, group at the Boston VA. In the months to come I learned that Nelson and I had quite disparate personalities and interests and politics, but our research styles, aspirations and goals meshed perfectly.

The prevailing theory of memory back then had been, and was continuing to be, one based on a dichotomy of Short-term Memory and Long-term Memory. Fed by the findings with H.M. who could retain material so long as he was permitted to recirculate it but could not place it into a permanent store, the modal model of memory considered temporary storage of material to be independent of permanent storage. Further evidence supporting this thesis had just been published by Baddeley and Warrington in the Journal of Verbal Learning and Verbal Behavior. They reported that amnesics not only could hold material by recirculating it, but could demonstrate normal retention following a brief distractor interval (the so-called Brown-Peterson distractor task) and could show normal recall from the recency portion of a serial task (the Waugh and Norman STM recency effect). Both these paradigms were felt to be tapping a Short-term store, so normal performance by amnesics was anticipated and was taken as further evidence for the distinction between Short and Long Term Memory. It pretty much seem to be all wrapped up, leaving little room for further research in the field. Some still see this as true.

ENCODING AND EXPLICIT MEMORY

At about this same time, there was a new movement in the field of normal human memory, one that was very much a favorite of mine and which I somehow convinced Nelson to embrace. However, as those who know him would readily attest, this convincing took time and many, many reiterations; but, embrace it he did. The new theory that I was asking him to absorb was one that was advanced by Craik and Lockhart (1972) dubbed "Levels of Processing". This theory placed the onus of probability of retrieval upon the processing achieved by the subject during the time that he was being presented with the stimulus materials. Such emphasis upon the initial stages of processing contrasted with the prevailing zeitgeist within memory theory that held to the notion that the characteristics of the store into which material was placed held the key to probability of retrieval. Those of us who advocated strongly for the levels of processing framework firmly believed, as a doctrine of the times taught, that "you are what you eat". Your probability of recall was a direct function of the extent to which you processed the information in the first place. If your processing was deep, that is contained semantic analysis of the to-be-remembered stimulus, then retrieval was enhanced over and above what would be the case were you to process only the shallow physical characteristics of the material. A study by Craik and Tulving (1975) in which subjects were directed to analyze only a particular feature of the information and then were given a surprise memory test confirmed this belief. Semantic analysis produced substantially better recall than orthographic or phonemic processing. Our subsequent test of this assumption with amnesics (Cermak, Butters and Moreines, 1974) revealed that alcoholic Korsakoff patients failed to improve as a consequence of instructions to analyze the semantic features of words leading us to conclude that they did not profit from such analysis. Precisely why was an area of concern for us in the years to come, but it was clear that the ability to base one's retention upon initial analysis was not something that was available to our amnesics. Thus, the material at retrieval was not as adequately represented as it was for normals. Instead something was truly going on at the time of input that affected output probability. Our original belief that "You are what you eat in memory" became "You reconstruct from whatever pieces you have available". Amnesics had little from which to reconstruct because the normal byproduct of initial analysis was not available to them at retrieval. Was this because of an initial deficit at input as we had expected, or was it a consequence of the storage system's inability to retain features of input as the STM/LTM dichotomy favored?

That it was a problem in initial processing became apparent as we continued to employ encoding tasks with our patients (Butters and Cermak, 1980). We had, as it happened, already demonstrated two instances in which our patients, left to their own devices and given no instructions, failed to utilize semantic levels of processing. In the first (Cermak and Butters, 1972), Korsakoff amnesics and alcoholic controls were asked to retain a short eight item list of words. Within the list of eight words there were two that were animal names, two that were names of tools, two were vegetables and two were articles of clothing. Immediately at the close of reading the list, the patients were asked for recall. Since the task was immediate and essentially a readout of the word span for the patients, they were normal. Retention for both groups was about 4.5 items. However, when the patients were asked to recall by category, in other words the patient was asked to first recall the tools, then the animals and etc., the amnesic patients retrieval ability tumbled. Now the patients recalled only about an average of one item, while the controls improved in recall probability because the categories cues were found to be facilitating. What we suspected was that the amnesics had not been encoding the semantic characteristics of the words "on-line" and so had to go back and try to do so at retrieval. Once the task went beyond merely spewing-out the information, the amnesics showed their analytic deficit.

Further evidence that the amnesics had trouble with on-line semantic analysis was provided by our adaptation of the Wickens (1970) release of PI technique. In this procedure (Cermak, Butters and Moreines, 1974), the patient is asked to retain three words from a specific taxonomic category, such as animals, across an eighteen second interval filled with distracting activity such as counting backwards by twos. The typical experience is that the patient can retain these three words but when he is faced with a subsequent, and immediate, second trial which also requires the retention of words from the same taxonomic category, recall fades fast. In fact, by a third trial retention is nearly nil for the amnesics and only around 40-50% for the controls. If the words presented on the fourth trial are taken from another taxonomic category (e.g. vegetables), the controls retention returns to nearly 100%; however, the amnesics' retention remains at its lowest ebb. This was interpreted, following the theorizing of Wickens, to mean that the patient had not utilized the change in class at the time of input to permit differential storage and facilitate later retrieval. Interestingly, later investigators (Winocur and Kinsbourne, 197) pointed out that a second trial given to amnesics did result in some release of the PI but only a very small increase in recall resulted. They assumed that this meant that the patients encoded the difference on the second trial, but they did not design the experiment to allow an interpretation based on decay of prior trials rather than differential encoding to be done. It is likely that time alone out of the taxonomic class may have allowed the increase to occur. At any rate, the fact remained that on-line the analysis was not performed and allowed us to conclude that it is not just the case that amnesics fail to profit from on-line analysis as was shown by the Craik and Tulving procedure, but that they probably failed to perform analysis in a automatic fashion at all.

All this meant that the encoding theory of interference was widely supported by the processing studies we had performed (Butters and Cermak, 1980). Studies from the Warrington and Weiskrantz group (1974, 1978) also began to lean in the direction of initial analytic deficits among amnesic patients but from a slightly different perspective, of course. They began to find that their patients had a great deal of difficulty learning a second list of paired-associate words when the stimuli between the two list was identical. They attributed this learning deficit to an inability to inhibit the prior learning during the subsequent learning, but regardless the conclusion still admitted that an initial processing deficit existed and that all amnesia was not solely a problem in retrieval. The difficulty was still that the patients were more susceptible to interference than were normals, but no one was debating that at the time; it was simply a matter of debate over the source of that interference. Was it at encoding or at retrieval? It appeared that to some extent the British group now agreed that it could affect the input stage as well. Not precisely the same way as we were imagining, but at least in the same stage. At the same time, we (Cermak and Stiassny, 1982) began to explore the possibility that our amnesic patients might be having trouble at the retrieval stage as well. Our emphasis was on processing deficits during this stage; specifically on reconstruction difficulties, but like the British group, we were at least admitting that the amnesic patients had processing impairments beyond the initial stages of processing and that this might occur in a stage where other theorists had already pinpointed the deficit.

Our initial experimental foray into this domain was based on a task introduced by Thomson and Tulving (1970) which emanated from Tulving's Encoding Specificity theory. Basically, this theory postulated that the best cue during retrieval is always the cue that was present during initial presentation of the material assuming, of course, that cue was incorporated into the processing of the critical word in the first place. What we proposed was that this encoding specificity would not hold for amnesics because they would not incorporate cues into their initial analysis of critical words so that during reconstruction of the desired material at the time of retrieval, such cues would not be useful.

In the actual experiment, patients were given a list of 12 words to try to remember. Above each word, as it was being presented, was another word which the patient was told may or may not be present at retrieval but could help him remember the critical word. After all words were presented, the patient was then shown 12 cue words and asked to write down the words from the list corresponding to each cue. Actually, there were five input-output relationships that were investigated: (1) S-S, in which the same strongly associated cue word occurred at input and again at output. (2) W-W in which the same weakly associated cue word occurred at input and output. (3) S-W in which a strong associate was presented at input, but a weak associate at output. (4) W-S, which was the reverse of S-W. (5) O-O, a control with no cues. The result was that the amnesics showed normal recall on the S-S condition (and well above the O-O), but below normal on the W-W (and this, in turn, was even below the O-O). Even the W-S condition (which also was no better that O-O) exceeded the W-W condition for the amnesics in direct violation of the encoding specificity principle. All this meant that anything less than a high associate of a desired word appearing at both input and output did not facilitate an amnesics' retrieval. Anything that seemed to require a reorganization of the patient's semantic network did not prove facilitating. Amnesics were cued successfully only under conditions that automatically regenerated a correct response, but fail to produce that same word to a cue which did not naturally elicit the desired response.

It seemed that the amnesic was responding to the word elicited to a strongly associated cue by stating that it was a member of the desired list of words largely because the fluency of producing it from the strong cue made it feel right. That this was indeed the case was demonstrated by a subsequent experiment in which the amnesics were given a different set of strong cues and asked to generate four items to each and then to circle the item that they remembered as being in a list that had been previously presented (when, actually, none had been presented). The patients generated four items and then circled the highest associate to that item. Usually, this item had also been the first one generated as well so it felt right to the patient and he went with it. The patients seemed to be confusing fluency with recency and attributing a feeling of being easily retrieved with its having just been presented. Such an attribution might lead to apparent normal retrieval under conditions where the cue elicited previously presented material, but it could also lead to misattribution when the material was not that which had just occurred. It occurred to us that this same fluency heuristic could be an explanation for amnesics' normal performance on so-called "implicit" tasks in a manner analogous to this demonstration of normal retrieval on an ostensibly explicit task. The investigation of this possibility formed the framework for our studies during the last ten years which incidentally began about the same time that Nelson departed for San Diego.

ENCODING AND IMPLICIT PERFORMANCE

The notion of implicit task performance is well known to the readers of this volume and need not be fully described again. Basically, this type of performance refers to changes in a patient's response behavior as a consequence of prior experience even though the patient is not explicitly aware of that prior experience. The two most frequently used paradigms to study this phenomenon are the perceptual identification task and the word-stem completion task. In the first, it is reported that amnesic patients identify words at short durations of exposure if that word has just occurred within a list of to-be-recalled words just prior to the threshold identification task. Since this "primed" identification occurs even for items that cannot be recognized as having been previously presented, it is assumed (Squire, 1987; Schacter, 1990) that it resides in an independent memory system. One system exists for explicit retrieval and one for implicit. The other paradigm is similar theoretically in that is requires that the patient complete an incomplete word with the first response that comes to mind and, since that response is often a word that was also just recently presented, it is proposed that it is drawn from an implicit memory system of which the subject is unaware.

That the subject is unaware of both this memory system and the fact that he is using the information present within the system is one of the hallmark characteristics of "implicit memory" regardless of the terminology (e.g. "procedural", "nondeclarative", "habit", etc.) that is used to describe it. Such nomenclature also exists in the domain of processing theories as well and provides a point of interaction between the two divergent encampments. Mandler (1980) and Jacoby (1984) were the first to suggest that awareness or nonawareness may be a characteristic of an individuals' memorial ability, but they emphasized that the awareness was of their initial processing and was not an emergent property of an explicit memory system. Jacoby has emphasized that awareness is more a property of the type of processing that an individual achieves and not so much a consequence of the memory store in which the item resides. Specifically, he suggested that processing of which we are aware is strategic and conceptual, producing a level of encoding that includes the knowledge of the existence of the episode of analysis itself. Unaware processing, on the other hand, is defined as being largely automatic and probably perceptually based. This latter type of processing, we have already projected as being available to amnesics, while the former seems beyond their reach. The automatic processing that amnesics perform may be sufficient to support their implicit performance, but strategic or conceptual processing, necessary for aware levels of retention, is not available to amnesics. Consequently their explicit performance is impaired while their implicit is not. The prediction is the same as the systems theorists would have it, but the emphasis is on the processing stages just as it had been for our research group since the early 1970s. In order to demonstrate our approach concretely we need next turn to a series of experiments performed at the Boston University Memory Disorders Research Center on amnesic patients' automatic perceptual and strategic conceptual processing during implicit task performance reported during the last ten years.

We begin with a perceptual identification task that we had used previously to show that pseudowords do not produce normal priming for amnesics. Our original interpretation of this below normal priming (Cermak, et. al., 1985) had been based on the belief that pseudowords lack semantic representation. However, it is also the case that pseudowords have unfamiliar orthography and phonology. So, in order to determine whether deficits in analyzing these features could account for amnesics' deficient pseudoword priming, we performed two further perceptual identification experiments (Cermak, Verfaellie, Milberg, Letourneau and Blackford, 1991). These studies used pseudohomonyms as stimuli since they do not have existing orthographic representation but do share phonology with real words (e.g., 'phaire'). We found that amnesics could demonstrate normal priming for these pseudohomonyms. As in our initial report (Cermak, et. al., 1985) priming for pseudowords was overshadowed by the control subjects' demonstration of a dramatic repetition effect for pseudowords. It was clear that, for control subjects, memory of the specific stimuli presented on the study list could be used to support their performance on the identification task. This occurred for pseudowords, as opposed to real words, since these stimuli were harder to identify initially and probably demanded more initial processing. Amnesics, less capable of this initial processing, had to rely only on implicit retention and, therefore, showed less priming. But, this still left us to explain why amnesics evidenced normal pseudohomonym priming.

One possibility was that the semantic connotation of a pseudohomonym mediated such priming more or less automatically. To investigate this possibility we conducted a second experiment in which pseudowords, pseudohomonyms and real words were presented within one single study list. We felt that if mediated activation occurred automatically then this mixed list design should produce the same pattern of results as that for an unmixed design. However, we discovered that priming for pseudohomonyms now became considerably less than normal; in fact, it was nearly nonexistent. In other words, when pseudohomonyms were mixed within the same list as pseudowords, Korsakoff patients' priming for pseudohomonyms (as well as pseudowords) was nonsignificant. The fact that pseudohomonyms have a familiar auditory word form appeared to be concealed by the unfamiliar orthography of all stimuli on the list. Clearly, the semantic processing of pseudohomonyms did not occur automatically simply because of their auditory correspondence with real words. Instead, such processing seemed critically to depend on the patients' "realization" that the orthographically unfamiliar stimuli in the study list corresponded phonemically to real words. This was more likely to occur when all the stimuli shared this characteristic than when stimulus types were mixed within a list. Thus, for pseudohomonyms, the presence and magnitude of priming effects was affected by contextual variables which influenced the manner in which information is processed. Left to their own devices, amnesic patients did not appear to perform the conceptual processing required for priming in this paradigm. When automatic processing is sufficient to support implicit performance, amnesics perform normally but when conceptual processing is required, amnesics may not demonstrate normal implicit performance.

In a similar investigation using another type of implicit task, we (Verfaellie, Cermak, Keane and Treadwell, 1994) found a similar outcome. Homonyms were presented concurrently with disambiguating context words (e.g. dollar-bank) during a lexical decision task. Upon a second presentation, these same homonyms were presented along with the same context word (dollar-bank), or with a different context word that biased the same meaning (teller-bank), or with a different context word that biased a different meaning (river-bank). We felt that the administration of this paradigm to a group of amnesic patients would help to determine the nature of contextual priming in amnesia. Our rationale was as follows; first, as a measure of repetition priming, we could compare response latencies for first presentations of a homonym with response latencies for homonyms repeated in the various context conditions. Then, as an index of contextual influences on priming, we could examine response latencies to homonyms upon their second presentation across the different context conditions. Specifically, we compared response latencies for homonyms presented with an identical or same meaning context word to those obtained for homonyms presented with a different context word. We hypothesized that if amnesic patients are sensitive to the prior conceptual interpretation of a target word, then their responses should be faster in the first (identical or same meaning) condition than in the second (different meaning) condition as it is for normals (Masson and Freedman, 1990). However, if priming for amnesics is solely perceptual in nature, then their response latencies should be equivalent across conditions.

We did find that the amnesic patients responded faster to the second presentation of a homonym than to its first presentation when the data was collapsed across context conditions. Furthermore, the magnitude of this benefit was equivalent to that obtained by control subjects, suggesting that amnesic patients show normal repetition priming effects in this task. On the other hand, we also found that the amnesic patients were not sensitive to the effects of contextual change. Their response latencies to the second presentation of a homonym did not differ as a function of the contextual relationship of the second presentation of the homonym relative to its first presentation. More interestingly, however, we also found that even though this lack of a normal contextual priming effect characterized the amnesic group as a whole, further analysis demonstrated the existence of two different patterns of performance among the amnesics; and, these two different patterns depended on how the individual patients encoded the homonyms upon their first presentation. Specifically, we found that the patients separated into two natural groups based upon the way in which they responded to the initial contextual biasing of each homonym. For one group of patients (CE+), responses to first presentations of homonyms were sensitive to homonym meaning, in that response latencies to homonyms presented with a context word biasing its dominant meaning were faster than those to homonyms presented with a context word biasing its subordinate meaning. This group of patients appropriately used the context to bias their interpretation of a homonym while the patients in the second group (CE-) did not. Upon the second presentation of a homonym, these CE+ patients responded faster when that homonym was repeated in a similar or identical meaning context than when it was repeated in a different meaning context. This means that, for these patients, the originally established conceptual interpretation of a homonym subsequently influenced the response to that homonym. Furthermore, like controls, they responded faster when the context word was identical across repetitions than when it merely biased the same meaning. This finding is important because it suggests that when amnesics' conceptual priming occurs in the present task it is not due to the activation of an abstract semantic representation. Instead, it appears that reinstatement of the specific processes engaged in during original presentation of a homonym is a critical factor in the occurrence of contextual repetition effects. When these processes do not occur during initial biasing, as is the case for the CE- group, then contextual repetition effects also do not occur.

The outcomes of these last two implicit tasks both suggest that priming, when it occurs, might be based, in part, upon the fluency with which items are processed through recruitment of the same processes that were applied to the same stimulus in the past. Reinstatement of processing may not require conscious recollection of the episode in which the processes were first applied, but could, perhaps, be invoked automatically by the stimulus. The more similar the re-recruitment, the more fluency may be generated by the task. In instances where perceptual features are repeated, fluency could be based on that feature. When conceptual features are emphasized, fluency may be based on conceptual repetition. The sensation of fluency may occur normally in amnesic patients (for a review, see Cermak and Verfaellie, 1992) and could be based not only on the reinstatement of perceptual processes, but on the reinstatement of conceptual processes for those patients capable of such processes as well. Thus, performance on an implicit task could be mediated by a combination of processes. Some may occur automatically and some may require conscious control. At any rate, it becomes clear that when amnesics and controls perform equivalently on any given memory task, their performance may be mediated differently. Therefore, it becomes exceedingly important to try to separate the effects of automatic processes and controlled processes within the same task, so as to isolate the contribution of each to the performance of amnesics and control subjects.

Following Jacoby and Kelley (1991), we have recently done so by creating a situation in which the effects of familiarity and conscious recollection are directly opposed to one another (Cermak, Verfaellie, Sweeney, and Jacoby, 1992). The patients participate in a word-stem completion task in which they are told not to use the words that had just been presented on the study list to complete the word stems. Under these instructions, amnesic patients complete more word stems with list items than do the alcoholic controls. In fact, comparing performance on this exclusion task with that on a standard word completion task, demonstrates that the exclusion instruction has very little effect on the performance of amnesics, while it sharply decreases the number of study words used as list completions for the alcoholic controls.

In a similar experiment (Cermak, Verfaellie, Jacoby and Butler, 1993), also designed to oppose fluency and recollection, names were randomly selected from a phone book and presented to patients. Initially, the patients were just asked to pronounce each name as it was presented. This was followed by a fame judgment task in which the previously presented nonfamous names were intermixed with new nonfamous names and with names which were indeed famous although not to the point of being immediately identifiable (e.g., Simon Bolivar, Henry Thoreau). The patients were first assured that the names they had just read were not famous since they were randomly drawn from a phone book and that they should respond "no" if one appeared. This task was considered to be an exclusion task because patients were instructed to exclude names which had just been presented. As in the word-stem completion task, the results showed that amnesic patients were much more likely to endorse an old, compared to a new, nonfamous name as being famous. Controls did not show this effect probably because their conscious recollection of the names presented on the study list allowed them to exclude them. From this, we concluded that amnesics must not be able to use conscious processes to oppose the automatic effects of memory. The fluency generated by the initial processing of a name and reflected during its subsequent processing was apparently misattributed (to use Jacoby's term) to the supposed fame of the name rather than to its true source. Controls, however, could correctly attribute this feeling to the correct source precisely because they could consciously remember its prior presentation.

We next asked the other side of the question of whether amnesics would use automatically generated fluency to "enhance" recall by testing for the effects of conscious recollection and fluency when they were not opposed. Patients were told that names just presented on the study list were indeed famous (but obscure), and ought now to be responded to positively in the fame judgment task (i.e., an inclusion task). In contrast to the results of the previous experiment, alcoholic patients endorsed significantly more old nonfamous names than did the amnesics. In fact, the amnesics' performance on the inclusion task was not higher than that on the exclusion task, whereas the alcoholics showed a striking and highly significant effect of task instructions. We concluded from these experiments that the amnesics' performance was mediated largely, maybe exclusively, by the effects of fluency of processing generated by repeated processing of the same stimulus in making judgments about a stimulus item. Alcoholic controls, in contrast, could use conscious recollection either to enhance or to counteract the effects of this processing fluency.

This entire series of investigations with amnesics suggests that the strategy of analysis utilized by the patient plays an important role in his implicit memory performance. This became clear when the mixed-list design experiment eliminated priming effects that had emerged when the patients were able to anticipate a relationship among list items and analyze them a particular way. Implicit priming for amnesics generally seems to be solely a product of the familiarity produced by fluency automatically generated by the repetition of processing itself except possibly for those instances where nonautomatic processing may be induced. Amnesics respond to fluency by producing the most easily processed word even when that word should have been explicitly excluded. They simply do not know how to attribute fluency to its source. In situations in which fluency of processing produces the correct response the patient appears to be primed; not simply because the processing has been repeated but because the repeated processing gives the amnesic the feeling of being correct. When this "feeling" is oppositional to the correct performance, it results in errors. This misattribution of fluency could even underlie many of the amnesic's other characteristics such as perseveration and source errors.

ACKNOWLEDGEMENTS. Most of the work reported in this chapter was funded by a grant (AA00187) from NIAAA which I have shared with Nelson Butters for 23 years. Recent work has also been funded by NINDS program project grant NS 26985 and by the Medical Research Service of the Department of Veterans Affairs.

REFERENCES

Butters, N. and Cermak, L.S. (1980). *Alcoholic Korsakoff's Syndrome: An Information Processing Approach to Amnesia*. New York: Academic Press.

Cermak, L.S. and Butters, N. (1972). The role of interference and encoding in the short-term memory deficits of Korsakoff patients. *Neuropsychologia, 10*, 89-96.

Cermak, L.S., Butters, N., and Moreines, J. (1974). Some analyses of the verbal encoding deficit of alcoholic Korsakoff patients. *Brain and Language, 1*, 141-150.

Cermak, L.S. and Stiassny, D. (1982). Recall failure following successful generation and recognition of responses by alcoholic Korsakoff patients. *Brain and Cognition, 1*, 165-176.

Cermak, L.S., Talbot, N., Chandler, K., and Wolbarst, L.R. (1985). The perceptual priming phenomenon in amnesia. *Neuropsychologia, 23*, 615-622.

Cermak, L.S. and Verfaellie, M. (1992). The role of fluency in the implicit and explicit task performance in amnesic patients. In L.R. Squire and N. Butters (Eds.), *Neuropsychology of Memory* (pp. 36-45). New York: Guilford.

Cermak, L.S., Verfaellie, M., Butler, T., and Jacoby, L.L. (1993). Fluency vs. recollection during fame judgment performance of amnesic patients. *Neuropsychologia, 7*, 510-518.

Cermak, L.S., Verfaellie, M., Milberg, W.P., Letourneau, L.L., and Blackford, S.P. (1991). A further analysis of perceptual identification priming in alcoholic Korsakoff patients. *Neuropsychologia, 29*, 725-736.

Cermak, L.S., Verfaellie, M., Sweeney, M., and Jacoby, L.L. (1992). Fluency vs. conscious recollection in the word completion performance of amnesic patients. *Brain and Cognition, 20*, 367-377.

Craik, F.I.M. and Lockhart, R.S. (1972). Levels of processing: A framework for memory research. *Journal of Verbal Learning Verbal Behavior, 11*, 671-684.

Craik, F.I.M. and Tulving, E. (1975). Depth of processing and retention of words in episodic memory. *Journal of Experimental Psychology: General, 104*, 268-294.

Jacoby, L.L. (1984). Incidental versus intentional retrieval: Remembering and awareness as separate issues. In L.R. Squire and N. Butters (Eds.), Neuropsychology of Memory, New York: Guilford Press.

Jacoby, L.L. and Kelley, C. (1991). Unconscious influences of memory: Dissociations and automaticity. In D. Milner and M. Rugg (Eds.), *Consciousness and Cognition: Neuropsychological Perspectives*, New York: Academic Press.

Mandler, G. (1980). Recognizing: The judgment of previous occurrence. *Psychology Review, 87,* 252-271.

Masson, M.E.J. and Freedman, L. (1990). Fluent identification of repeated words. *Journal of Experimental Psychology: Learning, Memory and Cognition, 16,* 355-373.

Schacter, D.L. (1990). Perceptual representation systems and implicit memory: Toward a resolution of the multiple memory systems debate. In A. Diamond (Ed.), Development and neural bases of higher cognition. *Annals of the New York Academy of Sciences, 608,* 543-571.

Squire, L.R. (1987). *Memory and Brain.* New York: Oxford University Press.

Thomas, D.M. and Tulving, E. (1970). Associative encoding and retrieval: Weak and strong cues. *Journal of Experimental Psychology, 86,* 255-262.

Warrington, E.K. and Weiskrantz, L. (1974). The effect of prior learning on subsequent retention in amnesic patients. *Neuropsychologia, 12,* 419-428.

Warrington, E.K. and Weiskrantz, L. (1978). Further analysis of the prior learning effect in amnesic patients. *Neuropsychologia, 16,* 169-177.

Wickens, D.D. (1970). Encoding strategies of words: An empirical approach to meaning. *Psychology Review, 22,* 1-15.

Verfaellie, M., Cermak, L.S., Keane, M.M. and Treadwell, J.R. (in press). Contextual priming in amnesia: Memory for context-specific interpretations of ambiguous words.

4

Verbal Priming and Semantic Memory in Alzheimer's Disease

Degraded Representation or Impaired Activation?

WILLIAM C. HEINDEL[1]

A major emphasis of Nelson Butters' research has been the application of the concepts and methodology of cognitive psychology to the cognitive and memory impairments seen in patients with different forms of dementia. These studies have had tremendous clinical impact, serving to more accurately characterize the nature and progression of the deficits displayed by different patient populations. These studies have also been instrumental in demonstrating that 'dementia' is not a homogenous entity, but rather that patients with different dementing illnesses display distinct neuropsychological profiles of preserved and impaired abilities which correspond to the distinctive neuropathology associated with each disorder. While these studies have largely supported, at a general level, the distinction between 'cortical' and 'subcortical' dementia (as typified by patients with Alzheimer's disease and Huntington's disease, respectively), they have also emphasized the uniqueness of each patient's cognitive and neurologic dysfunction.

Perhaps even more important than the clinical utility of Nelson's work, however, are the contributions his studies with demented populations have made

[1] WILLIAM C. HEINDEL, Ph.D. • Department of Psychology, Brown University

Neuropsychological Explorations of memory and Cognition: Essays in Honor of Nelson Butters, edited by Laird S. Cermak, Ph.D. Plenum Press, New York, 1994

to our understanding of the cognitive and neural architecture of normal memory. Nelson's comparative neuropsychological investigations of Alzheimer and Huntington patients have provided valuable insights into the psychological processes and neurological substrates mediating performance on tests of episodic memory, semantic memory, skill learning and priming. I feel extremely fortunate to have had the opportunity to participate, both directly and indirectly, in a number of these studies during the time I spent in Nelson's laboratory. The purpose of this chapter is to review one particular (and, in my mind, particularly interesting) story among the large array of topics pursued by Nelson; namely, the verbal priming performance of Alzheimer patients.

Priming refers to a wide variety of phenomena in which the presentation of a stimulus influences subsequent processing of either the same or a related stimulus. Previous exposure to verbal stimuli, for example, has been found to decrease reaction time to these words in lexical decision tasks, to decrease the exposure duration necessary to identify these words in perceptual identification tasks, and to increase the tendency to complete word fragments with these words. Priming has been considered by many investigators to be a form of implicit memory (Schacter, 1987), since the memory for the previously presented item is expressed unconsciously through performance of specific operations comprising a particular task. In contrast, traditional memory tests such as recall and recognition are considered explicit memory tests since they require the conscious recollection of previous study episodes.

Priming phenomena (and implicit memory in general) have generated considerable interest within the field of neuropsychology, primarily because of the demonstration that patients with circumscribed amnesic syndromes perform normally on these tasks despite their severe explicit memory deficits. For example, in a study by Graf and colleagues (Graf, Squire & Mandler, 1984), amnesic patients demonstrated as strong a tendency (relative to chance) as normal control subjects to complete three-letter word stems with previously presented words, despite the amnesic patients' failure to recall or recognize these words on standard memory tests. Amnesic patients apparently treat the stem-completion task as a word puzzle and report that the words seem to "pop" into mind in response to the stems even though the words are not recognized as familiar. This demonstration of preserved priming ability in the presence of severe explicit memory impairments have been observed across a wide variety of priming tasks (for a review, see Shimamura, 1986).

The repeated demonstration of normal priming performance by amnesic patients in the face of profound explicit memory impairments suggests that there may be a neurological as well as a psychological distinction between these two forms of memory. That is, explicit memory, but not priming, appears to be critically dependent upon the functional integrity of the medial temporal (hippocampal) and diencephalic brain regions known to be affected in amnesia. Investigations of amnesic patients have in fact been the critical source of information concerning our understanding of the psychobiological substrates of explicit memory.

Because priming is preserved in amnesics, however, little more can be learned from these patients about the brain structures that underlie this particular form of memory. A deeper and more extensive understanding of the psychobiological bases of priming phenomena can only be possible through careful investigations with patients whose brain damage extends beyond those regions involved in circumscribed amnesia. Studies of the priming performance of patients with different forms of dementing illnesses (and different sites of neural damage), therefore, may demonstrate unique patterns of preserved and impaired priming ability which reflect the particular brain pathology and corresponding processing deficits associated with each disease.

One of the first studies utilizing this approach (Shimamura, Salmon, Squire & Butters, 1987) compared the lexical priming performance of Alzheimer's disease patients, Huntington's disease patients, amnesic patients with alcoholic Korsakoff's syndrome, and normal control subjects on the word-stem completion task previously used by Graf et al. (1984). Subjects were first exposed to a list of 10 target words (e.g., MOTEL, ABSTAIN) and asked to rate each word in terms of its "likability." Subjects were shown three-letter stems (e.g., MOT, ABS) of words that were and were not on the presentation list, and simply asked to complete the stems with the "first word that comes to mind." Half of the stems could be completed with previously presented words, while the other half were used to assess baseline guessing rates (i.e., the tendency to complete word stems with target words if they had not been previously exposed to the target words). Other lists of words were used to assess the subjects' ability at free recall and recognition.

As expected, all three patient groups were found to be severely and equally impaired on their explicit memory (i.e., free recall and recognition) for the previously presented words in this experiment. However, significant differences were observed among the patient groups on the stem-completion priming task. Although all three groups demonstrated equivalent baseline guessing rates on this task, only the alcoholic Korsakoff and Huntington patients exhibited intact priming ability relative to normal control subjects. The Alzheimer patients, in contrast, showed significantly less tendency to complete the word stems with previously presented words compared to both the other patient groups and the controls. Although the Alzheimer patients did prime significantly above their baseline stem-completion rate, these patients were apparently unable to generate or activate memory traces to a level sufficient to support normal levels of priming in this task.

This initial finding of impaired stem-completion priming in Alzheimer patients has subsequently been replicated by a number of investigators (e.g., Bondi & Kaszniak, 1991; Heindel, Salmon, Shults, Walicke & Butters, 1989; Keane, Gabrieli, Fennema, Growdon & Corkin, 1991; Salmon, Shimamura,

Butters & Smith, 1988), and this study was among the first to demonstrate significant deficiencies in long-term priming in any neurologically impaired patient group. Of particular interest were the implications these findings had concerning the psychobiological substrates underlying verbal priming in the stem-completion task: These results suggested that stem-completion priming may be mediated at least in part by neural substrates selectively disrupted in Alzheimer patients but not in Huntington or amnesic patients.

SEMANTIC MEMORY

One of most striking differences between Alzheimer patients on the one hand, and Huntington and amnesic patients on the other, is their performance on tests of semantic memory.   Semantic memory contains the permanent representations of concepts, of words and their meanings, and in general knowledge about the world.   Semantic memories are considered to be independent of contextual cues, and can therefore be distinguished from episodic memories for personal experiences and events that do depend upon temporal and/or spatial cues for their retrieval (Tulving, 1983).   Of the three patient groups, only the Alzheimer patients seem to possess a marked disruption in the organization of semantic memory.

Evidence for a semantic memory impairment in Alzheimer but not Huntington or amnesic patients has come in part from verbal fluency studies in which subjects are required to generate words from specific categories. Butters and his colleagues (Butters, Granholm, Salmon, Grant & Wolfe, 1987) found that Huntington and alcoholic Korsakoff patients were impaired on both letter (i.e., F, A, S) and category fluency (i.e., animals) tasks, suggesting the presence of a general retrieval deficit which affects both fluency tasks equally.   In contrast, the performance of Alzheimer patients was directly related to the different demands the two fluency tasks place on the organization of the semantic network: They performed normally on the letter fluency task, but were severely impaired on the linguistically more demanding category fluency task. Alzheimer patients have also been found to generate (relative to normal controls) significantly fewer specific items per superordinate category and a larger ratio of superordinate category names to total words produced on the supermarket fluency task from the Dementia Rating Scale (Mattis, 1976) (Martin & Fedio, 1983; Tröster, Salmon, McCullough & Butters, 1989).

Consistent with these fluency findings, Alzheimer patients have also been shown to be much more likely than normal control subjects or patients with other dementing disorders to produce superordinate and within-category associative errors on tests of object naming (Bayles & Tomoeda, 1983; Huff, Corkin & Growdon, 1986; Smith, Murdoch & Chenery, 1989). Taken together, these results suggest that the Alzheimer patients' fluency and naming impairments reflect a disruption in the organization of semantic memory that is characterized by a loss of the specific attributes distinguishing items within a semantic category along with relative preservation of more general superordinate knowledge (Martin, 1987; Martin & Fedio, 1983).

Chertkow and Bub (1990) provide strong evidence that Alzheimer patients possess an actual loss of semantic knowledge rather than an inability to access a relatively intact semantic memory. In this study, Alzheimer patients were found to be markedly impaired on both a picture-naming test and a word-to-picture matching test (each comprising the same 150 pictorial stimuli), and showed little improvement with semantic cueing. Furthermore, the Alzheimer patients showed a remarkable consistency between the particular items correctly completed or failed, both across the naming and matching tasks, and on the same naming task across two different test sessions. The Alzheimer patients were also significantly impaired in their ability to answer probe questions concerning perceptual, functional and contextual aspects of items from the naming task, but had no difficulty identifying superordinate category membership. Finally, when asked to generate as many examplars as possible from the same eight semantic categories used in the picture naming test, fewer than 7% of all the items generated on this task were items that the patients had previously been unable to name.

Thus, the Alzheimer patients in the study by Chertkow and Bub (1990) were found to display first, a remarkable consistency in the particular items failed across the naming, matching and fluency tasks; second, a failure to benefit from semantic cueing; and third, a relative preservation of superordinate information along with a loss of detailed knowledge. According to the criteria developed by Warrington & Shallice (1979), this pattern of results is quite consistent with the presence of an actual loss of semantic knowledge in these Alzheimer patients, rather than simply a deficiency in accessing otherwise intact semantic information.

PRIMING AND SEMANTIC MEMORY

Since Alzheimer patients, and not Huntington or amnesic patients, evidence marked pathology in temporal, parietal and frontal association cortices (Brun, 1983; Terry & Katzman, 1983), their impaired priming may be the result of damage to those neocortical association areas involved in the storage of the representations underlying semantic memory. Neuronal loss in these regions may lead to a deterioration in the associative network which forms the skeletal structure of semantic memory. This deterioration may greatly limit the capacity of previously presented stimuli to activate the preexisting semantic representations necessary for verbal priming. That is, although Alzheimer patients are able to perform the stem-completion task by completing the stems with appropriate words, their semantic network may be sufficiently deteriorated to greatly limit the capacity of available cues to activate the representation necessary to display normal levels of priming. Because their semantic representations are intact, however, Huntington and amnesic patients are able to demonstrate normal verbal priming performance.

If the Alzheimer patients' stem-completion priming deficit is indeed related to deterioration in the organization of semantic memory, then these patients' priming performance should worsen as the semantic demands of the priming task increase. In order to examine this issue, Salmon and his colleagues (Salmon et al., 1988) compared the priming performance of Alzheimer, Huntington, and intact control subjects on a semantic priming test which employed a paired- associate procedure. In this task, subjects were first asked to judge categorically or functionally related word pairs (e.g., BIRD-ROBIN, NEEDLE-THREAD) and later to "free-associate" to the first words of the previously presented pairs as well as to words that were not presented as part of the paired-associates. Thus, priming is reflected in the greater tendency to produce the second word of semantically related pairs relative to baseline associative strengths. Presumably, the priming of semantic relationships places greater demand on the semantic network than does the priming of lexical relationships in stem-completion priming.

As with the stem-completion task, Alzheimer patients were found to be significantly less likely to produce the second word of the semantically-related pair than the other two patient groups. Unlike the stem-completion task, however, the priming score for the Alzheimer patients in the paired-associate task was not significantly greater than their baseline guessing rates. In other words, the priming performance of Alzheimer patients apparently worsened as the semantic demands increased from the stem-completion to the paired-associate task, suggesting that the priming deficits of the Alzheimer patients may in fact be related to a breakdown in the associative structure of semantic memory.

If the priming deficits described above reflect a deterioration in the structure of semantic knowledge, then a relationship should exist between performance on these tests of priming and performance on traditional measures of semantic knowledge, but not between priming performance and performance on tests assessing other "non-semantic" neuropsychological processes. To address this issue, stem-completion and paired-associate priming scores of 30 mildly to moderately demented Alzheimer patients were compared with their scores on traditional neuropsychological tests of episodic and semantic memory, language, attention and visuospatial processes (Salmon, Heindel and Butters, 1994). Correlational analyses revealed that the stem-completion priming score was not significantly related to any other neuropsychological measure, including scores on tests of semantic memory (e.g., Boston Naming Test, Number

Information Test, Letter and Category Fluency Tests, WAIS-R Vocabulary Subtest).

The lack of correlation between Alzheimer patients' priming performance and their performance on traditional tests of semantic memory would seem to cast doubt upon the notion that these patients' priming deficits are mediated by the disruption of their semantic memory, and instead suggests that the deficits in long-term priming exhibited by these patients may be due to, or at least influenced by, some factor other than the integrity of the semantic network. In particular, one possibility is that the priming deficits in Alzheimer patients may be related to a generalized disturbance in attention, arousal or activation which could lead to an inability to activate an otherwise intact representation in semantic memory to a level sufficient to support long-term priming. Although not as extensively studied as other cognitive functions, attentional disturbances have indeed been observed in Alzheimer patients, particularly in tasks concerned with the selective orientation of attention (Cossa, Della Sala, & Spinnler, 1989; Nebes & Brady, 1989; Grady, Grimes, Patronas, Sunderland, Foster & Rapoport, 1989; Freed, Corkin, Growden, & Nissen, 1989).

Freed et al. (1989) suggested that the selective attention impairments seen in some Alzheimer patients may be the behavioral manifestation of noradrenergic deficits resulting from damage to the locus coeruleus. Locus coeruleus neuropathology has been observed in a subset of Alzheimer patients at autopsy (Mann, Yates & Marcyniuk, 1986; Marcyniuk, Mann & Yates, 1986; Tomlinson, Irving & Blessed, 1981; Zweig, Ross, Hedreen, Steele, Cardillo, Whitehouse, Folstein & Price, 1988), and both animal and human studies have implicated noradrenaline in selective attention processes (Clark, Geffen & Geffen, 1989; Posner and Petersen, 1990; Sara, 1985a,b). Sara (1985a) has suggested that the locus coeruleus modulates selective attention by enhancing "cortical tonus", and therefore increasing the signal-to-noise ratio of cortical information processing. In this view, noradrenergic deficits in Alzheimer patients could lead to an inability to activate an otherwise intact representation in semantic memory at a level that would be sufficient to support priming.

This idea is consistent with a number of studies demonstrating normal priming in Alzheimer patients on very short-term, on-line priming tasks . In this view, traces may still be sufficiently activated to manifest intact priming over very short delay intervals, but not sufficiently activated to support long-term priming on tasks such as stem-completion and paired-associate priming. In a study by Nebes and colleagues (Nebes, Martin & Horn, 1984), for example, a given word was preceded (by approximately 500 msec) either by a semantically related word (primed trials) or by an unrelated word (unprimed trials). Both the Alzheimer patients and control subjects displayed a slight and equivalent facilitation in naming latency when a word was preceded by a semantic associate (i.e., semantic priming). Nebes et al. concluded that Alzheimer patients' semantic memory is normal when it is assessed with techniques which rely solely upon automatic information processing, and that the deficits these patients display on other tasks are due to the heavy attentional demands of these tasks rather to an impairment in semantic memory per se. Ober, Shenaut, Jagust and Sillman (1991) similarly concluded that the semantic memory structures and processes that support automatic semantic priming effects are intact in Alzheimer patients.

This idea is also consistent with a study by Partridge, Knight and Freehan (1990) which found that Alzheimer patients demonstrate normal levels of stem-completion priming when the nature of the orienting task was changed to increase the likelihood of semantic processing of the target words. Rather than judging the likability of the target words during the presentation phase of the task (as in the studies by Shimamura et al., 1987; and Salmon et al, 1988.), Alzheimer patients were required to supply the meaning of each word. Partridge and colleagues suggested that, due possibly to an attentional or controlled processing deficit, Alzheimer patients could be providing appropriate responses in the standard"likeability" orienting task without fully attending to the semantic aspects of the target word. In this view, forcing the Alzheimer patients to attend to the semantic aspects of the words by using the "meaning" task may have increased the activation of the semantic representations sufficiently to support long-term priming in these patients.

Despite the evidence reviewed above supporting the notion that the verbal priming impairment of Alzheimer patients is related to a general disturbance in attention or activation, one still cannot, for several reasons, completely rule out the possibility that this impairment is primarily caused by a semantic storage deficit. First, the stem-completion study by Partridge et al. (1990) failed to include a"likability" rating condition to directly compare with the more semantic "meaning" task within the same Alzheimer patients. Thus, it is not clear whether these particular Alzheimer patients actually improved their stem-completion performance from "likeability" to "meaning" orienting task conditions, and therefore whether differences in task orientation actually had any effect on these patients' priming performance.

Second, several studies have in fact reported abnormal performance by Alzheimer patients on short-term, on-line semantic priming tasks. In a study by Ober and Shenault (1988), for example, Alzheimer patients demonstrated impaired semantic priming but normal repetition priming effects within an on-line lexical decision task. Chertkow and his colleagues (Chertkow, Bub and Seidenberg, 1989) actually observed abnormally high levels of semantic priming (i.e., hyperpriming) relative to controls using a lexical decision task. Martin (1993) also recently demonstrated abnormally high levels of semantic priming in Alzheimer patients using pictorial stimuli within an on-line object/nonobject decision paradigm. Martin further argued that these results are quite consistent with a degraded store hypothesis in which the specific attributes distinguishing between exemplars within the same semantic category are lost, thereby creating underspecified and overgeneralized representations. In this view, since the overgeneralized representations of two items within the same semantic category in Alzheimer patients would be more similar to each other than the corresponding representations in intact control subjects, the amount of semantic priming using these two items should approach the higher level of direct repetition priming (i.e., prime and target are the same item) in the Alzheimer patients.

Finally, a recent study by Glosser and Friedman (1991) demonstrated normal lexical but impaired semantic priming in Alzheimer patients on a short-term priming task. Glosser and Friedman argued that the prime-target word pairs used in previous studies were related to each other both associatively and semantically, and therefore that the priming observed in Alzheimer patients in these studies could be due either to the activation of semantic relationships between the prime and the target, or to the activation of relationships at a lexical-associative (i.e., nonsemantic) level. When the effects of lexical and semantic facilitation were assessed independently, Glosser and Friedman found that Alzheimer patients showed no effects of priming for word pairs related only by semantic features (e.g., bed-sofa), but showed normal priming for word pairs associatively related only at the level of the lexicon (e.g., 'accidents of contiguity' such as cottage-cheese). These results are consistent with the notion that the priming impairments of Alzheimer patients are related to a disturbance of semantic processing in these patients, but that their ability to prime at the lexical level remains intact.

LEXICAL AND SEMANTIC PROCESSES

Thus, it is still not clear what factors contribute to the impaired stem-completion priming performance of Alzheimer patients initially demonstrated by Shimamura et al. (1987). Do Alzheimer patients (and normal controls) rely on lexical processes, semantic processes, or both when performing the standard stem-completion task?   What, if anything, changes in the processing of Alzheimer patients when they are forced to attend to the semantic relationships of the target words (e.g., Partridge et al., 1990)?

In order to directly examine this issue, we (Heindel & Rosenblum, 1994) recently completed a study which systematically manipulates, within the stem-completion paradigm, both the lexical and semantic set sizes of the target words and the degree to which attention is focused on the semantic aspects of the target words. Set size refers to the number of preexisting associates of a specified type linked to a particular stimulus (Nelson, Schreiber & McEvoy, 1992). The semantic set size of a target word, for example, is reflected in the number of different meaningfully related words generated in response to that target word. In contrast, lexical set size (in the case of stem-completion priming) is reflected in the number of different words generated in response to a particular word stem (i.e., word endings).

Nelson and his colleagues have demonstrated set size effects across a number of explicit and implicit memory conditions. For example, both cued recall (using word endings as cues) and stem-completion priming have been found to be inversely related to both lexical and semantic set size (Nelson & Freidrich , 1980; Nelson, Canas, Bajo & Keelen, 1987). That is, cued recall and stem-completion priming were both greater for words with smaller semantic set sizes, and for ending cues (i.e., stems) with smaller lexical set sizes. In contrast, significant lexical but not semantic set size effects were found on a word fragment completion task (Nelson et al., 1987), suggesting that priming tests may in fact differ in terms of the relative demands these tasks place on lexical and semantic processes.

The results of these studies with normal subjects also suggest that the systematic manipulation of the lexical and semantic set sizes of target words within the stem-completion paradigm should be useful in identifying the processes underlying the priming deficits of Alzheimer patients. That is, if Alzheimer patients are engaged in both lexical and semantic processes in their performance of the stem-completion task, then these patients, like normal controls, should display significant lexical and semantic set size effects. A failure to engage in one or both of these processes, however, should be reflected in the absence of a significant set size effect for the corresponding domain(s).

In our study (Heindel & Rosenblum, 1994), subjects were first asked to rate a list of 20 words using a five-point scale, and later asked to complete ending stems with the first word that came to mind. One half of the target words had small lexical set sizes (i.e., the corresponding stems could be completed with seven or less different words) and half had large lexical sets (i.e., stems could be completed with ten or more words). In addition, one half of the words had small semantic set sizes (i.e., words with ten or fewer meaningfully related associates) and half had large semantic sets (i.e., words with fourteen or more associates). Across these different set sizes, associative strength (i.e., the cue-to-target probability) was held constant in order to insure that the baseline tendency to complete the word-stem with the target word was the same for each lexical/semantic set size combination.

Two different conditions of this stem-completion task were administered to Alzheimer patients and age-matched normal control subjects. In the single-word condition, subjects studied words in isolation and were asked to rate the likeability of each word. This condition is modeled after the standard stem-completion paradigm utilized by Shimamura et al. (1987) and others in demonstrating impaired priming in Alzheimer patients. In the paired-word condition, subjects studied target words paired with a meaningful associate and were asked to rate how related they thought the two words were. This condition was intended to force subjects to attend to the semantic relationships of the words in a fashion analogous to those studies which demonstrated normal priming in Alzheimer patients (e.g., Partridge et al., 1990). Taken together, these two conditions were designed to examine first, whether Alzheimer patients display the same pattern of lexical and semantic processing on the stem-completion task as normal controls, and second, whether this pattern of processing changes when subjects are forced to attend to semantic relationships.

As expected from previous studies (Shimamura et al., 1987, Salmon et al.,1988 Heindel et al.1989), the overall priming performance of the Alzheimer patients in the single-word condition (i.e., standard stem-completion paradigm) was significantly impaired relative to the intact elderly control subjects. More interesting was the presence of a significant group by semantic set size interaction: The elderly control subjects but not the Alzheimer patients displayed a significant semantic set size effect on this task. In other words, in the standard likeability stem-completion rating task, elderly control subjects appeared to activate and engage in semantic processing of the target words to a degree sufficient to display significant semantic set size effects in their priming performance, whereas the Alzheimer patients did not. These results are consistent with the notion that the impaired priming performance of Alzheimer patients in the standard stem-completion paradigm is related to impaired semantic processing of target words by these patients relative to normal controls.

A different pattern of results was observed in the paired-word condition, in which subjects were explicitly told to attend to the semantic aspects of the target words. In this condition, the overall priming performance of the Alzheimer patients was not significantly different from intact control subjects, nor were the group by semantic or lexical set size interactions significant. There was, however, a highly significant main effect of semantic set size. Post-hoc analyses indicated that both the elderly controls and the Alzheimer patients demonstrated significant semantic set size effects in this condition. Thus, when forced to attend to the semantic relationships of the target words, Alzheimer patients were not significantly impaired in their stem-completion priming performance relative to elderly controls, and both groups appeared to engage in semantic processing sufficient to demonstrate significant semantic set size effects. Thus, the Alzheimer's patients' impaired priming performance in the single-word condition on the one hand, and their intact priming performance in the paired-word condition on the other, appear to be directly related to these patients' deficient semantic processing in the former but not the latter condition.

Taken together, these results seem to support the hypothesis that the priming deficits of Alzheimer patients may be primarily due to a general deficit in activating semantic representations rather than to a deterioration in the semantic representations themselves. Intact elderly control subjects appear to automatically engage in semantic processing of target words regardless of task demands at time of study (i.e., rating the likeability vs. the relatedness or words).

Alzheimer patients, in contrast, appear to have difficulty activating the semantic associates of isolated words in the standard likeability condition, leading to impaired priming performance with no effect of semantic set size. When their attention is properly directed to the semantic relationships of the target words, however, these patients can activate semantic associates and perform normally on the stem-completion priming task.

However, even these findings still do not necessarily preclude the hypothesis that the Alzheimer patients' priming deficit is primarily related to a degradation in the representations underlying semantic memory. It is possible, for example, that semantic degradation leads to greater difficulty activating semantic representations in Alzheimer patients compared to intact controls, such that, left to their own devices, these patients fail to fully process at a semantic level words presented in isolation. Attentional processes, however, may be able to potentiate the degree to which these representations are activated in response to stimuli. Thus, helping Alzheimer patients to focus their attention to the semantic aspects of target words may help them activate these degraded representation sufficiently to support long-term priming.

Indeed, viewed from a neural network perspective, activation and representation are in many ways two sides of the same coin, and it may be quite difficult (if not impossible) to ever differentiate between these two possibilities. From this view, representations are defined by the pattern of activation across a set of distributed nodes, and degraded representations would manifest themselves in the difficulty reactivating the corresponding distributed patterns. Thus, representations may be difficult to activate because they are degraded, and representations may appear to be degraded because of a difficulty in reactivating the corresponding pattern. Consistent with this notion, preliminary findings in our laboratory have in part replicated Chertkow et al.'s (1989) demonstration that the degree of short-term, on-line priming displayed by Alzheimer patients is influenced by the degree to which the semantic representations underlying the target items appear to be degraded (as assessed by off-line tests of semantic memory). Specifically, although unprimed degraded target items are more difficult to activate than unprimed intact items (as measured by latency to identify that item as a word or nonword), degraded items receive substantially greater benefit from priming than do intact items.

In summary, the early demonstrations of impaired verbal priming performance in Alzheimer patients, conducted in large part by Nelson Butters and his colleagues, have lead to an explosion of related studies utilizing a wide range of priming paradigms in a number of different laboratories. Although these studies have gone far in providing a taxonomic account of the boundary conditions under which priming is preserved or impaired in Alzheimer patients, a number of apparently conflicting findings still remain. It is likely that the priming deficits observed in Alzheimer patients are not simply attributable to an impairment in either activation or representation, but rather reflect in some way an interaction between impaired and intact cognitive processes and structures within these patients. Regardless of the final outcome, it seems clear that future studies of priming in Alzheimer's disease will serve not only to clarify the nature of the cognitive impairments associated with this particular disorder, but will also provide substantial insight into the cognitive architecture involved in the normal operation of implicit and semantic memory.

ACKNOWLEDGEMENT. The preparation of this manuscript was supported in part by NIMH grant MH-48819 to the University of California at San Diego.

REFERENCES

Bayles, K.A. and Tomoeda, C.K. (1983). Confrontation naming impairment in dementia. *Brain and Language, 19*, 98-114.

Bondi, M.W. and Kaszniak, A.W. (1991). Implicit and explicit memory in Alzheimer's disease and Parkinson's disease. *Journal of Clinical and Experimental Neuropsychology, 13*, 339-358.

Brun, A. (1983). In B. Reisberg (Ed.), *Alzheimer's Disease*. New York: The Free Press.An overview of light and electron microscopic changes.

Butters, N., Granholm, E., Salmon, D., Grant, I. and Wolfe, J. (1987). Episodic and semantic memory: A comparison of amnesic and demented patients. *Journal of Clinical and Experimental Neuropsychology, 9*, 479-497.

Chertkow, H. and Bub, D. (1990). Semantic memory loss in dementia of Alzheimer's type. *Brain, 113*, 397-417.

Chertkow, H., Bub, D. and Seidenberg, M. (1989). Priming and semantic memory loss in Alzheimer's disease. *Brain and Language, 36*, 420-446.

Clark, C., Geffen, G. and Geffen, L. (1989). Catecholamines and the covert orientation of attention in humans. *Neuropsychologia, 27*, 131-139.

Cossa, F., Della Sala, S. and Spinnler, H. (1989). Selective visual attention in Alzheimer's and Parkinson's patients: Memory- and data-driven control. *Neuropsychologia, 27*, 887-892.

Freed, D., Corkin, S., Growdon, J. and Nissen, M. (1989). Selective attention and Alzheimer's disease: Characterizing cognitive subgroups of patients. *Neuropsychologia, 27*, 325-339.

Glosser, G. and Friedman, R.B. (1991). Lexical but not semantic priming in Alzheimer's disease. *Psychology and Aging, 6*, 522-527.

Grady, C., Grimes, A., Patronas, N., Sunderland, T., Foster, N. and Rapoport, S. (1989). Divided attention, as measured by dichotic speech performance, in dementia of the Alzheimer type. *Archives of Neurology, 46*, 317-320.

Graf, P, Squire, L. and Mandler, G. (1984). The information that amnesic patients do not forget. *Journal of Experimental Psychology: Human Learning and Memory, 10*, 164-178.

Heindel, W. and Rosenblum, J. The role of lexical and semantic processes in the stem-completion priming performance of Alzheimer's disease patients. Submitted for publication.

Heindel, W., Salmon, D., Shults, C., Walicke, P. and Butters, N. (1989). Neuropsychological evidence for multiple implicit memory systems: A comparison of Alzheimer's, Huntington's and Parkinson's disease patients. *Journal of Neuroscience, 9,* 582- 587.

Huff, F.J., Corkin, S, and Growdon, J.H. (1986). Semantic impairment and anomia in Alzheimer's disease. *Brain and Language, 28,* 235-249.

Keane, M.M., Gabrieli, J.D.E., Fennema, A.C., Growdon, J.H. and Corkin, S. (1991). Evidence for a dissociation between perceptual and conceptual priming in Alzheimer's disease. *Behavioral Neuroscience, 105,* 326-342.

Mann, D.M.A., Yates, P.O. and Marcyniuk, B. (1986). A comparison of nerve cell loss in cortical and subcortical structures in Alzheimer's disease. *Journal of Neurology, Neurosurgery and Psychiatry, 49,* 310-312.

Marcyniuk, B., Mann, D.M.A. and Yates, P.O. (1986). The topography of cell loss from locus coeruleus in Alzheimer's disease. *Journal of Neurological Science, 76,* 335-345.

Martin, A. (1987). Representation of semantic and spatial knowledge in Alzheimer's patients: Implications for models of preserved learning in amnesia. *Journal of Clinical and Experimental Neuropsychology, 9,* 191-124.

Martin, A. (1993). Degraded knowledge representations in patients with Alzheimer's disease: Implications for models of semantic and repetition priming. In L.R. Squire & N. Butters (Eds.), *Neuropsychology of Memory, 2nd Edition.* New YorkL Guilford Press.

Martin, A. and Fedio, P. (1983). Word production and comprehension in Alzheimer's disease: The breakdown in semantic knowledge. *Brain and Language, 19,* 124-141.

Mattis, S. (1976). Mental status examination for organic mental syndrome in the elderly patient. In L. Bellack and T. Karasu (Eds.), *Geriatric Psychiatry,* New York: Grune & Stratton.

Nebes, R. and Brady, C. (1989). Focused and divided attention in Alzheimer's disease. *Cortex, 25,* 305-315.

Nebes, R., Martin, D. and Horn, L. (1984). Sparing of semantic memory in Alzheimer's disease. *Journal of Abnormal Psychology, 93,* 321-330.

Nelson, D.L., Canas, J., Bajo, M.T., and Keelean, P. (1987). Comparing word fragment completion and cued recall with letter cues. *Journal of Experimental Psychology: Learning, Memory, and Cognition, 13,* 542-552.

Nelson, D.L. and Friedrich, M.A. (1980). Encoding and cuing sounds and senses. *Journal of Experimental Psychology: Human Learning and Memory, 6,* 717-731.

Nelson, D.L., Schreiber, T.A., and McEvoy (1992). Processing implicit and explicit representations. *Psychological Review, 99,* 322-348.

Ober, B.A. & Shenaut, G.K. (1988). Lexical decision and priming in Alzheimer's disease. *Neuropsychologia, 26,* 273-286.

Ober, B.A., Shenaut, G.K., Jagust, W.J. and Stillman, R.C. (1991). Automatic semantic priming with various category relations in Alzheimer's disease and normal aging. *Psychology and Aging, 6,* 647-660.

Partridge, F., Knight, R. and Feehan, M. (1990). Direct and indirect memory performance in patients with senile dementia. *Psychological Medicine, 20,* 111-118.

Posner, M. and Petersen, S. (1990). The attention system of the human brain. *Annual Review of Neuroscience, 13,* 25-42.

Richardson-Klavehn, A, and Bjork. (1988). Measures of memory. *Annual Review of Pschology, 39,* 475-543.

Salmon, D., Heindel, W., & Butters, N. (1994). The relationship between neuropsychological deficits and impaired priming in Alzheimer's disease. Manuscript in preparation.

Salmon, D., Shimamura, A., Butters, N. and Smith, S. (1988). Lexical and semantic priming deficits in patients with Alzheimer's disease. *Journal of Clinical and Experimental Neuropsychology, 10*, 477-494.

Sara, S. (1985). The locus coeruleus and cognitive function: Attempts to relate noradrenergic enhancement of signal/noise in the brain to behavior. *Physiological Psychology, 13,* 151-162.

Sara, S. (1985). Noradrenergic modulation of selective attention: Its role in memory retrieval. *Annals of the New York Academy of Sciences, 444*, 178-193.

Schacter, D. (1987). Implicit memory: History and current status. *Journal of Experimental Psychology: Learning, Memory and Cognition, 13*, 501-517.

Shimamura, A.P. (1986). Priming effects in amnesia: Evidence for a dissociable memory function. *Quarterly Journal of Experimental Psychology [A], 38*, 619-644.

Shimamura, A., Salmon, D., Squire, L. and Butters, N. (1987). Memory dysfunction and word priming in dementia and amnesia. *Behavioral Neurosciences, 101*, 347-351.

Smith, S.R., Murdoch, B.E. and Chenery, H.J. (1989). Semantic abilities in dementia of the Alzheimer type: 1. Lexical semantics. *Brain and Language, 36*, 314-324.

Terry, R.D. and Katzman, R. (1983). Senile dementia of the Alzheimer type. *Annals of Neurology, 14,* 497-506.

Tomlinson, B.E., Irving, D. and Blessed, G. (1981). Cell loss in the locus coeruleus in senile dementia of the Alzheimer type. *Journal of Neurological Science, 11*, 205-242.

Troster, A.I., Salmon, D.P., McCullough, D. and Butters, N. (1989). A comparison of the category fluency deficits associated with Alzheimer's and Huntington's disease. *Brain and Language, 37*, 500-513.

Tulving, E. (1983). *Elements of Episodic Memory.* New York: Oxford University Press.

Warrington, E.K. and Shallice, T. (1979). Semantic access dyslexia. *Brain, 102*, 43-63.

Zweig, R., Ross, C., Hedreen, J., Steele, C., Cardillo, J., Whitehouse, P., Folstein, M. and Price, D. (1988). The neuropathology of aminergic nuclei in Alzheimer's disease. *Annals of Neurology, 24*, 233-242.

5

Semantic Memory Deficits Associated with Alzheimer's Disease

DAVID P. SALMON[1] and AGNES S. CHAN[2]

The characterization and analysis of the neuropsychological processes underlying the cognitive deficits associated with Alzheimer's disease and other dementing disorders is one of the many major contributions Nelson Butters has made to the study of brain-behavior relationships. Over the past 15 years, his research in this area has helped to define the relationship between specific neuropsychological deficits and regional neuropathological changes (e.g., synapse loss, neuritic plaque and neurofibrillary tangle formation) in Alzheimer's disease, demonstrated dissociations between various forms of procedural learning (e.g., priming and skill learning) in dementing disorders with different sites of neuropathology, delineated the neuropsychological features that differentiate the dementia syndromes associated with primarily cortical (e.g., Alzheimer's disease) and primarily subcortical (e.g., Huntington's disease) brain damage, and identified the neuropsychological characteristics that most effectively distinguish early Alzheimer's disease from the benign cognitive changes of normal aging.

We have been extremely fortunate to collaborate with Nelson, as students and colleagues, on many of these research efforts. We have benefitted greatly from his wisdom, scholarship and keen insight in these collaborations, and have also had the opportunity to work with the many excellent students, scholars and scientist who have been drawn to the Neuropsychology Laboratory

---

[1] DAVID P. SALMON, Ph.D.• Department of Neurosciences, School of Medicine, University of California, San Diego

[2] AGNES S. CHAN • Department of Psychiatry, School of Medicine, University of California, San Diego, and Department of Psychology, San Diego State University

Neuropsychological Explorations of Memory and Cognition: Essays in Honor of Nelson Butters, edited by Laird S. Cermak, Ph.D. Plenum Press, New York, 1994

in San Diego by Nelson's presence. One aspect of Nelson's research that we have been particularly involved in, and that we will focus on in this chapter, is the neuropsychological analysis of the language and semantic memory deficits associated with Alzheimer's disease.

Although memory impairment is usually the earliest and most prominent feature of dementia of the Alzheimer type (DAT) (Corkin, Davis, Growdon, Usdin and Wurtman, 1982; Moss and Albert, 1988), language disturbances often occur during the course of the disease (Bayles and Kaszniak, 1987; Hart, 1988; Nebes, 1989). The language impairment associated with DAT has been characterized as an anomia or word-finding deficit in which patients have difficulty naming common objects or in producing an appropriate word during speech. While these language disturbances have been attributed to an impairment of semantic memory (Abeysinghe, Bayles and Trosset, 1990; Huff, Corkin and Growdon, 1986; Martin and Fedio, 1983; Nebes, 1989), the exact nature of this deficit remains the source of considerable controversy (Nebes, 1989). The present chapter shall describe our research efforts to better characterize the language and semantic memory deficits associated with DAT, and to better understand the nature of the processes underlying these deficits.

Our studies of semantic memory deficits in patients with DAT were conceived in the context of constructs and models developed in cognitive psychology. In this context, semantic memory refers to our general fund of knowledge which consists of the meanings and representations of words, concepts and overlearned facts that are not dependent upon contextual cues for their retrieval (Tulving, 1983). Models of semantic memory (e.g., Collins and Loftus, 1975) usually assume that semantic knowledge is organized as a complex network of associated concepts, and that within the network, concepts that have many attributes in common are more strongly associated than those that share fewer attributes. These strongly related concepts are thought to form conceptual categories made up of exemplars which share many attributes. The attributes not only provide a means of grouping concepts into categories, but also provide a means of distinguishing among the various exemplars that constitute a given category. Thus, car and truck are both categorized as vehicles because they share attributes such as being mobile, having wheels and providing transportation; however, they can be distinguished from each other by such attributes as size, shape and use.

Two major hypotheses have been proposed to account for the language deficits of patients with Alzheimer's disease. The first is a structural hypothesis that proposes that DAT patients suffer a breakdown in the organization and structure of semantic knowledge (Butters, Salmon and Heindel, 1990; Grober, Buschke, Kawas and Fuld, 1985; Martin, 1987; Smith, Murdoch and Chenery, 1989). According to this point of view, semantic knowledge concerning concepts, and attributes of concepts, is actually lost during the course of the disease as a result of the degradation of the neocortical association areas that are presumed to store these representations (Squire, 1987; Warrington and Shallice, 1984). This loss of semantic knowledge results in concepts becoming less well defined as their distinguishing attributes are eliminated, and in a weakening of the formerly strong associations between related concepts in the semantic network.

The second hypothesis is a functional one that proposes that patients with Alzheimer's disease suffer from an impairment in retrieving or accessing semantic knowledge (Bayles, Tomoeda, Kaszniak and Trosset, in press; Nebes and Brady, 1988; Nebes, Brady and Huff, 1989; Nebes, Martin and Horn, 1984). According to this point of view, semantic knowledge remains intact in Alzheimer's disease patients, but they are unable to retrieve the information in an efficient and effective manner. The language deficits exhibited by patients with Alzheimer's disease, and particularly the anomia, are thought to result from the patients' inability to retrieve a desired word or name. According to this functional hypothesis, normal semantic knowledge can be expressed by DAT patients if effortful retrieval demands are eliminated or reduced.

Over the past five years our laboratory has conducted a number of studies of verbal fluency, confrontation naming and other semantic memory processes in patients with DAT. These studies have often compared the performances of DAT patients and patients with Huntington's disease (HD), a genetically transmitted disorder that produces a progressive degeneration of the caudate nucleus (Bruyn, Bots and Dom, 1979; Vonsattel, Myers, Stevens, Ferrante, Bird and Richardson, 1985) with a resultant movement disorder (i.e., chorea) and dementia (Brandt and Butters, 1986; Hayden, 1981). The results of these studies support the structural hypothesis and lead us to believe that patients with DAT suffer a loss of semantic knowledge and a breakdown in the organization of semantic memory. We will now review the evidence from our laboratory that has lead us to this conclusion.

One line of evidence supporting that notion that DAT patients suffer a breakdown in the organization of semantic memory is found in studies employing word generation, or verbal fluency, tasks. In an initial study from our laboratory, Butters and his colleagues (Butters, Granholm, Salmon, Grant and Wolfe, 1987) systematically examined the verbal fluency performance of 13 mildly demented DAT patients, using both letter and category fluency tasks, and compared their performance to those of 13 elderly normal control (NC) subjects and 12 patients with HD. In the letter fluency task, subjects orally generated words beginning with the letters F, A, and S, with one minute allowed for each letter category. In the category fluency task, subjects generated exemplars from the semantic category "animals" for one minute.

Although the subjects in both patient groups were matched for overall severity of dementia with the Dementia Rating Scale (DRS) (Mattis, 1976), the DAT and HD patients produced different patterns of performance on the two fluency tasks. Patients with HD demonstrated severe deficits (relative to NC subjects) on both fluency tasks, whereas the mildly demented Alzheimer's disease patients were impaired only on the category fluency task.

A recent study from our laboratory replicated and extended this finding with larger and more demented groups of DAT and HD subjects (Monsch, Bondi, Butters, Paulsen, Salmon, Brugger and Swenson, in press). In this study, 44 patients with DAT, 42 HD patients, and their respective age- and education-matched control subjects were administered the letter and category fluency tasks described above; however, in this case three semantic categories were sampled, animals, fruits and vegetables. As in the previous study, the DAT and HD patient groups were matched for overall level of dementia as measured by the DRS. When the performances of the two patient groups were expressed as fluency scores normalized to their respective control group scores, HD patients were severely and equally impaired on both letter and category fluency tasks. Patients with DAT were also clearly impaired on both tasks, but demonstrated a much greater impairment on the semantically-based category fluency task than on the letter fluency task.

The DAT patients' greater impairment on category than on letter fluency tasks demonstrated in these studies is consistent with the notion that they suffer a loss or breakdown in the organization of semantic memory rather than from a general inability to retrieve or access semantic knowledge. Letter fluency tasks do not place great demands on the organization of semantic memory since they can be performed using phonemic cues to search a very extensive set of appropriate exemplars within the lexicon. In contrast, category fluency tasks require the generation of words from a small and highly-related set of exemplars within a single, restricted semantic category. While normal control subjects are able to use the organization within a restricted semantic category to guide their responses on the category fluency task, Alzheimer's disease patients appear to be deficient in their knowledge of the attributes and/or exemplars that define the relevant semantic category and are thus unable to use this knowledge to generate specific category exemplars. When semantic organization is less salient or useful in the fluency task, as in the letter fluency task, DAT patients show less impairment relative to control subjects. If their fluency deficit was due simply to an inability to retrieve information from semantic memory, then letter and category fluency tasks would be equally affected. Indeed, such a general retrieval deficit has been proposed to explain the pattern of performance of the HD patients on the verbal fluency tasks (Butters, et al., 1987; Butters, Wolfe, Martone, Granholm and Cermak, 1985).

Direct evidence of a deficiency in DAT patients' knowledge of attributes and exemplars that define a specific semantic category is provided by studies examining the types of responses they produce on category fluency tasks (Martin and Fedio, 1983; Troster, Salmon, McCullough and Butters, 1989). For example, Troster and his colleagues (1989) classified DAT, HD and NC subjects' responses produced on the supermarket fluency task from the DRS into specific category items and more general category labels. This category fluency task required subjects to generate items that can be found in a supermarket as quickly as possible for one minute. The results of this analysis revealed that moderately demented DAT patients (mean DRS score=101.85) produced fewer exemplars (e.g., steak, carrots) per category sampled than NC subjects and HD patients (who had equivalent word generation deficits), and had a greater propensity to produce general category labels (e.g., meat, vegetables) than did either of the other subject groups. Thus, DAT patients were less likely than other groups to provide subordinate category information, but more likely to produce superordinate information. These findings appear to reflect an initial loss of subordinate knowledge about the most specific attributes of a semantic category, with relative preservation of more general superordinate knowledge. If the semantic representations of objects and categories are viewed as being organized in a hierarchical fashion with the most general aspects at the top and more specific features at the bottom, then, as Martin (1987) has proposed, the DAT patients in this study demonstrated a progressive "bottom-up" breakdown in the hierarchical organization of semantic knowledge.

In addition to its theoretical relevance, the disproportionately severe fluency deficit exhibited by DAT patients with semantic categories relative to letter categories has important clinical implications (Monsch, Bondi, Butters, Salmon, Katzman and Thal, 1992; Monsch et al., in press). For example, in the study described above, Monsch and his colleagues (Monsch et al., in press) compared the sensitivity and specificity of the letter and category fluency tasks for distinguishing between DAT and HD patients and their respective control subjects. Receiver Operating Characteristic (ROC) curves were plotted to compare sensitivity and specificity of diagnosis for every possible cut-off score for the two tests. The ROC curve analysis allows the most effective cut-off score to be determined in an objective fashion (Mossman and Somoza, 1991).

These analyses demonstrated that the most effective cut-off score for the category fluency task provided sensitivity of 100.0% and specificity of 90.9% for distinguishing between patients with Alzheimer's disease and elderly normal control subjects. On the other hand, the most effective cut-off score for the letter fluency task provided sensitivity of only 81.8% and specificity of 84.1% for differentiating these two groups. In contrast to the clearly superior discriminability of the category fluency task for DAT, the category and letter fluency tasks provided equivalent levels of sensitivity (category: 85.7%; letter: 95.2%) and specificity (category:97.6%; letter: 88.1%) for distinguishing HD patients from their controls.

One of the most prominent features of the language impairment associated with Alzheimer's disease is a deficit in object naming (for review, see Hart, 1988). This deficit has been well documented in numerous studies which have shown that DAT patients are much more likely than normal elderly individuals, or patients with other dementing disorders, to perform poorly on confrontation naming tasks (Bayles and Tomoeda, 1983; Bowles, Obler and Albert, 1987; Hodges, Salmon and Butters, 1991; Huff, et al., 1986; Martin and Fedio, 1983; Smith et al., 1989). In addition, the types of errors produced on confrontation naming tasks by patients with DAT suggests that their naming deficit reflects a loss of semantic knowledge and a breakdown in the organization of semantic memory rather than a general retrieval deficit (Bayles and Tomoeda, 1983; Hodges et al., 1991).

Our laboratory recently conducted a systematic comparison of the types of errors produced by DAT and HD patients on a modified version of the Boston Naming Test (Hodges, et al., 1991). Errors on the confrontation naming task were classified for this analysis as non-responses, visually-based errors (e.g., calling a pretzel a snake), and semantically-based errors. Semantically-based errors included producing the name of another item in the category (e.g., broccoli for asparagus), producing the superordinate category rather than the specific exemplar (e.g., animal for camel), providing an associated feature rather than the name (e.g., found in Egypt for pyramid) and circumlocutory errors. Several additional types of non-semantic and non-perceptual errors were also noted (e.g., repetitions, phonemic errors).

To avoid biasing the error analysis, DAT and HD patient groups were selected for comparison that were matched in terms of their overall naming performance. This procedure resulted in 21 DAT patients and 21 HD patients who were able to spontaneously name an average of 23.5 of a total of 30 items. The percentage of each type of error produced, as a function of the total number of errors, was calculated for the two patient groups.

The results of this detailed analysis revealed that DAT and HD patients differed in two ways. First, HD patients produced a significantly greater proportion of visually-based errors than did patients with DAT. Second, patients with DAT made a significantly greater proportion of semantic-superordinate errors than did HD patients. These results suggest that naming deficits in HD patients initially involves a significant disruption of perceptual analysis, whereas in DAT patients such naming impairments are due, to a large extent, to a breakdown in semantic processes.

It should also be noted that the particular type of semantically-based error produced to a greater extent by DAT than by HD patients (i.e., semantic-superordinate errors) is consistent with the notion that DAT patients undergo a "bottom-up" breakdown in the organization of their semantic knowledge. Although DAT patients have lost knowledge about the specific attributes and exemplars that constitute a given semantic category, they retain general category knowledge. Thus, when shown a picture of a camel and asked to name it, for example, they are likely to respond with the superordinate category name "animal".

In conjunction with their performance on verbal fluency tests, the pattern of performance and types of responses produced by patients with

Alzheimer's disease on object naming tasks strongly suggest that these patients suffer a loss of semantic knowledge and a breakdown in the structure of semantic memory, rather than a general deficit in retrieving intact semantic memory. However, to clearly distinguish between semantic storage and semantic access disorders, Warrington and Shallice (Shallice, 1988a; Shallice, 1988b; Warrington and Shallice, 1984) have outlined criteria that assume that if a particular item has been permanently lost from semantic memory, then a patient should: (1) demonstrate consistent failure in accessing that item across different tests and test sessions; (2) demonstrate a loss of detailed knowledge along with relatively preserved superordinate knowledge about the item; (3) derive no benefit from semantic cueing in accessing that item.

To determine if the performance of DAT patients on tests of semantic memory is indicative of a true loss of semantic knowledge, our laboratory recently conducted a study (Hodges, Salmon and Butters, 1992) in which semantic memory was examined in a group of 22 Alzheimer's disease patients using a battery of tests designed to probe for semantic knowledge for a particular item across different modes of access and output. The various tests in the battery all employed the same 48 stimulus items which were exemplars from three categories of living items (i.e., land animals, birds and water creatures) and three categories of non-living items (i.e., household items, vehicles and musical instruments). Knowledge of the items was assessed with fluency tasks, a confrontation naming task, a sorting task designed to test superordinate and subordinate knowledge, a word-to-picture matching task, and a definition task.

The results of this study were consistent with those of a similar study by Chertkow and Bub (1990) and showed that DAT patients were significantly impaired relative to NC subjects on all measures of semantic memory, regardless of method of access. Furthermore, DAT patients exhibited a disproportionately severe impairment when knowledge of subordinate information was assessed. This pattern of deficits was best illustrated in the results of the semantic sorting task. In this task, subjects first sorted the 48 stimuli into the global categories of living versus man-made, then sorted the living items and man-made items into three superordinate categories each (e.g., land animal vs. sea creature vs. bird), and finally sorted the stimuli on the basis of subordinate attributes (e.g., locality, size and fierceness). At the global level, knowledge about whether an item was living or man-made was preserved in Alzheimer's disease patients. At the superordinate level (e.g., land animal vs. sea creature vs. bird), DAT patients were impaired overall relative to NC subjects, but the impairment was relatively mild and evident in only certain categories. At the subordinate level, patients with Alzheimer's disease were severely impaired when they had to sort items on the basis of their specific attributes.

Further evidence for semantic memory loss was provided by an analysis of item-to-item correspondence produced on a number of the different tests used in the Hodges et al. (1992) study. This analysis sought to determine whether or not a particular stimulus item was likely to be missed on any or all tests, regardless of how the information was accessed. When comparing naming ability to performance on the other semantic memory tasks, Alzheimer's disease patients showed a striking correspondence across items. Patients were able to name about 78% of the items that they correctly matched on the word-to-picture matching task, but only named about 23% of the items they could not correctly match. Similarly, about 77% of the items correctly sorted could also be named, while only about 58% of incorrectly sorted items were named. The same pattern was also seen with the definition task, with about 59% of correctly defined items named and only 10% of non-defined items named.

The correspondence in items missed across tasks designed to access semantic knowledge through different modes of input and output, and the pattern of relatively preserved superordinate knowledge with a loss of subordinate information on the sorting task, suggests that patients with Alzheimer's disease do indeed suffer a loss of semantic knowledge rather than a disorder of semantic access. Furthermore, the pattern is consistent with the "bottom-up" breakdown in semantic memory discussed earlier.

Our laboratory has recently initiated a series of studies in which we attempted to model the organization of semantic memory in Alzheimer's disease patients using clustering and multidimensional scaling techniques (Romney, Shepard and Nerlove, 1972; Shepard, Romney and Nerlove, 1972; Tversky and Hutchinson, 1986). Multidimensional scaling provides a method for generating a spatial representation of the degree of association between concepts in semantic memory. The spatial representation, or cognitive map, generated in this manner clusters concepts along one or more dimensions according to their proximity, or degree of relatedness, in the patient's semantic network. The distance between concepts in the cognitive map reflects the strength of their association.

In an initial study in this series, Chan and her colleagues (Chan, Butters, Paulsen, Salmon, Swenson and Maloney, 1993) compared the organization of semantic memory for the category "animals" in DAT, HD and NC subjects. The strength of association between concepts, or their proximity, was estimated for each subject from the pattern of responses they produced on a category fluency task in which they generated names of animals for one minute. It was assumed that through spreading activation within the semantic network (Collins and Loftus, 1975; Meyer and Schvaneveldt, 1975), animals that are highly associated would tend to be produced closer together within a subject's sequential responses on the fluency task than animals that are not highly associated. Thus, the number of items that intervene between two target words, corrected for the total number of words produced, provides an estimate of the semantic proximity of the target words.

Proximity scores for each subject were generated in this manner for twelve target animal names which were selected for two reasons: 1) the names were among the 25 most frequent responses of DAT, HD and NC subjects, and

2) the animal names could be categorized within domestic-wild, carnivore-herbivore, and small-large dimensions. The proximity scores were subjected to multidimensional scaling and clustering analyses which produced a model, or cognitive map, of the organization of semantic memory for each of the subject groups.

The multidimensional scaling procedure resulted in cognitive maps for all three subject groups that were best represented by two dimensions, domesticity and size (see Figure 1). However, the cognitive map of the DAT patients differed considerably from that of the NC subjects in terms of the classification of individual exemplars. For example, in the cognitive map of DAT patients, but not NC subjects, bear appeared in the space representing domestic animals, zebra appeared in the space representing small animals, and dog was categorized as more representative of a large animal than elephant. Similarly, the cluster analyses revealed two global clusters for the NC subjects which were interpretable as wild and domestic, whereas three essentially uninterpretable clusters were derived for the DAT patients.

The results of the HD patients in this study are of particular interest because these subjects produced as few exemplars in the fluency task as the DAT subjects, but their poor fluency performance is presumed to be due to a general retrieval deficit rather than a breakdown in the organization of semantic memory. Interestingly, the HD subjects cognitive maps and clusters of animal names were virtually identical to those of the NC subjects. Thus, the abnormal cognitive maps of the DAT patients are not likely to be an artifact of poor fluency performance per se, but are likely to be indicative of a true breakdown in the structure of semantic memory.

Although the automatic spread of activation reflected in the verbal fluency task used by Chan and her colleagues (Chan et al., 1993) allows the structure of semantic memory to be explored, the saliency of a particular dimension for categorizing concepts, and individual differences in the semantic network, cannot be examined with this task because of the variance in the total number of responses produced by each subject. To circumvent these deficiencies, Chan and her colleagues (Chan, Butters, Salmon and McGuire, 1993) recently completed a second study of the structure of semantic memory in DAT patients using a more systematic procedure to estimate semantic relations. The strength of association between concepts, or their proximity, was estimated using a triadic comparison task in which subjects chose, from among three concepts (i.e., among three animals), the two that are most alike. Every possible combination of three animal names, from a total sample of twelve animals, was presented. This procedure produced a proximity score reflecting strength of association for each pair of animals in relation to all of the other animal names; that is, how frequently those two animals were chosen as most alike.

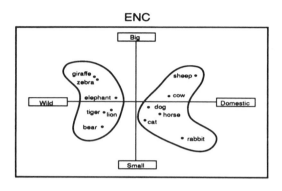

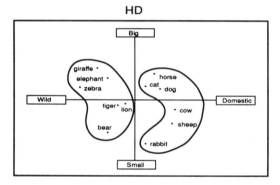

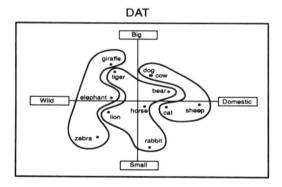

Figure 1. The cognitive maps of normal elderly normal control (ENC) subjects (upper panel), patients with Huntington's disease (HD) (middle panel), and patients with dementia of the Alzheimer type (DAT) (lower panel) obtained from multidimensional scaling and clustering analyses performed on data from a verbal fluency task. The position of each animal name is determined by multidimensional scaling; animals in the same cluster are encircled together. (Adapted from Chan, Butters, Paulsen, Salmon, Swenson and Maloney, 1993).

The proximity data produced on the triadic comparison task formed a 12 X 12 half matrix which was subjected to a multidimensional scaling statistic. This technique produced a spatial representation, or cognitive map, of the structure of the subjects' semantic network. The dimensions used to categorize concepts, the strength of the various dimensions for categorizing concepts (dimension weights), and the subjects' degree of reliance on one or more of the dimensions (skewness index), were also generated.

The semantic networks of the DAT and elderly NC subjects revealed with this procedure were best represented by three dimensions that appeared to correspond to domesticity (i.e., wild vs. domestic), predation (herbivore vs. carnivore) and size (large vs. small) (see Figure 2). Although a three-dimensional solution provided the best spatial representation of the semantic network of both DAT and NC subjects, several significant alterations in the semantic networks of the Alzheimer's disease patients were evident.

First, Alzheimer's disease patients focused primarily on concrete conceptual information (size) in categorizing animals, whereas control subjects stressed abstract conceptual knowledge (domesticity). Second, a number of animals that were highly associated and clustered together for control subjects were not strongly associated for patients with Alzheimer's disease. For example, DAT patients tended to cluster cat with small wild carnivores, whereas, control subjects clustered cat with small domestic carnivores. Third, patients with DAT were less consistent than NC subjects in utilizing the various attributes of the animals (predation, domesticity and size) in categorization. This was indicated by a significantly lower skewness index for the patients than for the controls.

In a subsequent ongoing study, Chan and her colleagues (in preparation) have examined the structure of semantic memory in patients with Huntington's disease and their age-matched control subjects using these same multidimensional scaling techniques. In contrast to the Alzheimer's disease patients, the semantic networks of HD patients and middle-aged NC subjects were best represented by two dimensions. The cognitive maps of these two groups were almost identical, and for both groups domesticity was the most salient dimension for categorizing animals. Furthermore, the HD patients and their control subjects did not differ in the importance applied to the various dimensions or in their reliance on a particular dimension for categorization.

The findings from these multidimensional scaling studies are consistent with the notion that patients with Alzheimer's disease suffer a breakdown in the structure and organization of semantic memory. The DAT patients' abnormal categorization and clustering of concepts most likely reflects both a deterioration in associations between formally highly-related concepts and a relative strengthening of associations between formally non-related or only slightly-related concepts. Because of the semantic deterioration, patients with DAT tend to rely heavily on a concrete perceptual dimension (i.e., size) in categorizing animals rather than the more semantically-demanding abstract conceptual

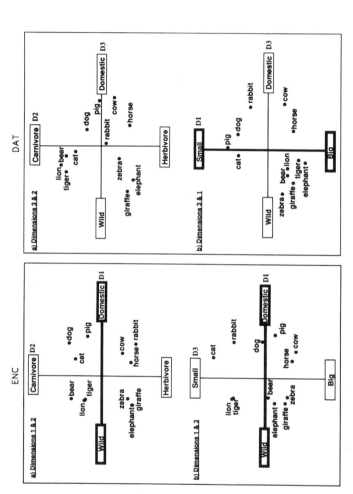

Figure 2. The cognitive maps of elderly normal control (ENC) subjects and patients with dementia of the Alzheimer type (DAT). The maps were obtained with multidimensional scaling analysis performed on data from a triadic comparison task. The most salient dimension (D1, D2 or D3) used in categorizing concepts is represented in bold type. Domesticity is the dominant dimension used for the categorization of animals by ENC subjects, whereas, size is the dominant dimension used by patients with DAT. (Adapted from Chan, Butters, Salmon and McGuire, 1993).

dimension (i.e., <u>domesticity</u>) used by NC subjects. The interpretation that the alterations in the DAT patients' semantic network is due to a breakdown or loss of semantic knowledge rather than to a retrieval deficiency is strengthened by the fact that these abnormalities in the semantic network are not observed in HD patients who are thought to have a general deficit in retrieving information from semantic memory.

In conclusion, the studies of semantic memory in patients with Alzheimer's disease that have emanated from our laboratory over the past five years have generated a number of important findings that can be summarized as follows. First, patients with DAT exhibit a disproportionately severe fluency deficit when generating exemplars from a semantic category as compared to generating words from a lexical or phonemic category. Second, the category fluency performance of DAT patients is characterized by an increased propensity to produce category labels relative to specific exemplars. Third, DAT patients are impaired on object naming tasks and produce a significantly greater proportion of semantically-based errors than HD patients and elderly NC subjects, and tend to refer to specific objects by their superordinate category name. Fourth, patients with DAT demonstrate a deficit in sorting items on the basis of subordinate, but not superordinate, attributes. Fifth, there is a correspondence in items missed by Alzheimer's disease patients across tasks designed to access semantic knowledge through different modes of input and output. Finally, there is a deterioration in the organization of semantic knowledge in DAT patients that can be consistently demonstrated by alterations in cognitive maps which reflect the semantic relationships used in categorizing concepts.

Taken together, these findings suggest that there is a true loss of semantic knowledge in patients with Alzheimer's disease, and that the nature of their semantic memory deterioration is consistent with a "bottom-up" breakdown in which specific attributes of a semantic category are lost before more general superordinate knowledge. This loss of semantic knowledge disrupts the normal organization of semantic memory in Alzheimer's disease patients and results in aberrations in their network of semantic representations. The breakdown in the structure of semantic knowledge evident in these patients does not occur in all dementias, and in particular does not appear to occur in subcortical dementias such as Huntington's disease.

ACKNOWLEDGEMENTS. We would like to acknowledge the contributions of the many investigators who collaborated on the studies of semantic memory described in this chapter. We are particularly grateful for the major contributions of Drs. John R. Hodges and Andreas U. Monsch. The preparation of this chapter was supported in part by NIA grant AG-05131 and NIMH grant MH-48819 to the University of California at San Diego.

REFERENCES

Abeysinghe, S.C., Bayles, K.A. and Trosset, M.W. (1990). Semantic memory deterioration in Alzheimer's subjects: Evidence from word association, definition, and associate ranking tasks. *Journal of Speech and Hearing Research, 33*, 574-582.

Bayles, K.A. and Kaszniak, A.W. (1987). *Communication and cognition in normal aging and dementia.* Boston: Little-Brown.

Bayles, K.A. and Tomoeda, C.K. (1983). Confrontation naming impairment in dementia. *Brain and Language, 19*, 98-114.

Bayles, K.A., Tomoeda, C.K., Kaszniak, A.W. and Trosset, M.W. (in press). Alzheimer's disease effects on semantic memory: loss of structure or impaired processing? *Journal of Cognitive Neuroscience.*

Bowles, N.L., Obler, L.K. and Albert, M.L. (1987). Naming errors in healthy aging and dementia of the Alzheimer type. *Cortex, 23*, 519-524.

Brandt, J. and Butters, N. (1986). The neuropsychology of Huntington's disease. *Trends in Neurosciences, 9*, 118-120.

Bruyn,. G.W., Bots, G. and Dom, R. (1979). Huntington's chorea: Current neuropathological status. In: T. Chase, N. Wexler N. and A. Barbeau (eds.), *Advances in neurology, Vol. 23: Huntington's disease.* New York: Raven Press.

Butters, N., Granholm, E., Salmon, D., Grant, I. and Wolfe, J. (1987). Episodic and semantic memory: A comparison of amnesic and demented patients. *Journal of Clinical and Experimental Neuropsychology, 9*, 479-497.

Butters, N., Salmon, D.P. and Heindel, W.C. (1990). Processes underlying the memory impairments of demented patients. In E. Goldberg (ed.), *Contemporary neuropsychology and the legacy of Luria* (pp. 99-126). Hillsdale, NJ: Erlbaum.

Butters, N., Wolfe, J., Martone, M., Granholm, E. and Cermak, L. (1985). Memory disorders associated with Huntington's disease: Verbal recall, verbal recognition and procedural memory. *Neuropsychologia, 23*, 729-743.

Chan, A.S., Butters, N., Paulsen, J.S., Salmon, D.P., Swenson, M.R. and Maloney, L.T. (1993). An assessment of the semantic network in patients with Alzheimer's disease. *Journal of Cognitive Neuroscience, 5*, 254-261.

Chan, A.S., Butters, N., Salmon, D.P. and McGuire, K.A. (1993). Dimensionality and clustering in the semantic network of patients with Alzheimer's disease. *Psychology and Aging, 8*, 411-419.

Chertkow, H. and Bub, D. (1990). Semantic memory loss in dementia of Alzheimer's type. *Brain, 113*, 397-417.

Collins, A.M. and Loftus, E.F. (1975). A spreading activation theory of semantic processing. *Psychological Review, 82*, 407-428.

Corkin, S., Davis, K.L., Growdon, J.H., Usdin, E. and Wurtman, R.J. (1982). *Alzheimer's disease: A report of research and progress.* New York: Raven Press.

Grober, E., Buschke, H., Kawas, C. and Fuld, P. (1985). Impaired ranking of semantic attributes in dementia. *Brain and Language, 26*, 276-286.

Hart, S. (1988). Language and dementia: A review. *Psychological Medicine, 18*, 99-112.

Hayden, M.R. (1981). *Huntington's chorea*. New York:Springer-Verlag.

Hodges, J.R., Salmon, D.P. and Butters, N. (1991). The nature of the naming deficit in Alzheimer's and Huntington's disease. *Brain, 114*, 1547-1558.

Hodges, J.R., Salmon, D.P. and Butters, N. (1992). Semantic memory impairment in Alzheimer's disease: Failure of access or degraded knowledge? *Neuropsychologia, 30*, 301-314.

Huff, F.J., Corkin, S. and Growdon, J.H. (1986). Semantic impairment and anomia in Alzheimer's disease. *Brain and Language, 28*, 235-249.

Martin, A. (1987). Representation of semantic and spatial knowledge in Alzheimer's patients: Implications for models of preserved learning in amnesia. *Journal of Clinical and Experimental Neuropsychology, 9*, 191-124.

Martin, A. and Fedio, P. (1983). Word production and comprehension in Alzheimer's disease: The breakdown in semantic knowledge. *Brain and Language, 19*, 124-141.

Mattis, S. (1976). Mental status examination for organic mental syndrome in the elderly patient. In: L. Bellack and T. Karasu (eds.), *Geriatric psychiatry*. New York: Grune & Stratton.

Meyer, D.E. and Schvaneveldt, R.W. (1975). Meaning, memory structure, and mental processes. In C.N. Cofer (ed.), *The structure of human memory* (pp. 54-89). San Francisco: W.H. Freeman.

Monsch, A.U., Bondi, M.W., Butters, N., Paulsen, J.S., Salmon, D.P., Brugger, P. and Swenson, M.R. (in press). A comparison of category and letter fluency in Alzheimer's and Huntington's disease. *Neuropsychology*.

Monsch, A.U., Bondi, M.W., Butters, N., Salmon, D., Katzman, R. and Thal, L.J. (1992). Comparisons of verbal fluency tasks in the detection of dementia of the Alzheimer type. *Archives of Neurology, 49*, 1253-1258.

Moss, M.B. and Albert, M.S. (1988). Alzheimer's disease and other dementing disorders. In M.S. Albert and M.B. Moss (eds.), *Geriatric neuropsychology* (pp. 145-178). New York: Guilford Press.

Mossman, D. and Somoza, E. (1991). ROC curves, test accuracy, and the description of diagnostic tests. *Journal of Neuropsychiatry and Clinical Neuroscience, 3*, 330-333.

Nebes, R. (1989). Semantic memory in Alzheimer's disease. *Psychological Bulletin, 106*, 377-394.

Nebes, R. and Brady, C.B. (1988). Integrity of semantic fields in Alzheimer's disease. *Cortex, 24*, 291-299.

Nebes, R., Brady, C.B. and Huff, F.J. (1989). Automatic and attentional mechanisms of semantic priming in Alzheimer's disease. *Journal of Clinical and Experimental Neuropsychology, 11*, 219-230.

Nebes, R., Martin, D. and Horn, L. (1984). Sparing of semantic memory in Alzheimer's disease. *Journal of Abnormal Psychology, 93*, 321-330.

Romney, A.K., Shepard, R.N. and Nerlove, S.B. (1972). *Multidimensional scaling: Theory and applications in the behavioral sciences* (Vol. II). New York: Seminar Press.

Shallice, T. (1988a). *From neuropsychology to mental structure*. Cambridge: Cambridge University Press.

Shallice, T. (1988b). Specialization within the semantic system. *Cognitive Neuropsychology,, 5*, 133-142.

Shepard, R.N., Romney, A.K. and Nerlove, S.B. (1972). *Multidimensional scaling: Theory and applications in the behavioral sciences* (Vol. I). New York: Seminar Press.

Smith, S.R., Murdoch, B.E. and Chenery, H.J. (1989). Semantic abilities in dementia of the Alzheimer type: 1. Lexical semantics. *Brain and Language, 36*, 314-324.

Squire, L. (1987). *Memory and Brain.* New York: Oxford University Press.

Troster, A.I., Salmon, D.P., McCullough, D. and Butters, N. (1989). A comparison of the category fluency deficits associated with Alzheimer's and Huntington's disease. *Brain and Language, 37*, 500-513.

Tulving, E. (1983). *Elements of Episodic Memory.* New York: Oxford University Press.

Tversky, A. and Hutchinson, J.W. (1986). Nearest neighbor analysis of psychological spaces. *Psychological Review, 93*, 3-22.

Vonsattel, J.P., Myers, R.H., Stevens, T.J., Ferrante, R.J., Bird, E.D. and Richardson, E.P. (1985). Neuropathological classification of Huntington's disease. *Journal of Neuropathology and Experimental Neurology, 44*, 559-577.

Warrington, E.K. and Shallice, T. (1984). Category specific semantic impairments. *Brain, 107*, 829-854.

6

Exploring Disorders of Semantic Memory

JOHN R. HODGES[1]

My strongest and most enduring memory of Nelson has been his generosity and enthusiasm which pervaded our initial professional relationship as well as our subsequent friendship. My first encounter with Nelson was in about 1986. At this time my thesis work (on transient global amnesia) was coming to an end and I was contemplating a period of post-doctorate research in North America. Clearly no one can make transient global amnesia a life's work. Since Alzheimer's disease is by far the commonest cause of memory impairment likely to be seen by a behavioural neurologist, it seemed obvious to consider working on the neuropsychology of dementia. With this in mind, I wrote to a number of eminent neuropsychologists in the field to explore the possibility of joining their research group for a year. Nelson replied, by return, with a pressing invitation to come to UCSD for a year (or two!), suggestions for research grant applications, a list of people I should contact, and a sheaf of recent publications. After this, it was only a matter of time before I arrived in San Diego.

Of the areas under investigation by Nelson's group, the one that caught my interest the most was the nature of the semantic memory loss in patients with dementia of Alzheimer's type (DAT). Although impairment in episodic memory clearly predominates in the early stages of DAT, it seemed to me that a loss of vocabulary and general knowledge is the fundamental cognitive deficit which separates patients with even early DAT from those with the amnesic syndrome. The studies of semantic memory which I began under the direction of Nelson and David Salmon at the Alzheimer's Disease Research Centre

[1] JOHN R. HODGES, M.D., FRCP • University, Neurology Unit, Addenbrooke's Hospital, Cambridge

Neuropsychological Explorations of Memory and Cognition: Essays in Honor of Nelson Butters, edited by Laird S. Cermak, Ph.D., Plenum Press, New York, 1994

(ADRC) at UCSD turned out to have a major impact on my subsequent research career: the study of disorders of semantic memory has continued to be the focal point of my research. Moreover, the stimulation provided by spending a year with Nelson and his group also convinced me to pursue a predominately research based career on returning to the UK.

When I arrived at UCSD in the summer of 1988 I had only the roughest of research plans: to do something related to memory in Alzheimer's disease following the general strategy applied by the UCSD group of comparing patient groups with different forms of dementing disease. After talking to Nelson and reading around the area, I decided to attempt a synthesis of the large group study approach prevalent in dementia research and the single-case based method which predominates in European cognitive neuropsychology. At this time, it had been established that patients with DAT are impaired on tests of semantic memory (see below) but it was unclear whether this impairment reflected an actual loss of knowledge or an disorder of access. In fact, these general concepts --which had been developed largely by Elizabeth Warrington and Tim Shallice (eg Warrington and Shallice, 1984; Shallice, 1988) -- had not been applied to patients with DAT and other dementing illnesses. The general goal of the research which I started in San Diego was to bring together the two research traditions.

SEMANTIC MEMORY: THEORETICAL ISSUES

The term semantic memory refers to the component of long-term memory containing knowledge of objects, facts and concepts as well as words and their meaning (Tulving, 1972; 1983). In short, semantic memory gives meaning to our sensory experience. In contrast to episodic memory, semantic memory is culturally shared, not temporally specific and to a large extent acquired early in life. Tasks dependent on intact semantic memory include object naming, generation of definitions for spoken words, word-picture and picture-picture matching and the generation of exemplars on category fluency tests (e.g., animals, vegetables etc.). Particular attention has been devoted to three theoretical issues: i) the question of whether impairment on tests of semantic memory reflects an actual loss of information, or an accessibility of that information, ii) the internal architecture of semantic memory, for instance whether there is separate representation of knowledge relating to different sensory modalities, or to different conceptual categories, or both (e.g., Allport, 1985; Caramazza, Hillis, Rapp & Romani, 1990; Saffran & Schwartz, in press; Warrington & McCarthy, 1987; Warrington & Shallice, 1984), and iii) the inter-relationship of semantic memory and other closely related, but arguably separate cognitive modules (e.g., the syntactic system, phonological and orthographic lexicons, stored structural descriptions of objects etc. [Hodges,

Patterson and Tyler, in press a]). It was the first of these issues on which I began work with Nelson, while the latter two are topics which now dominate our research in Cambridge. I shall briefly outline the research undertaken at USCD, then the more recent work performed jointly with Karalyn Patterson from the MRC Applied Psychology Unit in Cambridge.

SEMANTIC MEMORY IMPAIRMENTS

Impairment on tests of semantic memory can result from a lack of access to item specific knowledge from a particular sensory modality of input, or actual loss of representational knowledge. For instance, in some patients with associative visual agnosia the defect in object recognition is confined to the visual domain with preservation of visual semantics (e.g. , Humphreys & Riddoch, 1987), and similar access disorders limited to written or spoken language have also been documented (see Shallice, 1988). By contrast, in other patients with visual agnosia the impairment is not modality specific and represents an actual breakdown in representational knowledge (Warrington & Shallice, 1984).

A number of studies prior to 1989 had shown that patients with DAT are impaired on a range of tests conventionally considered as measures of semantic memory. For instance, early in the course of the disease DAT patients show impairment on verbal fluency tests (Butters, Granholm, Salmon, Grant & Wolfe, 1987; Martin & Fedio, 1983). However, verbal fluency is a complex task dependent upon several cognitive processes including attention and retrieval strategies, working memory, intact semantic stores and phonological processes. Clearly impairment in any of these could occur in DAT. The disproportionately severe reduction in category as opposed to initial letter fluency in DAT found by a number of workers (including a comparative study of patients with DAT and Huntington's disease which I was involved with while working in San Diego [Hodges, Salmon & Butters, 1990]), suggests breakdown in the semantic component of the task.

Further evidence for impaired semantic memory in DAT emanates from the consistent demonstration of impaired object naming. A number of claims have been made regarding the nature of the naming deficit in DAT; while early studies suggested a primary perceptual deficit as the major cause of the naming disorder, other more recent investigators have favoured a central semantic defect (for review see, Hodges, Salmon & Butters, 1991). The evidence supporting the latter hypothesis derives, to a large extent, from the analysis of the types of error produced. Prior to our investigation of the underlying cause of the semantic memory deficit in DAT, we analysed the performance of a large group of patients with DAT as well as patients with HD and normal control subjects on the Boston Naming Test . This test had been given serially to all

DAT patients and controls enrolled in the San Diego ADRC project as part of their routine annual neuropsychological work-up. We found that although both spontaneous and cued naming were significantly impaired in the two patient groups, the pattern of errors differed: DAT patients made a significantly greater proportion of semantic-superordinate (e.g. vegetable for asparagus) and semantic-associative (e.g. sea for octopus, green for asparagus) errors, while the Huntington's disease patients made a significantly greater proportion of visually-based (e.g. pen or snake for asparagus) errors. We were also able to document that the pattern of naming errors made by the DAT patients changed over time. Not only did their overall performance fall, but the proportion of both semantically-based and visually-based errors increased. These findings suggested that in the early stages of DAT the anomia reflects breakdown in semantic memory, but as the disease progresses, perceptual problems also begin to occur. Although other studies of naming in DAT had been performed, ours was perhaps the most comprehensive in terms of the number of patients studied, the availability of comparative patient groups (DAT and Huntington's disease) and the use of an error classification system which attempted to separate truly visual from ambiguous and various forms of semantically-based error.

The evidence from error analyses points to a defect within the semantic system, but this evidence is rather indirect . We felt that it was necessary to show consistent impairment of knowledge for the same items across tests which access knowledge via different modalities (e.g., picture naming, picture-name matching, generating verbal descriptions in response to the item's name etc.). The technique of testing knowledge of items across a range of semantic categories, both within and across modalities, has been applied in detail to individual cases with semantic memory loss (both generalised and category-specific), mostly resulting from Herpes Simplex encephalitis (e.g., Sartori & Job, 1988; Warrington & Shallice, 1984). But at the start of our investigation in 1988-89 such techniques had not been applied systematically to patients with DAT. The studies of Warrington (1975) and Schwartz, Marin and Saffran (1979) are clearly exceptions to this, but their patients almost certainly did not have DAT and would, in retrospect, now be considered as cases of semantic dementia (see below). In the context of DAT, Huff, Corkin and Growden (1986) had shown a positive correlation between anomia and word comprehension for the same exemplars in a selected group of patients. Chertkow and Bub (1990) extended these findings and confirmed a significant item-by-item correspondence between comprehension (picture-word matching) and name production. Their patients also showed a significantly greater inability to answer detailed probe questions concerning items whose pictures they named incorrectly.

Against this background, the aims of our study (Hodges, Salmon & Butters, 1992) were to investigate further the nature of the semantic memory deficit in DAT and particularly to study the co-occurrence of deficits on a broad range of semantic memory tasks using the same target items in each test. Warrington and Shallice (1984) had proposed the following criteria for a semantic storage disorder: i) consistency of performance across test sessions and between tests within a sensory modality, ii) preservation of superordinate with loss of subordinate information, iii) loss of priming effects and iv) disproportionate loss of information about low frequency items. In addition, we postulated that a central loss of semantic knowledge should result in item-by-item consistent across test modalities.

In order to investigate the hypothesis that the semantic memory disorder in DAT results from an actual loss of semantic knowledge we designed the following test battery with was then given to a group of 22 well documented DAT patients and 26 age and education matched controls. The test battery has subsequently been modified for use in British subjects and is being used in our studies of patients with DAT and semantic dementia in Cambridge (see Patterson, Graham & Hodges in press a; Hodges, Patterson, Oxbury & Funnell, 1992).

THE SEMANTIC TEST BATTERY

This battery of tests, all employing one consistent set of stimulus items, and designed to assess input to and output from central representational knowledge about the same group of items via different sensory modalities, has been described in detail elsewhere (Hodges, Patterson, Oxbury & Funnell, 1992; Hodges, Salmon & Butters, 1992). It contains 48 items from three categories of animals (land animals, sea creatures and birds) and three categories of man-made items (household items, vehicles and musical instruments) matched for category prototypicality and word frequency. They were chosen from the corpus of line drawings by Snodgrass and Vanderwart (1980). In brief, the original five sub-tests consisted of
1. Category fluency for each of the 6 main categories plus two lower order categories (breeds of dog and types of boat).
2. Naming of all 48 line drawings with cueing.
3. Picture sorting at superordinate (living vs manmade), category (land animal vs bird vs water creature; household item vs vehicle vs musical instrument) and subordinate (e.g., fierce vs non fierce animal; native vs foreign; kitchen vs non kitchen item; electrical vs non electrical etc.) levels.
4. Picture pointing to spoken word using within-category arrays (the original battery used arrays of 6 items all from the same category, such as land animals, but in the subsequent version we now use arrays of 8 which contain two foils not otherwise included in the test battery).
5. Generation of verbal definitions in response to the spoken name of the item (e.g., "tell me everything you can about a rhinoceros"; penguin; guitar etc.).

The following two sub tests have been added since the battery was developed:
6. Naming in response to the verbal description (e.g. "what do you call the large African animal with a curved horn on its head").
7. Semantic feature questions for each item we designed 8 questions such that 4 questions explore knowledge of physical features (size, shape, colour etc.) and 4 knowledge of more abstract attributes (habitat, ferocity, diet, uses etc.).

APPLICATION OF THE SEMANTIC MEMORY TEST BATTERY TO PATIENTS WITH DAT

As predicted, the 22 DAT patients given the semantic memory test battery showed significant impairment on all subtests (see Hodges, Salmon & Butters, 1992). The pattern of the results suggested a loss of semantic knowledge rather than a disorder of semantic access. This conclusion was based upon three lines of evidence. Firstly, the finding of preserved superordinate knowledge on the picture sorting and definitions tests, together with the suggestion of a disproportionate reduction in the generation of exemplars from the lower order categories on the fluency test (i.e. relatively greater impairment for the category dogs than for the category animals). Secondly, the finding of a marked frequency effect, in that DAT patients were more impaired at naming less familiar items. Third, and perhaps most persuasively, the demonstration of item-by-item correspondence across a number of subtests. In other words, the DAT patients showed a significant correspondence between the individual items that they were unable to name and those that produced errors on the picture matching-to-spoken word test. Similarly there was item-specificity between naming and sorting, and between naming and the ability to generate adequate definitions in response to spoken names. Analysis of the exemplars produced on the category fluency tests and performance on the naming test showed that unnamed items were very rarely produced in the free recall condition. This combined evidence offered, we argued, strong evidence in favour of semantic memory loss in DAT.

This work is being extended in a study funded by the Medical Research Council in which we are following up a larger group of around 50 DAT patients to examine the longitudinal pattern of the semantic memory impairment and its relationship to other cognitive impairments. We are also interested to find out just how early in the course of DAT loss of semantic memory occurs, and which are the most sensitive tests for its detection.

SEMANTIC DEMENTIA

Although semantic memory impairment in DAT has continued to be a major area of interest of our memory and language research group in Cambridge, we have also turned our attention to the closely related, but separate, syndrome of semantic dementia. In DAT, the semantic memory impairment is invariably accompanied by other cognitive deficits which make it less than ideal as a model for investigating the theoretical issues raised above. For instance, the deficits in episodic and working memory which occur from an early stage in DAT make it impossible to investigate the inter-relationship of semantic memory and other cognitive modules or the neural basis of these subcomponents of memory.

This work derives from that started at UCSD. At a fundamental level, the studies of memory and other cognitive abilities in patients with progressive degenerative disease pioneered by Nelson and his co-workers over the past 15 years have had an enormous impact. Their application of the models and test methods developed in the setting of experimental psychology to patients with Huntington's and Alzheimer's disease (who had previously been considered to have "global dementia" of little interest to neuropsychologists) was clearly a ground-breaking step which paved the way to understanding the cognitive dysfunction in these disorders. Recognising the patterns of impairment in these more common disorders has been important for identifying rarer syndromes such as semantic dementia. At a more practical level, our application of the semantic memory test battery described earlier has helped in the identification and understanding of this subgroup of patients with a severe but selective loss of semantic memory

Selective impairment of semantic memory was, in fact, first clearly delineated almost 20 years ago by Elizabeth Warrington (1975), who described three patients with cerebral atrophy presenting with progressive anomia and impaired word comprehension. Detailed neuropsychological testing revealed a loss of receptive and expressive vocabulary, and impoverished knowledge of a wide range of living things and inanimate objects affecting particularly specific subordinate attributional knowledge. Other aspects of spoken language (e.g., phonology and syntax) and perceptual skills appeared relatively intact. Such a deficit would previously have been assimilated under the rubric of associative agnosia. Warrington, drawing a distinction made by Tulving (1972; 1983), identified the deficit as one of semantic memory. The famous patient, WLP, shown by Schwartz, Marin and Saffran (1979) to have a progressive disintegration of semantic memory could, in retrospect, also be regarded as an example of semantic dementia.

Since these seminal early reports, a number of other patients with selective semantic memory impairment have been reported. The majority have occurred in the context of extensive temporal lobe damage, for instance following herpes simplex virus encephalitis (e.g., De Renzi, Liotti and Nichelli, 1987; Sartori and Job, 1988; Warrington and Shallice, 1984). In Japan, the syndrome of Gogi (word meaning) aphasia, first described in 1943 by Imura (see Sasanuma & Monoi, 1975) and later studied by Tanabe et al. (1993) has all the features of selective semantic memory breakdown, together with relatively spared phonological and syntactic aspects of language.

Other examples of semantic memory impairment have been subsumed within the category of primary progressive aphasia. The latter term was originally introduced by Mesulam (1982) to describe a syndrome, clearly distinct from semantic memory loss, characterised by non-fluent language output with phonemic paraphasic errors progressing in many instances to complete mutism, but sparing comprehension. As is often the case following the description of an apparently "new" syndrome the term progressive aphasia has been widened to embrace a range of progressive disorder of language. Hence, patients very different to the original cases of non-fluent aphasia have been reported under the title of progressive aphasia (e.g. Basso, Capitani & Laiacona, 1988; Poeck & Luzzatti, 1988; Tyrrell, Warrington, Frackowiak & Rossor, 1990). The pattern of deficits in these latter cases has been one of undoubted semantic memory loss causing deficits both in word production and comprehension, but with relative sparing of other components of language (i.e., syntax and phonology).

The introduction of the term semantic dementia (first coined by Snowden, Goulding & Neary, 1989) may be thought to add further to the nosological confusion. It does, however, have the advantage of brevity, avoids pathological assumptions and implies a cognitive deficit affecting fundamental aspects of language, memory and object recognition. In our first paper (Hodges, Patterson, Oxbury & Funnell, 1992), we described five cases with semantic dementia which, we suggested, is a clinically recognisable syndrome with the following characteristics: i) selective impairment of semantic memory causing severe anomia, impaired spoken and written single-word comprehension, reduced generation of exemplars on category fluency tests and an impoverished fund of general knowledge, ii) relative sparing of other components of language output and comprehension, notably syntax and phonology, iii) normal perceptual skills and non-verbal problem solving abilities, iv) relatively preserved autobiographical and day-to-day (episodic) memory and, v) a reading disorder with the pattern of surface dyslexia. It should be noted that the inclusion of the latter feature has been questioned by Saffran and Schwartz (in press) as their patient WLP was proficient at reading irregular words, at least at in the earlier stage of the disease.

Although semantic dementia is a relatively rare condition, it provides an ideal model for the investigation of the issues outlined above. Patients with other causes of semantic memory loss such herpes simplex virus encephalitis almost invariably have additional complicating cognitive deficits, making them less than ideal candidates for addressing the question of the independence of semantic memory from other putative modules. In addition, the progressive nature of semantic dementia makes it possible to explore the internal organisation of semantic memory; the investigation of patients with acute stable brain injury is complicated by the fact that it is never possible to establish what an individual subject knew before the insult. In semantic dementia patients can act as their own controls in longitudinal studies.

THE NATURE OF THE SEMANTIC MEMORY IMPAIRMENT IN SEMANTIC DEMENTIA

Among the issues that we are currently addressing in these patients are the following: Is the loss of knowledge about individual items consistent over time? Is there evidence that physical properties of objects are stored differently to more abstract properties? Is there really sparing of category/superordinate information or does this reflect test artefact? Many of these questions stem from the basic issue of whether there is a unitary system of semantic representation, as some have claimed (e.g., Caramazza, Hillis, Rapp & Romani, 1990; Riddoch, Humphreys, Coltheart & Funnell, 1988), as opposed to an organisation comprised of subsystems specialised for particular aspects of semantic knowledge (e.g. Allport, 1985; Saffran & Schwartz, in press; Warrington & McCarthy, 1987). Although it has been shown that some patients with semantic memory impairment show a disproportionate loss of knowledge about living as opposed to man-made items, theoretical interpretations of this finding differ. Furthermore, it has been argued that such dissociations may reflect test artefacts due to a failure to match stimulus items appropriately. Through longitudinal study of a number of patients with semantic dementia, we hope to determine whether there is a consistent pattern of differential loss of knowledge about specific categories of items (living, man-made etc.) or specific attributes (e.g. physical features such as colour, shape, size vs more abstract features such as habitat, diet, uses etc.) using a range of verbal and visually-based tasks.

To date, our studies have failed to show category-specific effects. All of the patients have shown a loss of knowledge about a wide range of living and manmade things. One of the striking findings has been the highly consistent drop out of items as illustrated by performance of one of our patients, JL, on the category fluency and naming subtests from the semantic battery (see Table 1).

A related topic is the status of subordinate, basic-level and superordinate knowledge. It has frequently been observed that patients with semantic dementia as well as DAT (as discussed earlier) appear to have lost knowledge concerning the finer-grained attributes but nevertheless retain higher-order information such as category membership for the same items (e.g.,

Table 1. Longitudinal performance of patient JL (reported by Hodges, Patterson, Oxbury & Funnell, 1992) on the semantic memory test battery showing data from the category fluency (animals) and naming subtests.

Animal Fluency

April 91	Sept 91	March 92	Oct 92	March 93
cow	horse	horse	dog	----
bullock	cows	cows	cats	
sheep	bullock	birds	horses	
lamb	duck	birds (P)		
pig	cats			
dog	dog			
horse	bullocks (P)			
cat	cows (P)			
birds				
geese				

P = perseverative response

Naming Test: Items ever correctly named

	April 91	Sept 91	March 92	Oct 92	March 93
1. telephone	+	+	+	+	-
2. fish	+	+	+	-	-
4. chicken	+	-	-	-	-
5. lorry	+	+	+	+	+
10. deer	+	-	-	-	-
12. rabbit	+	-	-	-	-
13. bus	+	+	+	-	-
16. duck	+	+	-	-	-
17. cooker	+	-	-	-	-
18. monkey	+	+	-	-	-
20. tiger	+	-	-	-	-
21. aeroplane	+	+	+	+	-
25. bicyle	+	+	+	+	+
29. kettle	-	+	-	-	-
31. helicopter	+	-	-	-	-
32. mouse	+	-	-	-	-
35. motorbike	+	+	+	-	
41. toaster	+	-	-	-	-
Total correct max = 48	17	9	7	5	2

+ = correct, - = incorrect

all other items incorrect on each test session

Hodges, Patterson , Oxbury and Funnell, 1992; Warrington, 1975). For instance, a patient may fail on questions about the size, colour, and typical habitat of a tiger, but still know that it is an animal. Such observations have been taken as evidence in favour of a hierarchically organised semantic memory system in which information is accessed from "top down". This type of model conflicts, however, with connectionist theories in which a item or concept is represented by a conjunction of overlapping or connected features rather than a single node (McClelland & Rumelhart, 1985). It is possible that the type of experimental evidence discussed above is, in fact, misleading since the ability to answer questions like "Is a tiger fierce" requires the subject to comprehend the concept of "fierce" and then to apply this knowledge to the item. The question "is a tiger an animal" merely relies upon retention of the general concept "animal". We are currently exploring this aspect more systematically.

THE IMPACT OF SEMANTIC DEMENTIA ON OTHER COGNITIVE SYSTEMS

We have been particularly concerned with the following questions: Is syntactic processing spared in semantic dementia? What is the effect of semantic disintegration on the integrity of phonological and orthographic representations? Are the units responsible for object recognition (stored structural descriptions) represented independently of semantic memory?

The status of syntactic operations in patients with semantic dementia relates to the controversial question of modularity within the language system (Fodor, 1983) to what extent do syntactic operations function independently of semantic knowledge? Early assertions of highly modular organisation have been challenged by evidence of interaction between semantics and syntax in "on-line" sentence processing tasks (see Tyler, 1992). Evidence from patients with semantic dementia would lead to a contrary opinion. In contrast to the progressive breakdown in the semantic components of language, syntax is preserved, at least as assessed by conventional explicit tasks. Even in the advanced stages sentences are well articulated and grammatically correct although simplified and repetitious in content. Similarly, comprehension of even fairly complex syntax can be normal. This is illustrated by patient JL's near perfect performance on the Token Test (De Renzi & Faglioni, 1978) and on the Test for the Reception of Grammar TROG (Bishop, 1983) in the face of progressive decline on all semantically-based tasks (see Table 2). Schwartz, Marin and Saffran (1979) reported a similar preservation of syntax and phonology in their patient WLP, and have subsequently extended these finding in a more recent patient, dB, with semantic dementia (Saffran and Schwartz, in press) both of whom show severe semantic memory impairment.

Table 2. Performance of patient JL (reported by Hodges, Patterson, Oxbury & Funnell, 1992) on the shortened version of the Token test and Bishop's Test for the Reception of Grammar (TROG) over a time when he showed progresive and profound impairment on the semantic battery (maximum scores shown in parentheses).

	June 1991	Dec 1991	March 1992	Oct 1992
Semantic battery				
Naming (48)	17	9	8	5
Category fluency (3 living categories)	20	13	4	3
Picture-word matching spoken (48)	31	27	25	16
Syntactic comprehension				
Token Test (36)	30	30	28	-
TROG (80)	76	73	76	65

English-speaking patients with semantic dementia typically exhibit a pattern of reading disorder known as surface alexia, in which reading aloud of regular words (like *mint*) is virtually normal, but there is a marked disadvantage for words with an exceptional spelling-sound correspondence. An exception word like *pint* (compare *pint* with *mint, hint, print, glint*, etc.) is very likely to be "regularised" when surface alexic patients read aloud. This finding is illustrated by the performance of three of our patients on a reading list consisting of 126 pairs of regular and exception words matched for length, frequency and initial phoneme (see Table 3).

An account of the relationship between semantic deterioration and surface alexic reading in semantic dementia has been one of the major theoretical interests of the our group (Patterson & Hodges, 1992). According to our hypothesis, two factors provide coherence among the elements making up individual words. The first of these factors operates within the level of the speech lexicon itself: whenever a person utters a word, its individual phonological elements will be activated concurrently and, by notions of Hebbian associative learning, will establish strong auto-associative links. The second factor operates between the level of the speech lexicon and semantic memory: the appropriate semantic representation is also active when a person uses a word since the specification of a phonological word in spontaneous speech must begin

Table 3. Performance of three patients with semantic dementia on the surface reading list described by Patterson and Hodges (1992) showing the proportion correct word reading for REG (regular) and EXC (exception) words in three frequency bands (Hi, Med, Lo). The results show a marked effect of regularity and word frequency.

Patient	REG			EXC		
	Hi	Med	Lo	Hi	Med	Lo
F.M.	0.98	1.0	0.95	0.95	0.81	0.62
J.L.	1.0	0.93	0.93	0.9	0.86	0.74
P.P.*	0.98	0.9	0.62	0.36	0.18	0.08

*P.P. was also a letter-by-letter reader and was tested, therefore by identication from oral spelling

with its meaning. We argue that this link from a word's meaning to the set of phonological elements comprising its pronunciation serves a prominent role in binding those elements into a unitised whole. Therefore, if representations of meaning deteriorate, as in progressive dementing diseases like semantic dementia, a major source of coherence for individual phonological representations will gradually be lost.

Along with Shallice (Shallice, 1988; Shallice, Warrington & McCarthy, 1983), we assume that when the normal reader pronounces a written word, the process of computing phonology from orthography occurs at multiple levels, including whole words, syllables, sub-syllabic components (especially the onset -- that is, the initial consonant or consonant cluster of a syllable such as the *m* of *mint* or the *fl* of *flint* , and the rime -- the remainder of the syllable, *int* in both of these cases), and even individual graphemes and phonemes. How these various levels of translation co-operate, or compete, and eventually result in a single fluent pronunciation is, of course, a complex and incompletely understood process. The only point that is crucial to the present story is that, like Shallice and his colleagues, we argue that the highest (whole-word) level of translation is the one most vulnerable to brain injury; and we extend their argument by hypothesising that the reason for the specific vulnerability of whole-word translation to semantic deterioration is that -- as indicated above -- part of what makes a phonological (and orthographic) word whole is its link to semantic memory.

The tendency to misread exception words follows as a direct consequence of this vulnerability of whole-word representations. If the process of computing phonology from orthography is dominated by segments smaller than the whole word, then words with regular spelling-sound correspondences (like *mint* and *flint*) will still tend to be pronounced correctly, because the pronunciation of a whole regular word corresponds to the sum of the typical pronunciations of its component segments as they occur in the vocabulary at large. The same treatment accorded to the exception word *pint*, however, will yield a pronunciation rhyming with *mint*, i.e. a regularization error.

The difficulty in reading irregular words has practical implications for the interpretation of the widely used National Adult Reading Test, NART (Nelson, 1982). The ability to read irregular words is usually regarded as a retained skill, even in moderately advanced dementia (for review see, Patterson, Graham & Hodges, in press a), which can therefore be used to predict premorbid verbal IQ. Since the NART consists almost exclusively of irregular words, the surface dyslexia typically seen in semantic dementia means that the NART may lead to erroneously low predictions of pre-morbid intellectual level if the examiner does not recognise the dyslexia.

Further evidence that the loss of semantic memory has a destablising effect on phonological representations comes from our studies of word repetition (Patterson, Graham and Hodges, in press b). In these, we adapted a task used by McCarthy and Warrington (1987) in which subjects are asked to repeat short lists of 'known' and 'unknown' words. 'Unknown' items are words that patients had specifically failed to comprehend in picture-pointing tests. 'Known' words are those that had been produced appropriately in spontaneous speech and/or had been understood on word comprehension tasks. There was a striking effect of the known/unknown manipulation, with adequate reproduction of lists of known words but very poor performance on lists of unknown words. The majority of the errors involved migrations of phonemes from words within the current sequence being repeated, particularly the substitution of a different consonant (or consonant cluster) as the onset of the word; a number of these onset errors were perfect "Spoonerisms" such as *mint, rug*-->"rint, mug". Normal speakers make frequent errors of this type when asked to repeat nonsense words (Treiman and Danis, 1988). These findings support the hypothesis that meaning is essential for the integrity of phonological representations and also has a bearing on our understanding of the form in which words are stored in the speech output lexicon.

Turning to the processes involved in object recognition. The ability to recognise possible objects as real objects is thought to depend upon the operation of a module containing the "stored structural descriptions" of familiar objects. This module is usually conceived of as separate from the semantic system. Hence it is possible that disintegration of semantic memory would have no impact on ability to perform an object decision test; indeed Sheridan and Humphreys (1993) have argued for just this position. Alternatively, one might predict that structural descriptions of objects share with phonological representations of words the fact that, in normal processing, they are always active in conjunction with the relevant semantic representations. Evidence to address this issue is at present limited, but our initial studies suggest that the stored structural descriptions of objects are disrupted by semantic memory loss

(Hodges, Patterson & Tyler, in press); a patient (PP) with semantic dementia was administered an object decision test (Riddoch & Humphreys 1987) consisting of drawings of real objects (e.g. a pair of scissors, a tiger) and chimeric objects (e.g. the body of a tiger with the head of a mouse). PP's performance was at chance, which contrasted with her near perfect performance on an "unusual views" test, which requires matching a photograph of a target object, photographed from a conventional angle, with one of two response alternatives: i) the same target object photographed from an unusual view, and ii) a photo of a different but visually similar object. PP performed at a normal level on this task, despite the fact that she could not name, identify or describe the use of the objects in the test. This result suggests that the kind of object-centred analysis which is essential for recognising that two different views represent the same object is a separate process from knowing what the object is, or even whether it is familiar.

THE NEURAL BASIS OF SEMANTIC MEMORY

The neural basis of episodic memory has been a topic of intense investigation over the past decade; as a result there have been considerable advances in understanding of the structures involved in episodic memory (Squire, 1992). By comparison, we know very little about the neural substrate of semantic memory. Our patients with semantic dementia, as well as those reported by Tanabe et al. (1993) under the label of Gogi aphasia, have all had structural and/or functional changes in the temporal lobe(s). On MRI, the areas most involved appeared to be the lateral temporal neocortex, with an emphasis on the middle and inferior temporal gyri. More medial temporal structures (the hippocampus, parahippocampal gyrus and subiculum) were relatively spared. Pathological data from patients with semantic dementia are extremely limited, but in recently reported cases the distribution of atrophy and of neural loss corresponded closely to that found on MRI (Neary, Snowden & Mann, 1993; Graff-Radford et al., 1990). It is worth emphasising that in neither case were changes of Alzheimer's disease present; in the former patient there was non-specific neuronal loss with spongiosis and gliosis, while the latter had the typical inclusions of Pick's disease. Two earlier cases reported by Warrington (1975) also had the changes of Pick's disease largely confined to the temporal lobe (personal communication).

There is converging evidence that the temporal lobe plays a critical role in semantic memory. Beyond this gross assertion much remains uncertain; it is still unclear, for instance, exactly which temporal lobes structures are consistently involved in semantic dementia, and whether there is regional or lateralised specialisation of function. Some cases have had bilateral temporal lobe atrophy while in others the atrophy has been confined to the left (Hodges,

Patterson, Oxbury & Funnell, 1992). It is possible, for instance, that left-sided pathology causes impairment in verbal semantic knowledge with relative preservation of non-verbally based knowledge, while for right-sided disease, the opposite pattern might be found.

ACKNOWLEDGEMENTS. The research undertaken by the author both in San Diego and in Cambridge has been supported by the Medical Research Council. All of the recent work has been conducted in collaboration with Karalyn Patterson who has contributed enormously to the development of the theoretical ideas expressed in this chapter.

REFERENCES

Allport, A. (1985) Distributed memory, modular subsystems and dysphasia. In S. K. Newman & R. Epstein (Eds.), *Current perspectives in dysphasia*. Edinburgh: Churchill Livingstone.

Basso, A., Capitani, E., & Laiacona, M, (1988) Progressive language impairment without dementia: a case with isolated category specific semantic defect. *Journal of Neurology, Neurosurgery and Psychiatry, 5*, 1201-1207.

Bishop, D.V.M. (1983) *Test for the reception of grammar*. Manchester, UK: University of Manchester, England.

Butters, N., Granholm, E., Salmon, D.P., Grant, I., & Wolfe, J. (1987) Episodic and semantic memory: A comparison of amnesic and demented patients. *Journal of Clinical Experimental Neuropsychology, 9*, 479-97.

Caramazza, A., Hillis, A.E., Rapp, B.C., & Romani, C. (1990) The multiple semantics hypothesis: multiple confusions. *Cognitive Neuropsychology, 7*, 161-189.

Chertkow, H., & Bub, D. (1990) Semantic memory loss in dementia of Alzheimer's type. *Brain, 113*, 397-417.

De Renzi, E., Liotti, M., & Nichelli, P. (1987) Semantic amnesia with preservation of autobiographic memory. A case report. *Cortex, 23*, 575-597.

DeRenzi, E., & Faglioni, P. (1978) Normative data and screening power of a shortened version of the Token Test. *Cortex, 14*, 41-49.

Fodor, J.A. (1983) *The modularity of mind*. Cambridge, MA: MIT Press

Graff-Radford, N. R., Damasio, A.R. , Hyman, B. T., Hart, M. N., Tranel, D., Damasio, H., Van Hoesen, G. W., & Rezai, K. (1990) Progressive aphasia in a patient with Pick's disease. *Neurology, 40*, 620-626.

Hodges, J. R., Patterson, K. E., & Tyler, L. K. (in press) Loss of semantic memory: implications for the modularity of mind, *Cognitive Neuropsychology*.

Hodges, J. R., Salmon, D.P., & Butters, N. (1990) Differential impairment of semantic and episodic memory in Alzheimer's and Huntington's disease: a controlled prospective study. *Journal of Neurology Neurosurgery and Psychiatry, 53*, 1089-1095.

Hodges, J. R., Salmon, D.P., & Butters, N. (1991) The nature of the naming deficit in Alzheimer's and Huntington's disease. *Brain, 114*, 1547-1558.

Hodges, J. R., Salmon, D.P., & Butters, N. (1992) Semantic memory impairment in Alzheimer's disease: Failure of access or degraded knowledge? *Neuropsychologia, 30,* 301-314.

Huff, F .J., Corkin, S., & Growden, J. H .(1986) Semantic impairment and anomia in Alzheimer's disease. *Brain and Language, 28,* 235-249.

Humphreys, G.W., & Riddoch, M.J. (1987) *To see but not to see: a case study of visual agnosia.* Hove, Suffolk: Lawrence Erlbaum Associates.

McCarthy, R.A. , & Warrington, E.K. (1987) The double dissociation of short-term memory for lists and sentences. *Brain, 110,* 1545-1563.

McClelland, J. L., & Rumelhart, D. E .(1985) Distributed memory and the representation of general and specific information. *Journal Of Experimental Psychology: General, 14,* 159-188.

Martin, A., & Fedio, P. (1983) Word production and comprehension in Alzheimer's disease: the breakdown of semantic knowledge. *Brain and Language, 19,* 124-141.

Mesulam, M.M. (1982) Slowly progressive aphasia without dementia. *Annals of Neurology, 11,* 592-598.

Neary, D., Snowden, J .S., & Mann, D. M. A. (1993) The clinical pathological correlates of lobar atrophy. *Dementia, 4,* 154-159

Nelson, H.E. (1982) *National Adult Reading Test (NART): for the assessment of premorbid intelligence in patients with dementia.* Windsor: NFER-Nelson.

Patterson, K. E., Graham, N., & Hodges, J. R. (in press a) Reading in Alzheimer's type dementia: a spared ability? *Neuropsychology*

Patterson, K. E., Graham, N., & Hodges, J. R. (in press b). The impact of semantic memory loss on phonological representations. *Journal of Cognitive Neuroscience,* in press.

Patterson, K. E., & Hodges, J .R. (1992) Loss of word meaning: Implication for reading. *Neuropsychologia., 30,* 1025-1040

Poeck, K., & Luzzatti, C. (1988) Slowly progressive aphasia in three patients: The problem of accompanying neuropsychological deficit. *Brain, 111,* 151-168.

Riddoch, M. J., Humphreys, G. W., Coltheart, M., & Funnell, E. (1988) Semantic system or systems? Neuropsychological evidence re-examined. *Cognitive Neuropsychology, 5,* 3-26.

Sartori, G., & Job, R. (1988) The oyster with four legs: A neuropsychological study on the interaction of visual and semantic information. *, 5,* 105-132.

Saffran, E. M., & Schwartz, M. F. (in press) Of cabbages and things: semantic memory from a neuropsychological perspective - A tutorial review *Attention and Performance XV* Hove and London: Lawrence Erlbaum

Sasanuma, S., & Monoi, H. (1975) The syndrome of Gogi (word meaning) aphasia. *Neurology, 25,* 627-632

Schwartz, M. F., Marin, O. S. M., & Saffran, E. M. (1979) Dissociations of language function in dementia: a case study. *Brain and Language, 7,* 277-306.

Shallice, T. (1988) *From neuropsychology to mental structure.* Cambridge, UK: Cambridge University Press.

Shallice, T., Warrington, E. K., & McCarthy, R. (1983). Reading without semantics. *Quarterly Journal of Experimental Psychology, 3 5A,* 111-138.

Sheridan, J ., & Humphreys, G. W. (1993) A verbal-semantic category specific recognition impairment. *Cognitive Neuropsychology, 10*, 143-185.

Snodgrass , J. G., & Vanderwart. M. (1980) A standardised set of 260 pictures: normal for name agreement, familiarity and visual complexity. *Journal of Experimental Psychology: General, 6,* 174-215.

Snowden , J. S., Goulding, P. J., & Neary, D. (1989) Semantic dementia: a form of circumscribed cerebral atrophy. *Behavioural Neurology., 2*, 167-182.

Squire, L.R. (1992) Memory and the hippocampus: a synthesis from findings with rats, monkeys and man. *Psychological Review, 99*, 195-231.

Tanabe, H., Nakagawa, Y., Ikeda, M., Kazui, H., Yamamoto, H., Ikejiri, Y., & Hashikawa, K. (1993) The neural substrate of the semantic memory for words. *Journal of Clinical and Experimental Neuropsychology, 15*, 395.

Treiman, R., & Danis, C. (1988) Short-term memory errors for spoken syllables are affected by the linguistic structure of the syllables. *Journal of Experimental Psychology: Learning, Memory and Cognition, 14*, 145-152, 1988.

Tulving, E. (1972) Episodic and semantic memory. In E. Tulving & W. Donaldson (Eds.), *Organisation of Memory*. New York and London: Academic Press.

Tulving, E. (1983) *Elements of episodic memory.* Oxford, UK: Oxford University Press.

Tyler, L.K. (1992) *Spoken language comprehension*. Cambridge, Mass: MIT Press.

Tyrrell, P. J,. Warrington, E. K., Frackowiak, R. S. J., & Rossor, M. N. (1990) Heterogeneity in progressive aphasia due to focal cortical atrophy. A clinical and PET study. *Brain, 113,* 1321-1336.

Warrington, E.K. (1975) Selective impairment of semantic memory. *Quarterly Journal of Experimental Psychology, 27*, 635-657.

Warrington, E.K., & McCarthy, R.A.(1987) Categories of knowledge: Further fractionation and an attempted integration *Brain, 110,* 1273-1296.

Warrington, E.K., & Shallice, T. (1984) Category specific semantic impairments. *Brain, 107*, 829-854.

7

Amnesia, Aging and Alzheimer's Disease

FELICIA A. HUPPERT[1]

Coming to work at the Boston VA Hospital was an exhiliarating experience after the studious atmosphere of Cambridge University. I have vivid recollections of the corridors resounding with laughter, with teasing and jokes and the bouncing around of ideas. It was the summer of 1972. At the suggestion of Susan Iversen, whose rats I trained and nurtured, I had written to her friend from NIH days, Nelson Butters. Testing hypotheses derived from my animal-based PhD research, I had begun working with human amnesic patients. Where better to advance this work than in Boston, amid the intellectual ferment of Butters and Cermak and their colleagues.

PUTTING MEMORY DISORDER INTO CONTEXT

Just before this first of many visits to Nelson and the VA, Malcolm Piercy and I had developed an experimental paradigm whose results challenged one of the prevailing theories of amnesia. According to the theory, amnesia was the consequence of retrieval failure; the evidence adduced in support of this theory (which is interpreted very differently today) was that memory was normal when amnesic patients were prompted with partial information, such as fragmented forms of pictures or words, or word stems (Warrington & Weiskrantz, 1968; Weiskrantz & Warrington, 1970). While it was true that the patients showed severe impairment of recall and recognition on standard tests, we

---

[1] FELICIA A. HUPPERT, PH.D. • Department of Psychiatry, University of Cambridge, and Addenbrooke's Hospital, Cambridge

Neuropsychological Explorations of Memory and Cognition: Essays in Honor of Nelson Butters, edited by Laird S. Cermak, Ph.D., Plenum Press, New York, 1994

demonstrated that they obtained very high levels of recognition performance when the material used was magazine pictures. Clearly, such high performance without prompting was inconsistent with the theory of retrieval failure. In trying to understand why the recognition failure was material-specific, we eventually developed a theory of the role of context in memory which is the forerunner of much recent work. In the process, we also gained a disturbing insight into academic politics.

But back in 1972, I arrived with a carefully planned experiment to compare recognition memory for pictures and for high and low frequency words in amnesic and control subjects. In his office, Nelson interrogated me on every detail of the experimental design and the underlying hypotheses. Somewhat to my chagrin, he made various improvements to my 'perfect' study. My respect increased still further when I found that his intellectual rigour was matched by his skill with patients. Nelson was a superb clinician - humorous and empathic, able to demonstrate deficits without causing distress. I learned from him how to get the best out of the precious cohort of Boston amnesics - and enjoy myself in the bargain.

Using large sets of material (80 pictures and 80 words to be remembered), I showed high levels of performance by the amnesic patients on yes-no recognition for both pictures and low frequency words over intervals as long as 7 weeks. By contrast, their performance on high frequency words was at chance after 10 minutes. This suggested that when material was familiar, they had difficulty in differentiating between target and distractor items. In another study, I checked this out by familiarizing subjects with a set of pictures one day prior to the learning trial. When targets and distractors were both familiar, although only the targets had been seen on the test day, the performance of amnesic patients was grossly impaired, while controls had no difficulty. These data are all reported in Huppert & Piercy (1976).

PUTTING CONTEXT INTO MEMORY DISORDER

From these and other findings, we hypothesised that amnesic patients were unable to utilize contextual information to aid their memory. The hypothesis was tested more directly by varying systematically the recency and frequency of picture presentation prior to testing, then testing subjects by asking them explicitly to judge how recently (today vs. yesterday) and how frequently (once or three times) each picture had been presented. The Korsakoff patients, unlike the controls, showed no ability to discriminate between recency and frequency; their recognition performance was based entirely on the overall strength of the trace (Huppert & Piercy, 1978a). In today's parlance, we might say their memory was determined by fluency (Cermak & Verfaellie, 1992).

The question still remained, however, whether the amnesics' problem with context was the result of an inability to retrieve contextual information or to encode such information because of their generally impaired processing ability. So in a further series of investigations in which we varied the duration and number of pretest exposures, we showed that (a) recognition memory is a function of total presentation time, and (b) amnesic patients require about four times as long as controls to attain a given level of performance (Huppert & Piercy, 1977). This simple and robust finding provided support for the encoding hypothesis, and also the key to undertaking the first true comparison of retention in amnesic and control subjects. By comparing the rate of forgetting of amnesics and controls when their initial level of performance was the same, we overcame the scaling problems inherent in previous comparisons of forgetting from different starting points. Accordingly, we equated initial level of performance by presenting the 120 target pictures for 1 sec each to control subjects and 4-8 secs each to the amnesic patients. This produced a mean initial performance of around 78% correct in both groups. When we tested subsequent retention, we found a progressive decrease in memory after intervals of 1 and 7 days for both groups, and superimposed forgetting curves, i.e. identical performance for the amnesic and control groups (Huppert & Piercy, 1978b). We concluded that once amnesic patients had succeeded in acquiring information, their subsequent retention was normal, at least when assessed by picture recognition tests.

It has been pointed out that this matching procedure resulted in the mean item-presentation-to-test delay at initial testing being shorter for controls, which may have exaggerated control forgetting relative to amnesics (e.g. Mayes, 1986). However, this assumes that forgetting rate is a function of mean item-presentation-to-test delay which is unlikely; for example, forgetting curves are parallel when the delay is identical for amnesic and control subjects (Huppert & Piercy, 1976). The argument also loses its force when forgetting curves of the two groups are superimposed over intervals as long as one week, which provides ample time for differential rates of forgetting to become evident. All our studies clearly pointed towards amnesia being primarily a defect of encoding. Nelson Butters, Laird Cermak and their co-workers had for some time been providing persuasive support for an encoding hypothesis (e.g. Cermak & Butters, 1974). The retrieval hypothesis was on very shaky ground.

It was at this point that science became entangled with politics. As a post-doctoral student, I had naively believed that scientific progress involved testing hypotheses and discarding or revising them if they were found wanting. I now learnt that discarding one's own hypotheses was acceptable, but discarding someone else's was another matter. In the ensuing nightmare, Nelson tried valiantly to act as a peacemaker, inviting all parties to Boston to settle their differences by assessing the same group of patients. However, the atmosphere in the UK remained charged. I decided that I preferred neuropsychology to politics, and moved to a different area of research.

FROM AMNESIA TO ALZHEIMER'S DISEASE

The transition from studying the 'pure' memory defect of amnesic patients to the more global cognitive deficits in dementia, has proved to be quite fascinating. First, there are the public health implications of the high prevalence of dementia in our aging societies, which gives the research practical relevance as well as scientific importance. Second, there are the methodological and neurobiological considerations which arise from the contrast between the two disorders. The amnesic syndrome occurs typically in middle-aged people and is categorically distinct from their previous state of functioning. Alzheimer's disease and most other forms of dementia occur typically in the elderly, and because they are progressive, neurodegenerative disorders, they are much more difficult to distinguish from the person's previous level of functioning, at least until the dementia becomes moderately severe. Since the normal aging process is also associated with progressive cognitive decline, issues of diagnosis and the neurobiological correlates of cognitive aging and dementia provide a major challenge.

IS ALZHEIMER'S DISEASE DISTINCT FROM NORMAL AGING

While most neuropsychologists involved in dementia research adopt a classical approach where well-defined patient groups are compared with selected controls, I have preferred to work in the borderline area, examining the relationship between the early stages of dementia and normal cognitive aging by studying typical, rather than highly selected elderly samples. This approach has led to a new type of research which could be called 'cognitive epidemiology', in which the cognitive changes in elderly population samples are studied prospectively. This enables us to examine normal patterns and rates of change as well as the emergence of dementia, and the extent to which genetic, environmental and lifestyle factors influence each type of outcome.

While there is evidence that Alzheimer's disease can be genetically determined, this has been demonstrated in only a very small proportion of cases; the vast majority of Alzheimer's disease appears to be sporadic. Chronological age is by far the strongest risk factor, and age-specific prevalence rates suggest that everyone may develop AD if they live long enough (Katzman & Saitoh, 1991). Data such as these, together with the absence of qualitative differences in cognition, behaviour, neuropathology or histochemistry, when subjects with mild dementia are compared with the normal elderly population, have led to the continuum model of dementia (e.g. Brayne & Calloway, 1988). According to this model, dementia is the tailend of a normal distribution of cognitive decline. It is a linguistic convenience to apply a disease label once impairment has progressed to a level where independent functioning is no longer possible (Storandt et al, 1988).

This view is congruent with contemporary approaches to understanding a wide range of diseases; by shifting the focus from individuals with disease to the population from which they come, it has become apparent that the proportion of individuals with the disease is related to the mean of the underlying risk factors in the population. For example, the prevalence of stroke or coronary heart disease is related to the mean blood pressure in the population, and the prevalence of lung cancer to the mean number of cigarettes smoked in the population (Rose, 1992). Most important of all, this conceptual shift has moved the emphasis away from the treatment of people with disease, to the prevention of disease by reducing the mean of the risk factors in the population.

But do these new ideas apply to dementia? I have recently edited a multi-disciplinary volume in which each author has discussed the evidence for and against the continuum model. The consensus across a wide range of disciplines, is that the data are best fitted by the continuum model. Where there appear to be categorical differences between dementia and normal aging, this is usually explained in terms of sampling bias, where severely demented patients and/or highly selected controls are examined. The book is entitled 'Dementia and Normal Aging' (Huppert, Brayne & O'Connor, 1994) and it includes a section on the profound implications for public health and the possible prevention of dementia, if the continuum model is sustained.

INDIVIDUAL DIFFERENCES

This foray into epidemiology has greatly widened my horizons although the drawback with population-based, longitudinal research is that the results are very slow in coming. Sometimes I feel a little envious of my neuropsychology colleagues, who can publish papers on a handful of cases, or even a single case. On the other hand, my experience of the extraordinary variety in the profiles of performance of normal individuals, makes me wary of over-generalizing when one sees an unusual pattern of deficits in a pathological conditition. It is worth considering whether such individuals may have had unusual structure or function pre-morbidly.

RETURNING TO ROOTS

Nelson's move to La Jolla and his involvement with the Alzheimer's Disease Research Center provided the opportunity to work with him once more. This was in the summer of 1986, exactly 20 years after I first arrived in La Jolla as a graduate student. Nelson looked wonderful, tanned, fit and beardless, and his hospitality was as gracious as ever, as was that of Robert Katzman, David Salmon and other stimulating colleagues. Once again, there was much to admire and learn from Nelson, including his skill at working effectively in a large, multi-disciplinary team, and especially the way in which he nurtured students and post-docs.

In the few weeks of my visit, I was given access to the excellent ADPC database, and began to explore verbal fluency and the cognitive and other variables associated with level of performance. This interest has continued in the longitudinal collection of data on letter and category fluency in elderly population samples in the UK.

This visit also provided the opportunity to meet Igor Grant, whose seminal work on depression and immune function in the elderly has provided a cornerstone of my current research. The aim is to understand cognitive ageing in a broad biological and psycho-social context. I believe this will enable us to determine not only the risk factors for cognitive decline and dementia, but also the protective factors for the maintenance of cognitive health.

In recent years, my encounters with Nelson were limited to international conferences where he delivered marvellous lectures on a wide variety of topics, and where there was also time for the informal exchange of ideas and academic gossip. Boston delis, Grecian ruins and Australian beaches provided the memorable backdrop. I valued these exchanges, which were in their way as important for scientific progress as publications and lectures. On the last such occasion, the Queensland sun was low on the horizon as we strolled along the beach at Surfers' Paradise, discussing the importance of synaptic loss, delayed recall and environmental factors such as education for understanding Alzheimer's disease. Our footprints mingled with the myriad of other footprints casting deep shadows in the sand, as the tide ebbed slowly away. Looking back over 21 years, I recognise that it is the special blend of Nelson's wisdom, humour and humanity which will provide a lasting inspiration to me, and a goal for which to strive.

REFERENCES

Brayne, C. and Calloway, S.P. (1988) Normal ageing, impaired cognitive function, senile dementia of the Alzheimer's type: a continuum? *The Lancet,* June, 1265-1267.

Cermak, L.S., Butters, N. and Moreines, J. (1974) Some analyses of the verbal encoding defect in alcoholic Korsakoff patients. *Brain and Language, 1*, 141-150.

Cermak, L.S. and Verfaellie, M. (1992) The role of fluency in the implicit and explicit task performance of amnesic patients. In: L.R. Squire and N. Butters (Eds) *Neuropsychology of Memory, Second Edition*, 3, 36-45. The Guilford Press, New York.

Huppert, F.A. and Piercy, M. (1976) Recognition memory in amnesic patients: effect of temporal context and familiarity of material. *Cortex, 12*, 3-20.

Huppert, F.A. and Piercy, M. (1977) Recognition memory in amnesic patients; A defect of acquisition? *Neuropsychologia, 15*, 643-652.

Huppert, F.A. and Piercy, M. (1978a) The role of trace strength in recency and frequency judgements by amnesic and control subjects. *Quarterly Journal of Experimental Psychology, 30*, 347-354.

Huppert, F.A. and Piercy, M. (1978b) Dissociation between learning and remembering in organic amnesia. *Nature, 275*, 317-318.

Huppert, F.A., Brayne, C. and O'Connor, D. (1994) *Dementia and Normal Aging*. Cambridge University Press, Cambridge, UK.

Katzman, R. and Saitoh, T. (1991) *Advances in Alzheimer's Disease*. FASEB J, 5, 278-286.

Mayes, A.R. (1986) Learning and memory disorders and their assessment. *Neuropsychologia, 24*, 25-39.

Rose, G. (1992) *The Strategy of Preventive Medicine*. Oxford University Press, New York.

Storandt, M., Aufdembrinke, B., Backman, L., Baltes, M.M., Blass, J.P., Braak, H., Gutzmann, H., Hauw, J-J, Hoyer, S., Jorm, A.F., Kauss, J., Kliegl, R. and Mountjoy, C.Q. (1988) Group Report: Relationship of normal aging and dementing diseases in later life. In: A.S. Henderson and J.H. Henderson (Eds) *Etiology of Dementia of Alzheimer's Type*. John Wiley & Sons, Chichester. Life Sciences Research Report 43: Report of the Dahlem Workshop, Berlin 1987, 231-239.

Warrington, E.K. and Weiskrantz, L. (1968) A new method of testing long-term retention with special reference to amnesic patients. *Nature, 217*, 972-974.

Weiskrantz, L. and Warrington, E.K. (1970) Verbal learning and retention by amnesic patients using partial information. *Psychonomic Science, 20*, 210-211.

8

Identification of Neuropsychologically Defined Subgroups of Alzheimer's Disease Patients

JAMES T. BECKER[1]

A diagnosis of Alzheimer's disease can only be made in the presence of significant impairments in at least two areas of cognitive function (APA, 1987; McKhann, Drachman, Folstein, Katzman, Price, & Stadlan, 1984), and memory loss is one of the most common symptoms early in dementia. Nevertheless, analyses of groups of patients with Alzheimer's disease (AD) has revealed the existence of subgroups of patients (Martin, 1990). These subgroups are characterized on the basis of the pattern of their neuropsychological deficits such that, for example, some may have pronounced defects in visuospatial functions, others may have focal lexical/semantic impairments, and still others may have profound dysexecutive syndromes; all of these patients nevertheless meet the criteria (Baddeley, Della Salla, & Spinnler, 1991; Becker, 1988; Martin, Brouwers, Lalonde, Cox, Teleska, Fedio, et al., 1986) for Probable AD. Analysis of the cognitive functions of these patients has revealed important features of their neuropsychological impairments (Martin, Cox, Brouwers, & Fedio, 1985), as well as correlations with cerebral glucose metabolism (Martin, Brouwers, Cox, & Fedio, 1985). Further, follow-up of these patients has

---

[1] JAMES T. BECKER, Ph.D.• Alzheimer's Disease Research Center, Departments of Psychiatry and Neurology, University of Pittsburgh Medical Center

Neuropsychological Explorations of Memory and Cognition: Essays in Honor of Nelson Butters, edited by Laird S. Cermak, Ph.D. Plenum Press, New York, 1994

revealed differential rates of decline among some of the subgroups (Becker, Bajulaiye, & Smith, 1992).

In 1983, the National Institute on Aging funded the Alzheimer Research Program at the University of Pittsburgh under the direction of Francois Boller (Becker, Boller, Lopez, Saxton, & McGonigle, in press). The purpose of this program was to evaluate the full spectrum of cognitive, neurological, and behavioral factors which could relate to the differential diagnosis and natural history of the disease. At that time, there was no clear consensus on the clinical diagnosis of AD, and diagnostic accuracy was considered important in light of the new directions in research and treatment. Critical to the program was the ability to identify signs or symptoms which could aid in the differential diagnosis and in determining prognosis of the dementia.

Early in the study, we reported on the functional dissociation of the visuospatial and lexical/semantic impairments associated with AD (Becker, Huff, Nebes, Holland, & Boller, 1988), following on the reports by Martin and colleagues (Martin, et al., 1986). We confirmed the earlier report that there were subgroups of patients with either relatively preserved language functions and impaired visuospatial skills, and a groups with impaired language functions and normal visuospatial skills. However, we failed to confirm other studies that reported that language impaired patients were at risk for a more rapid rate of decline (Filley, Kelly, & Heaton, 1986; Kaszniak, Fox, Gandell, Garron, Huckman, & Ramsey, 1978; Seltzer & Sherwin, 1983).

Our research group was also interested in the nature and extent of the memory impairment in AD. Morris and Kopelman (Morris & Kopelman, 1986) had argued that the memory loss in AD was due to a profound amnesic syndrome similar to that seen in patients with focal amnesic disorders, with the addition of another information processing defect which had an impact on their memory. We suggested that this additional deficit might be a dysexecutive syndrome (Becker, 1988), using the model of Working Memory developed by Baddeley and Hitch (Baddeley & Hitch, 1974). A cross-sectional analysis of the data demonstrated the existence of two subgroups of AD patients based on this model - one with a profound amnesic syndrome and normal executive functions, and the other with a significant dysexecutive syndrome and normal secondary memory. A subsequent longitudinal analysis (Becker, et al., 1992) revealed that the pattern of decline in these two subgroups of patients differed, with the dysexecutive patients demonstrating a dramatic loss of secondary memory functions over a one year period.

The purpose of this chapter is to describe our recent investigations of these two functional dichotomies. In the case of the lexical/semantic and visuospatial defects, we will describe the patterns of performance of the entire group of 181 patients with Probable or Definite AD. In the case of the analysis of the memory functions, we will report on a different analytical strategy which reveals important features of the memory loss in AD.

MATERIALS AND METHODS

Patient and control subjects enrolled into the Alzheimer Research Program (ARP) between March 1983 and March 1988. Details of the recruitment and assessment procedures have been published previously (Becker, et al., in press). Each subject, patients and controls alike, completed an extensive battery of neuropsychological tests which evaluated a wide range of cognitive functions. These evaluations were completed on an annual basis up through the ending of the ARP in 1988.

Of critical importance for this report was our method of reducing the extensive neuropsychological data into manageable units. As our goal was to reduce the data into composite variables with both face and construct validity, we have used factor analytic strategies to aid in this process (Becker, 1988; Becker, et al., 1992; Becker, et al., 1988). For the present study we focused on four specific composite scores reflecting Memory and Learning, Executive Functions, Visuoconstructional Skills, and Lexical/ Semantic Functions.

To create the composite scores, several steps were taken. First, the individual test scores were transformed into standard scores using the mean and standard deviations of the control group. In the event that a subject was missing a particular test score, the mean value for the study group was substituted. In the event that a subject (usually a patient) was unable to complete a particular test due to the severity of their dementia, then the maximum error score was substituted. The total number of data substitutions comprised less than 1% of the total dataset.

These standard scores were then averaged, using the appropriate sign, to create a score reflecting the subject's observed performance on the tasks. The data from the control group were then entered into a multiple regression analysis to evaluate the effects of age, education, and sex on the particular summary score. We then used these regression equations to *predict* individual performance based on age, education, and sex. The arithmetic difference between the observed and predicted scores constituted the composite variable. Thus, the composite scores can be interpreted as reflecting the deviation of an individual's performance from that expected based on their age, education, and sex. The mean value of these composite scores among the controls subjects varies about zero, while those of the patients were in the negative range, indicating performance worse than that expected (Becker, et al., in press)

To address the questions posed in this report, the data from the AD patients were then subjected to K-Means Cluster Analysis (Norusis, 1993) to identify groups of patients. Two analyses were completed - one included the lexical/semantic and visuoconstructional composite scores, and the other included the memory and learning and executive scores.

RESULTS

Lexical/Semantic and Visuoconstructional Functions
        Figure 1 shows the scatterplot of the visuoconstructional and language composite scores among the AD patients at study entry. The cluster analysis revealed five groups of patients, and these are also indicated in the figure. There are three groups of patients with relatively equivalent impairments in these two areas of function, and these are referred to as "non-focal" groups with regard to this dichotomy, and they are of increasing severity of impairment.
        There are two additional groups of patients which we refer to as having a "focal" impairment with regard to these two dimensions of cognitive function. One has significant abnormalities in visuoconstructional function, with relatively normal language functions, while the other has impaired language function with relatively normal visuoconstructional skills. The patterns of performance of these patients is shown in Table 1.

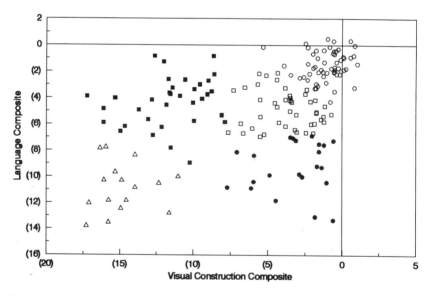

Figure 1. A scatterplot of the performance of 181 Probable AD patients as assessed by Language and Construction Composite scores. The open symbols correspond to the three non-focal groups: Mild (circles), Moderate (squares), and Severe (triangles) impairments. The filled symbols correspond to the Language Impaired (circles) and Construction Impaired (squares) subgroups.

TABLE 1

Characteristics and Neuropsychological Test Performance
of AD Patients as a Function of Language/Construction Dichotomy

	Non-Focal Groups			Focal Groups	
	Mild	Moderate	Severe	Language	Construction
N=	59	49	16	22	34
Age=	70.56	74.08	71.76	71.94	68.68
	(8.1)	(8.1)	(7.9)	(7.8)	(8.8)
Education	12.76	12.00	11.13	12.09	11.56
	(2.9)	(3.6)	(2.6)	(2.8)	(2.2)
Sex (%Male)	42.4	32.6	31.3	27.3	20.6
Mini Mental State	22.6	18.0	12.3	14.9	16.5
	(3.7)	(3.8)	(2.7)	(2.5)	(3.7)
Language	-1.54	-4.78	-10.88	-9.27	-4.32
Composite	(1.1)	(1.3)	(1.9)	(1.9)	(1.9)
Naming	31.64	21.24	14.1	14.41	20.62
	(5.4)	(6.7)	(7.0)	(9.3)	(6.9)
Fluency	8.36	5.37	2.31	3.05	5.48
	(4.0)	(3.5)	(2.7)	(2.1)	(4.9)
Easy Pairs*	10.52	15.87	29.81	25.41	14.87
	(2.1)	(3.8)	(4.4)	(5.2)	(5.6)
Construction	-1.06	-3.74	-14.82	-3.23	-11.59
Composite	(1.2)	(1.7)	(1.8)	(2.2)	(2.5)
Drawing	14.48	11.93	7.09	12.26	9.19
	(1.8)	(1.9)	(2.8)	(1.9)	(2.7)
Blocks	41.57	34.81	2.43	36.76	11.26
	(3.0)	(7.9)	(4.2)	(7.3)	(6.6)
Memory	-2.37	-3.24	-3.93	-3.33	-3.59
Composite	(0.9)	(0.7)	(0.3)	(0.7)	(0.6)
Perception	-1.09	-2.38	-7.73	-2.41	-4.92
Composite	(1.1)	(1.8)	(3.0)	(2.0)	(3.1)
Attention	-1.09	-2.55	-9.42	-3.71	-4.05
Composite	(2.0)	(2.5)	(5.4)	(3.1)	(3.5)
Executive	-4.10	-6.79	-17.93	-10.88	-9.09
Composite	(4.0)	(4.7)	(7.0)	(7.5)	(6.2)

*error score

The scores on the Mini-Mental State exam by these groups of patients are presented in Figure 2. Although the patients with the mildest degree of dementia had higher scores overall, there was no significant difference in the rate of decline in scores over a two year period. Furthermore, an analysis of the time until death revealed that while group membership did account for an increased risk for death, this was entirely accounted for by the patients in the moderate and severe groups. The Language Impaired subgroup had the *lowest* rate of death among the five patient groups. Thus, as we have noted previously, among AD patients of this age group (e.g., mean age = 71.4 years, range = 50.0 - 88.7) the presence of a profound impairment in language relative to other cognitive domains is *not* a risk factor for more rapid progression of dementia or shorter time until death.

Memory and Executive Functions
    The scatterplot of the memory and executive composite scores are shown in Figure 3. The K-Means cluster analysis revealed four clusters of patients. Three of the groups appeared to be related to increasing severity of the dysexecutive syndrome with a relatively constant score on the memory composite. These groups are described as Mild, Moderate, and Severely impaired on the executive score (See Table 2). The fourth group of patients appeared at first to correspond to the "amnesic" group noted earlier. However, further inspection of the performance by these patients revealed that they were impaired in only two areas of cognitive function, those related to memory and to language. There were no significant impairments in Perception, Construction, or Attention. Thus, these patients are described as having "Temporal Lobe" impairments - verbal and nonverbal memory are impaired, as are naming,

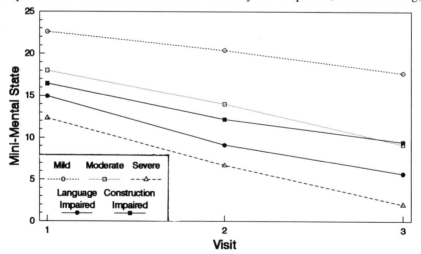

Figure 2. Scores on the Mini-Mental State Exam.

fluency, and the ability to associate highly related words (i.e., easy paired associates).

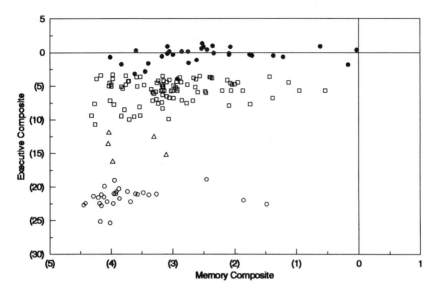

Figure 3.A scatterplot of the performance of the patients on the Memory and Executive Composite scores. The open symbols correspond to the three non-focal groups: Mild (squares), Moderate (triangles), and Severe (circles) impairments. The Temporal Lobe subgroup is shown in filled circles.

The performance of these groups of patients on the Mini-Mental State exam over a two year period is shown in Figure 4. These data demonstrate that the rate of decline among the patients in the Temporal Lobe group is significantly slower than that of the other three groups of patients. After two years of evaluation, the mean MMS score remains in the mildly impaired range (mean = 20.44, s.d. = 5.49), and is significantly different from that of the patients in the Mild group (mean = 10.77, s.d. = 6.37). In terms of physical survival, however, these patient groups did *not* differ in time until death during the follow-up period.

We compared the classification of these 181 patients with regard to these two functional dichotomies. There was a significant difference between these distributions (X^2 = 82.2, Phi = .67, p < .001, df = 12) indicating independence between these two dimensions. Among the patients classified as having a Language Impairment, only 1 (4.5%) was also included in the Temporal Lobe group. Indeed, it was generally the case that when a patient was classified in a subgroup on one dimension (e.g., Language vs. Construction) they were classified as Mild on the other (i.e., Memory vs. Executive) (65/88, 73.9%).

TABLE 2

Characteristics and Neuropsychological Test Performance
of AD Patients as a Function of Memory/Executive Dichotomy

	Mild	Moderate	Severe	Temporal Lobe
N=	114	5	29	32
Age	70.69	67.10	71.68	74.57
	(8.2)	(8.1)	(8.2)	(8.4)
Education	11.82	13.40	11.72	13.25
	(3.1)	(1.7)	(2.6)	(2.7)
Sex (%Male)	34.2	.0	24.1	40.6
Mini Mental State	18.2	14.6	14.83	22.5
	(4.4)	(4.5)	(4.3)	(3.7)
Memory Composite	-3.08	-3.70	-3.74	-2.47
	(0.8)	(0.5)	(0.7)	(1.0)
Story Recall	1.59	.60	.65	2.92
	(1.4)	(0.7)	(0.8)	(2.8)
Figure Recall	5.93	3.90	2.56	8.20
	(4.8)	(2.5)	(4.3)	(5.0)
Executive Composite	-5.89	-13.91	-21.58	-1.37
	(1.9)	(1.8)	(1.4)	(1.0)
Trails B*	233.8	240.0	236.8	174.5
	(20.1)	(0.0)	(17.3)	(52.3)
Reaction Time*	.68	1.33	2.02	.45
	(0.2)	(0.2)	(0.1)	(0.1)
Language Composite	-4.38	-7.95	-8.24	-2.24
	(2.9)	(2.5)	(3.5)	(2.1)
Naming	23.0	14.4	17.1	30.2
	(8.8)	(6.5)	(9.2)	(6.5)
Fluency	5.79	4.0	2.48	9.25
	(3.9)	(4.2)	(2.0)	(4.3)
Easy Pairs*	15.47	21.6	23.4	12.19
	(6.6)	(7.1)	(7.9)	(4.3)
Perception Composite	-2.88	-1.84	-5.72	-.69
	(2.5)	(1.1)	(3.7)	(1.0)
Construction Composite	-5.28	-5.56	-9.63	-1.18
	(4.6)	(6.5)	(5.7)	(1.7)
Attention Composite	-2.49	-1.96	-8.71	-.43
	(2.1)	(0.6)	(5.2)	(1.3)

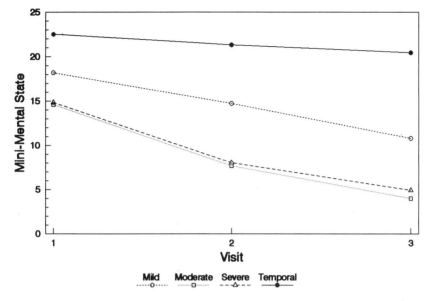

Figure 4. Scores on the Mini-Mental State Exam.

DISCUSSION

These data make several points relevant to our understanding of Alzheimer's disease. First, they reinforce the point, if it needs reinforcing at all, that Alzheimer's disease can present with relative sparing and impairment of specific cognitive functions. Second, as we have noted previously, the presence of a focal language impairment in AD patients over the age of 50 does not increase the risk to die relative to other AD patients. However, it must be noted, that while the time until death may not be shorter relative to other AD patients, it is clearly shorter than that for non-demented age- and medical status-matched healthy individuals (Martin, Miller, Kapoor, Arena, & Boller, 1987). Third, we identified a group of patients with impaired episodic and semantic memory, with few additional cognitive impairments, who had a slower rate of intellectual decline than other AD patients. These patients are felt to have a focal impairment in the functions of the temporal lobes, bilaterally, in the context of Probable AD.

With regard to the first point, it seems clear that while the most common pattern of impairment includes loss of episodic memory function early in the course of the disease, this may be accompanied by differential sparing and impairments of function. These patterns of impairment correspond to the altered regional CNS function as revealed by Positron Emission Tomography (Haxby, Duara, & Grady, 1985; Haxby, Grady, Koss, Horwitz, Hexton, Schapiro, et al., 1990), demonstrating a close link between loss of brain function and abnormal cognition.

With regard to the second and third points, the specific pattern of impairment is important. That is, the identification of a "Temporal Lobe" pattern of dysfunction appears to have significance for predicting a slower rate of decline in function, while the presence of neither a Language nor Construction deficit do not have the same predictive value. This suggests that when the cognitive dysfunction associated with AD begins with processes ascribed to the temporal lobes, and not, for example, the parietal lobes, then the rate of spread of these abnormalities may be different. This observation may have implications for understanding the nature of the progression of AD-related neuropathological changes throughout the brain.

One question that arises is why we (Becker, et al., 1988) and others (Selnes, Hart, & Gordon, 1989) have not reproduced earlier findings regarding the increased risk of progression and death in patients with pronounced language impairments (Filley, et al., 1986; Kaszniak, et al., 1978; Seltzer & Sherwin, 1983). Among the different possibilities are two which seem particularly important. First, some of these studies were conducted prior to the time that strict, rigorous diagnostic criteria were adopted (e.g., (APA, 1987; Lopez, Swihart, & Becker, 1990; McKhann, et al., 1984)). Thus, some of those data may represent the inclusion of other disease entities such as progressive fluent aphasia (Hodges, Patterson, Oxbury, & Funnell, 1992; Snowden, Neary, Mann, Goulding, & Testa, 1992) into a group of AD patients. Second, the use of tests with high verbal components may have confounded the analyses. Thus, if the selection criteria or outcome measures include, for example, the Mini-Mental State exam which has a significant verbal component, then a loss of verbal functions greater than other impairments may *appear* to result in more rapid decline. However, were other areas of cognition to be tested, we would suggest that the overall level of impairment would not be greater than the mean. In the present study we may have reduced these two difficulties by relying on strict diagnostic criteria (>90 % accuracy relative to autopsy (Becker, et al., in press; Lopez, et al., 1990)), and by using different tests for baseline classification and for tracking outcome.

These data make an important point about clinical pharmacological trials in AD. At the present time, there are no criteria for entry into studies based on the *pattern* of impairment. The assumption appears to be that in a large study, random assignment of patients to treatment or placebo conditions should eliminate any potential problems related to subgroup classification. This is probably true in terms of determining efficacy provided that the samples are large enough. However, in small studies (e.g., <20 per group), a bias in terms of patient characteristics could have important effects in terms of determining efficacy.

Perhaps more important, however, is that fact that these characteristics are not taken into account when designing these studies. The scientific and clinical merits of these pharmacological trials would be increased dramatically if these sorts of patient characteristics were used as blocking variables, and as outcome measures. It may be the case, for example, that while Drug X has only a marginally important effect on cognition when measured by summary variables, specific aspects of cognition are affected more than others, and certain subgroups of patients show marked improvement relative to other subgroups. The interaction between neuropsychology and psychopharmacology in the context of treating dementia syndromes seems to be potentially an important source of information on brain mechanisms in cognition.

AFTERWORD

When I was planning my postdoctoral experience, I had the opportunity to speak with Paul McHugh, Chairman of the Department of Psychiatry and Behavioral Sciences at The Johns Hopkins University School of Medicine. I was looking for a job, but also had an application pending for an individual fellowship to work with Nelson Butters at the Boston V.A. Dr. McHugh's advice was concise: forget the job search, go work with Nelson - even if I had to do so for free. I took his advice, although I was fortunate that the N.I.A.A.A. saw fit to provide financial support. From 1980 until Nelson left for San Diego in 1984, I was actively involved in research with him. I learned many important lessons from Nelson, many of them concerning science. Perhaps the most important, however, were those having to do with his intense sense of personal and professional loyalty. Nelson is pathologically incapable of having an unhappy student, and we all continue to rely on him for support and counsel.

The research that I reviewed here, quite literally would not have been possible without Nelson. It was through him that I first met Francois Boller and had the opportunity to come to Western Psychiatric Institute and Clinic. Using some ideas that we had discussed in Boston about rates of forgetting in amnesia and dementia, I began our research efforts in Pittsburgh (Becker, Boller, Saxton, & McGonigle-Gibson, 1987). We have continued to use the models of double and single dissociation that Nelson has applied so well (Martone, Butters, Payne, Becker, & Sax, 1984), and believe that it will lead to important understanding of brain function and behavior. In Nelson's Presidential Address to Division 40 of the American Psychological Association, he stressed the links between clinical and cognitive neuropsychology, arguing that the dichotomy was probably false. My own work has tried to live up to that goal of using (and testing) models of cognitive processing (Becker, 1988) to increase our understanding of clinical syndromes.

Throughout my career, I have had many excellent teachers who directed, instructed, or trained me by example or experience. I have also known several individuals from whom I could seek advice. It is in Nelson that I also find a close, trusted, experienced counselor and guide through the tracks of my career. He is good at what he does because he holds up a mirror in which we can see ourselves clearly, and learn from what we see. The success of Nelson's students, which is due largely to this skill, is perhaps the truest measure of his remarkable career.

ACKNOWLEDGMENTS. The preparation of this chapter was supported in part by funds from the National Institute on Aging (AG05133) and the National Institute of Mental Health (MH45311). I was assisted in this work by O.L. Lopez, K. Doyle, and D. Galeza. I am grateful to the Department of Psychiatry at the University of California - San Diego, for allowing me to participate in this Festschrift, and especially to Nelson for asking me to deliver a talk.

REFERENCES

APA (1987). *Diagnostic and statistical manual on mental disorders (DSM-III)* (3 (Revised) ed.). Washington, D.C.: American Psychiatric Press.

Baddeley, A. D., Della Salla, S., & Spinnler, H. (1991). The two-component hypothesis of memory deficit in Alzheimer's disease. *Jour Clin Exp Neuropsychol, 13*, 372-380.

Baddeley, A. D., & Hitch, G. (1974). Working memory. In G. H. Bower (Eds.), *The Psychology of Learning and Motivation* New York: Academic Press.

Becker, J. T. (1988). Primary memory and secondary memory deficits in Alzheimer's disease. *J Clin Exp Neuropsychol, 10*, 739-753.

Becker, J. T., Bajulaiye, O., & Smith, C. (1992). Longitudinal analysis of a two-component model of the memory deficits in Alzheimer's disease. *Psychol Med, 22*, 437-446.

Becker, J. T., Boller, F., Lopez, O. L., Saxton, J., & McGonigle, K. (in press). The natural history of Alzheimer's disease: Description of study cohort and accuracy of diagnosis. *Arch Neurol.*

Becker, J. T., Boller, F., Saxton, J., & McGonigle-Gibson, K. (1987). Normal rates of forgetting of verbal and non-verbal material in Alzheimer's disease. *Cortex, 23*, 59-72.

Becker, J. T., Huff, F. J., Nebes, R. D., Holland, A., & Boller, F. (1988). Neuropsychological functioning in Alzheimer's disease: Pattern of impairment and rates of progression. *Arch Neurol, 45*, 263-268.

Filley, C. M., Kelly, J., & Heaton, R. K. (1986). Neuropsychological features of early- and late-onset Alzheimer's disease. *Arch Neurol, 43*, 574-576.

Haxby, J. V., Duara, R., & Grady, C. L. (1985). Relations between neuropsychological and cerebral metabolic asymmetries in early Alzheimer's disease. *J Cereb Blood Flow Metab, 5,* 193-200.

Haxby, J. V., Grady, C. L., Koss, E., Horwitz, B., Hexton, L., Schapiro, M., Friedland, R., & Rapoport, S. I. (1990). Longitudinal study of cerebral metabolic asymmetries and associated neuropsychological patterns in early dementia of the Alzheimer type. *Arch Neurol, 47,* 753-760.

Hodges, J. R., Patterson, K., Oxbury, S., & Funnell, E. (1992). Semantic dementia: Progressive fluent aphasia with temporal lobe atrophy. *Brain, 115,* 1783-1806.

Kaszniak, A. W., Fox, J., Gandell, D. L., Garron, D. C., Huckman, M. S., & Ramsey, R. G. (1978). Predictors of mortality in presenile and senile dementia. *Ann Neurol, 3,* 246-252.

Lopez, O. L., Swihart, A. A., & Becker, J. T. (1990). Reliability of NINCDS-ADRDA clinical criteria for the diagnosis of Alzheimer's disease. *Neurology, 40,* 1517-1522.

Martin, A. (1990). Neuropsychology of Alzheimer's disease: The case for subgroups. In M. F. Schwartz (Eds.), *Modular deficits in Alzheimer's-type dementia* Cambridge, MA: Bradford/MIT.

Martin, A., Brouwers, P., Cox, C., & Fedio, P. (1985). On the nature of the verbal memory deficit in Alzheimer's disease. *Brain and Language, 25,* 323-341.

Martin, A., Brouwers, P., Lalonde, F., Cox, C., Teleska, P., Fedio, P., Foster, N. L., & Chase, T. N. (1986). Towards a behavioral typology of Alzheimer's patients. *Jour Clin Exp Neuropsychol, 8,* 594-610.

Martin, A., Cox, C., Brouwers, P., & Fedio, P. (1985). A note on the different patterns of impaired and preserved cognitive abilities and their relation to episodic memory deficits in Alzheimer's patients. *Brain and Language, 25,* 323-341.

Martin, D. C., Miller, J. K., Kapoor, W., Arena, V. C., & Boller, F. (1987). A controlled study of survival with dementia. *Arch Neurol, 44,* 1122-1126.

Martone, M. A., Butters, N., Payne, M., Becker, J. T., & Sax, D. S. (1984). Dissociations between skill learning and verbal recognition in amnesia and dementia. *Arch Neurol, 41*(9), 965-970.

McKhann, G., Drachman, D. A., Folstein, M. F., Katzman, R., Price, D. L., & Stadlan, E. (1984). Clinical diagnosis of Alzheimer's disease: Report of the NINCDS-ADRDA Work Group under the auspices of the Department of Health and Human Services Task Force on Alzheimer's disease. *Neurology, 34,* 939-944.

Morris, R. G., & Kopelman, M. D. (1986). The memory deficits in Alzheimer-type dementia: A review. *Quart Jour Exp Psychol, 38,* 575-602.

Norusis, M. J. (1993). *SPSS for Windows, Release 6.0.* Chicago: SPSS, Inc.

Selnes, O. A., Hart, J., & Gordon, B. (1989). Early Alzheimer's disease: Aphasia is not a consistent finding (Abstract). *Ann Neurol, 26,* 136.

Seltzer, B., & Sherwin, I. (1983). A comparison of clinical features in early- and late-onset primary degenerative dementia. *Arch Neurol, 40,* 143-146.

Snowden, J. S., Neary, D., Mann, D. M. A., Goulding, P. J., & Testa, H. J. (1992). Progressive language disorder due to lobar atrophy. *Ann Neurol, 31,* 174-183.

9

Contributions of Cognitive Psychology to the Study of Impaired Memory and Attention

ERIC GRANHOLM[1]

One of Nelson Butters' most important contributions to the field of neuropsychology has been to promote the use of experimental paradigms and concepts developed in cognitive psychology in studies of disordered cognition. In his Presidential Addresses to the International Neuropsychological Society (INS) and to Division 40 of the American Psychological Association, Butters (see Butters, 1984) presented a strong argument for greater interdependence of clinical and cognitive-experimental approaches to neuropsychological research. He noted that, although studies using standardized fixed or flexible clinical neuropsychological batteries have reliably described different patterns of impairment in different patient populations, the clinical battery approach has contributed little to our understanding of the nature of these impairments. Butters encouraged the application of cognitive psychology methods to the assessment of disordered cognition in order to move beyond simple descriptions of quantitative decline beyond normal limits. A more precise qualitative description of specific processing impairments underlying quantitative deficits can be achieved through the application of concepts and paradigms from cognitive psychology to neuropsychological studies.

Throughout his career, Nelson Butters has attempted to promote a more "symbiotic relationship" (Butters, 1984) between cognitive-experimental and

[1] ERIC GRANHOLM, Ph.D., • Psychology Service, San Diego Department of Veterans Affairs Medical Center; Department of Psychiatry, University of California, San Diego

Neuropsychological Explorations of Memory and Cognition: Essays in Honor of Nelson Butters, edited by Laird S. Cermak, Ph.D. Plenum Press, New York, 1994

clinical neuropsychological research. During his tenure as president of the INS, the *Journal of Clinical Neuropsychology* was selected to serve as the Society's official journal, and the name of the journal was changed to the *Journal of Clinical and Experimental Neuropsychology*, reflecting his emphasis on the complementary contributions of clinical and experimental approaches. Nearly ten years later, as editor of *Neuropsychology*, the first American Psychological Association journal dedicated to the discipline of neuropsychology, Butters (1993) continued this message in his editorial on the goals and direction of the journal. He stressed the importance of cognitive-experimental neuropsychological approaches to our understanding of clinical disorders, as well as the importance of clinical neuropsychological approaches to our understanding of normal cognition.

   As a student and colleague of Nelson Butters for the past ten years, I have learned the value of applying cognitive psychology concepts and experimental tasks to the study of disordered memory and attention. To illustrate this approach, studies carried out during my work in Butters' lab will be described. These studies apply concepts such as "episodic and semantic memory" and "encoding specificity" from cognitive psychology to examine the encoding, storage and retrieval abilities of Alzheimer's Disease (AD) and Huntington's Disease (HD) patients. To illustrate the impact of this work in the Butters' lab on my subsequent research with schizophrenic patients, studies which examine attentional impairments and the automation of processing in schizophrenia will then be described. These studies apply concepts such as "attentional resources" and "automatic and controlled processing" from cognitive psychology. I am just one of many researchers who has learned the value of this approach from Nelson Butters' work, as any glance at the neuropsychology literature will reveal.

IMPAIRED MEMORY IN ALZHEIMER'S AND HUNTINGTON'S DISEASE

   Our investigations of the memory disorders of patients with HD and AD provided evidence that HD patients are impaired in the retrieval of information from episodic and semantic memory, while AD patients fail to use semantic information to facilitate encoding of episodic memories (Butters et al., 1986; 1987; Granholm & Butters, 1988).

Episodic and Semantic Memory
   Tulving (1983) described a dichotomy between episodic and semantic memory. Episodic memories are defined as those dependent upon temporal and/or spatial cues for their retrieval. Examples of episodic memories include attempts to recall yesterday's activities or the name of someone you just met at a party. These events require the use of temporal and spatial contextual cues and,

thus, represent retrieval from episodic memory. Most standardized clinical memory measures are episodic memory tasks (e.g., list learning, story recall). In contrast, retrieval from semantic memory does not require contextual cues. Examples of semantic memories include a wide variety of well-learned factual information, such as historical (e.g., Who was president of the U.S. during the Civil War?), numerical (e.g., How many pennies in a dollar?), and geographic (e.g., What is the capital of New Jersey?) facts. Due to repetition and over-learning, memories which are initially episodic in nature may become context-free and part of an individual's semantic fund of knowledge.

This dichotomy was applied to studies of AD and HD, by examining performance on word-list and story recall (episodic memory) and verbal fluency (semantic memory) tasks (Butters et al., 1985; 1986; 1987). On list learning tests and tasks involving memory for prose passages, HD patients performed as poorly as amnesic, alcoholic Korsakoff patients when recall measures were employed, but the HD patients were superior to amnesic patients when recognition tests were introduced. On letter fluency tasks, HD patients generated fewer correct responses than did Korsakoff patients. This double dissociation between HD and Korsakoff patients on verbal recognition and verbal fluency tasks suggested that HD patients were impaired in the initiation of systematic strategies for searching and retrieving information from both episodic and semantic memory. As the retrieval demands were reduced (e.g., with recognition rather than recall measures) or increased (e.g., with letter fluency measures), the performance of HD patients changed dramatically relative to Korsakoff patients.

These investigations of episodic (story recall) and semantic (verbal fluency) memory disorders were then extended to early-stage AD patients (Butters et al., 1987). The performance of AD and HD patients (matched for severity of dementia), alcoholic Korsakoff patients, and age- and education-matched normal controls were compared on these tasks. On the story recall task, subjects recalled four thematically neutral stories composed of 23 arbitrarily designated phrases, which were similar to the Logical Memory Passages of the Wechsler Memory Scale. The AD patients, like HD and amnesic patients, showed severe impairments in comparison to controls. The major differences between AD, HD and Korsakoff patients were found when the numbers of prior-story intrusion (i.e., correctly recalled items from one story which are recalled as part of a subsequent story) and extra-story intrusion errors (i.e., ideas recalled which were never presented in any story) were examined. Both the Korsakoff and AD patients made more intrusion errors than did their age-matched controls and the HD patients. These intrusions reflect the AD and Korsakoff patients' increased sensitivity to proactive interference and confirms other reports that intrusion errors are an important characteristic of the episodic memory disorder of AD patients (Fuld, 1983). The HD patients' pattern of error scores, in contrast, did not suggest a special role for proactive interference in their episodic memory impairment.

On the verbal fluency tasks, subjects were read the letters 'F', 'A', and 'S' and asked to produce as many different words "as they could think of" that began with the given letter (letter fluency) and to name as many different animals (category fluency) in one minute. The total number of words reported on the fluency tasks is displayed in Figure 1 for each of the four 15-second quadrants of the one-minute letter (F+A+S total) and category fluency trials. As anticipated on the basis of previous studies (Martin & Fedio, 1983; Ober et al., 1986) all subject groups displayed their greatest fluency in the first 15-second quadrant, and their production tended to decrease as a function of time.

The HD patients were equally impaired on both letter and category fluency tasks. Of the three patient groups, the HD patients were the most consistently and severely impaired in their attempts to retrieve information from semantic memory. The Korsakoff patients showed a mild-to-moderate impairment on both fluency tasks, and like the HD patients, the severity of their

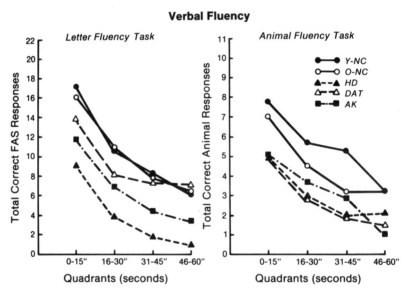

Figure 1. Performance of "young" (Y-NC) and "old" (O-NC) normal controls and patients with Huntington's Disease (HD), dementia of the Alzheimer's type (DAT), and alcoholic Korsakoff's (AK) syndrome on the letter (FAS) and category (animal) fluency tasks. (Reproduced with permission from Butters et al., *Journal of Clinical and Experimental Neuropsychology*, Vol. 9, copyright 1987 by Swets & Zeitlinger).

fluency problem was not related to the linguistic constraints (i.e., letter v. category fluency) of the semantic memory task. In contrast, the performance of the AD patients was directly related to the linguistic demands of the two fluency tasks. On the letter fluency task, the number of words generated by patients with AD did not differ significantly from their matched normal controls and was significantly better than HD patients. However, on the category fluency task, the performance of the patients with AD was severely impaired. The AD patients generated significantly fewer correct animal names than did their elderly age-matched controls, and their performance was indistinguishable from that of the severely impaired HD patients.

The finding that the HD patients' performance was severely impaired on *both* letter and category fluency test is consistent with the hypothesis that HD patients' episodic and semantic memory disorders reflect a general retrieval deficit. An impairment in retrieving stored information should be evidenced on virtually all fluency tasks, regardless of their linguistic demands. In contrast, the AD patients' fluency deficits were most apparent when they had to search for exemplars of an abstract category (animals). This finding is consistent with the hypothesis of Martin and Fedio (1983) and Ober and colleagues (1986) that AD patients' language problems involve a reduction in the number of exemplars comprising an abstract category, because the category fluency task should be a more sensitive measure of deficiencies in semantic memory than the letter fluency task. Letter fluency tasks can be performed using phonemic cues to search a very extensive set of appropriate exemplars, so impairments in AD involving a shrinkage or breakdown of the semantic memory network may not be apparent on letter fluency tasks until the disease has progressed beyond its earliest stages. The findings of these investigations demonstrate that the processes underlying disordered episodic and semantic memory systems may vary from one patient population to another, despite quantitative similarity in level of severity of memory impairment.

Encoding Specificity

The above evidence for a breakdown or shrinkage of the semantic memory network in AD raised the question of whether AD patients are capable of performing semantic analyses to facilitate encoding novel episodic memories. The principle of encoding specificity was used in one study (Granholm & Butters, 1988) to answer this question. The principle of encoding specificity states that "specific encoding operations performed on what is perceived determine what is stored, and what is stored determines what retrieval cues are effective in providing assess to what is stored" (Tulving & Thomson, 1973; p. 369). In a demonstration of this principle in college students, Thomson & Tulving (1970) showed that, on a word-list recall task, cue words presented with to-be-remembered (TBR) words at both input and output, whether strong or weak semantic associates of the TBR words, were the most effective retrieval cues.

Individuals benefiting from retrieval cues that were paired with TBR words at presentation are presumably capable of performing semantic analyses during encoding, because they utilize the product of their analyses when cued recall is attempted.

The encoding specificity task designed by Thomson and Tulving (1970) and used by Cermak and colleagues (1980) was used to compare early-stage HD and AD patients (matched for severity of dementia) and age- and education-matched normal controls. Subjects were presented a list of 12 word pairs, consisting of a capitalized TBR word and an associated cue word printed in lowercase letters and enclosed in parentheses above it. Four encoding/retrieval cue conditions were generated by varying the types of cues (i.e., strong: S; weak: W; or no cues: O) present at presentation and recall: O-O (standard free recall), S-S, W-W, W-S, and S-W. At recall, subjects were presented with the associate cue words and instructed that these were cues to aid recall of one of the capitalized TBR words from the list.

If AD patients have a limited ability to perform adequate semantic encoding during presentation, then they should not show improvement in recall performance with the introduction of retrieval cues which were the verbal associates shown at presentation (i.e., in S-S and W-W conditions). In contrast, if HD patients' memory disorder is not due to breakdowns in their semantic network, but to a general retrieval problem, then they should have poor recall overall, but their pattern of performance should be qualitatively similar to that of controls.

Figure 2 presents the total number of correctly recalled words for the four subject groups in each of the five experimental conditions. The overall recall of each patient group was significantly impaired relative to controls, but the overall recall of the HD and AD patient group did not differ significantly. The most relevant findings are apparent when one looks at the various cue conditions individually. The normal controls' performance followed the pattern predicted by the encoding specificity principle. Their recall was the best when cues were identical at presentation and recall (S-S; W-W) and was worse when cues were mixed (W-S; S-W), although the trends for facilitation of recall in the W-W condition relative to the W-S and free recall conditions were not statistically significant. In the mixed-cue conditions, the strength of the retrieval cues clearly influenced recall: When strong cues were present at retrieval (W-S), recall was much better than when weak retrieval cues were present (S-W).

The major finding of this study was that the AD and HD patients were dissociated by their pattern of performance across cue conditions. As anticipated on the basis of their general retrieval problem, the pattern of performance shown by HD patients across conditions was identical to that of controls. As predicted by the encoding specificity hypothesis, the HD patients were most successful at recalling words when the cues were identical at presentation and output. Thus, their impaired performance in total recall does not necessarily reflect any

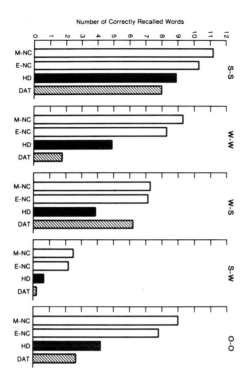

Figure 2. Total number of correctly recalled words in each of the five encoding specificity task cue conditions (Strong-Strong, S-S; Weak-Weak, W-W; Weak-Strong, W-S; Strong-Weak, S-W; and free recall, O-O) for the middle-age (M-NC) and elderly (E-NC) normal controls, Huntington's Disease (HD) and dementia of the Alzheimer type (DAT) patients. (Reproduced with permission from Granholm & Butters, *Brain and Cognition,* Vol. 7, copyright 1988 by Academic Press).

limitations in encoding. Rather, the HD patients were less able than normal subjects at initiating retrieval, regardless of how well the relationship between cue and TBR words was encoded.

In contrast, for the AD patients, a very different pattern of performance emerged. Although recall was significantly better in the S-S condition than in the mixed-cue conditions, surprisingly, the AD patients recalled significantly more words in the W-S condition, where cues were mixed, than in the W-W condition, where cues were identical. In addition, the recall performance of the AD patients was significantly worse than that of the HD patients in the W-W condition. These findings suggest that, unlike the HD and control subjects, the AD patients did not adequately utilize semantic information present at encoding to facilitate recall performance. Rather, the AD patients appeared to simply free-associate to the cues present at retrieval, which is a strategy that is only likely to result in enhanced performance when strong, rather than weak, cues are present at retrieval (S-S and W-S). An additional finding that the AD patients produced a greater number of extra-list intrusion errors than did any other group supports this free-association interpretation. These results are consistent with the notion that a breakdown or shrinkage of the semantic memory network may lead to reduced sensitivity to the semantic properties of stimuli and thus, to impaired semantic encoding of novel episodic memories in AD.

IMPAIRED ATTENTION IN SCHIZOPHRENIA

Since leaving the Butters lab, I have continued to apply cognitive psychology concepts and paradigms to the study of disordered attention in schizophrenia. These studies (Granholm, et al., 1991; 1993) have focused on processing resources limitations and the development of automatic processing skills in patients with schizophrenics.

Information-Processing Resources

When processing stimuli in the environment, one is generally concerned with analyzing inputs and then acting upon them. Since the processes by which these goals are accomplished occur at a limited rate (i.e., our information processing system can analyze, decide about and transform a limited number of items per unit of time), certain channels or subsets of stimuli impinging upon us must be selectively attended to for processing to avoid information overload.

In order to capture this notion of processing limitations, the human brain as an information-processor has been conceptualized as possessing a "pool of processing resources" which are available for the performance of cognitive tasks (e.g., Kahneman, 1973). Like "arousal" and "activation," "resources" are not directly observable entities. Resources represent a hypothetical commodity to be utilized and consumed for the purpose of information processing. There is no current consensus about which metaphor best captures the concept of resources, but resources have been broadly conceptualized as the limited pools of fuels, processes, skills and structures that are available at a given moment to enable performance of cognitive tasks (Hirst & Kalmar, 1987). Placing cognitive systems under time pressure (e.g., increasing the amount of information that must be processed in a fixed unit of time) makes greater demands on processing resources (Kahneman, 1973). The use of this concept simply provides a means of describing the human brain as a resource-dependent system; in that, there are clear limits on its ability to perform. Within this framework, cognitive deficits are expected to occur on a wide variety of tasks tapping a variety of stages of processing, whenever the resource demands of the task exceed the overall amount of processing resources available to the system.

Automatic and Controlled Processing

In discussing resource limitations, it is crucial to consider the mode of information processing employed on a task, because not all types of processing are subject to the constraints of a limited-resource system. Several investigators (e.g., Schneider, Dumais & Shiffrin, 1984; Posner & Snyder, 1975; Hasher & Zacks, 1979) draw a distinction between a resource-demanding, controlled mode of processing and a relatively resource-free, automatic mode of processing. Controlled processing, is a relatively slow, generally serial processing mode, which is resource-limited. By contrast, automatic processing is a relatively fast, generally parallel processing mode, which requires few or no resources. Processes which are widely believed to be controlled processes include rehearsal, serial search, and mental arithmetic. Automatic processes include simple recognition and encoding of spatial and frequency information about stimuli.

Work by Schneider and colleagues (1984) indicates that automatic processes can be broken down into "informational processes," which are responsible for the parallel encoding of input stimuli to various code levels in short-term store (e.g., visual features and category codes), and "actional processes," such as operations that direct attention and controlled processes to specific inputs without utilizing resources in the act (i.e., "automatic attention responses") or that produce overt responses (e.g., push a button). Actional processes develop through practice with consistent stimuli that always give rise to a relevant, non-conflicting response. For example, on a visual detection task where a target stimulus (e.g., "T") does not appear on any trial as a distractor letter that should be ignored, the target always receives a positive response (e.g., always push a button for "T"). In this example, the target stimulus ("T") is "consistently-mapped" onto the button-push response, so sufficient practice should lead to the development of automatic attention responses for the target stimulus. Squire's (1986) description of "procedural memory" as the learning of general rules or procedures through practice provides another description of the automation of processes, such as motor skills and perceptual discriminations. One of the most beneficial features of practice and skill development is that the processing of information can become resource-free through the development of automatic operations; thus, increasing the human brain's capacity to process information.

Resource-Limitations and Automatic Processing

To account for the wide variety of cognitive impairments observed in schizophrenic patients, which range from deficient icon formation to poor abstract thinking, studies of information processing in schizophrenia have typically attempted to identify a specific dysfunctional processing stage. More recently, however, several researchers (e.g., Gjerde, 1983; Nuechterlein & Dawson, 1984) have refuted the notion of a specific defective processing stage underlying schizophrenic patients' nearly global cognitive dysfunctions. These researchers have observed that, across cognitive domains, patients with schizophrenia perform poorly only when processing loads (i.e., resource demands) are high. For example, on the span of apprehension task, subjects must report whether a 'T' or 'F' target letter is among an array of distractor letters flashed briefly in a visual display. Numerous studies (Asarnow et al., 1991) have shown that patients with schizophrenia detect significantly fewer targets on this span of apprehension task than do control subjects when 10 letters are in the arrays (higher load), but their detection rates are normal with three letters in the arrays (lower loads). Processing demands are higher in the 10-letter condition, because subjects must carry out an increased number of repetitions of controlled serial search and discrimination operations per unit of time with 10-letter arrays, relative to 3-letter arrays. The frequent result on numerous cognitive tasks (Granholm, 1992; Nuechterlein & Dawson, 1984) that patients with schizophrenia are more adversely affected by higher resource demands than are controls is consistent with the hypothesis that these patients reach the limits of their available resources at lower processing loads (i.e., have fewer resources mobilized and available) than do nonpsychiatric individuals.

Normal amounts of processing resources may not be _available_ to schizophrenic patients for at least four possible reasons (Nuechterlein & Dawson, 1984): (1) The actual pool of resources may be smaller or more limited in schizophrenics; (2) Resources may not be mobilized and allocated efficiently in accordance with task demands, despite intact resource pools; (3) Excessive resources might be wasted on processing of task-irrelevant stimuli, leaving fewer resources available (remaining) for task-relevant operations; and/or (4) Automatic processes might be disrupted, which would require that resource-demanding controlled processing be utilized to carry out processing normally accomplished through resource-free automatic operations.

A recent investigation (Granholm, et al., 1991), was designed to examine this resource-limitation hypothesis and to begin to identify which of the above four possible explanations might account for resource deficiencies in schizophrenics. Two procedures were borrowed from cognitive psychology for this study. First, the secondary-task or dual-task procedure, which was developed in cognitive psychology specifically to examine resource-limitation hypotheses (Gophor & Donchin, 1986; Norman & Bobrow, 1975) was used. In the dual-task paradigm, subjects are asked to favor performance of a primary task, but to simultaneously perform a secondary task. Findings of decrements in overall performance on both tasks during dual-task relative to single-task performance are taken to reflect resource limitations (Gophor & Donchin, 1986). If subjects can perform each of the two tasks separately, but are unable to perform them together in the dual-task condition, what accounts for the decline in performance?

The notion of a stage deficit or impairment in a specific cognitive operation cannot account for successful single-task performance. Thus, the dual-task paradigm allows one to more directly conclude that task performance declines because insufficient resources are available for adequate dual-task performance.

Second, a hybrid memory and visual search task called the multiple-frame search task (MFST; Schneider & Shiffrin, 1977) was used to examine the automatic processing abilities of schizophrenics. On the MFST, one trial consisted of a series of twelve 2 X 2 letter arrays (frames) which were sequentially flashed briefly (80 msec exposure per frame) on a computer monitor. Subjects were asked to search the series of frames for either a "T" or "F" target letter, under two processing load conditions: two or four letters per frame (FS2; FS4). Since the targets never appeared as distractors on any trial (consistent-mapping), sufficient practice on this task should result in the development of automatic detection responses for the targets. At the beginning stages of practice, subjects use controlled serial search to compare display set letters with memory (target) set letters to find targets. This is reflected in a processing load effect (i.e., FS2>FS4 detection rates). The development of automatic detection responses is inferred when, with practice, detection accuracy becomes independent of processing load (i.e., FS2 = FS4 detection rates; Schneider & Shiffrin, 1977).

The MFST results are shown in Figure 3. At the beginning blocks of practice (64 trials per block), chronic schizophrenic patients showed a significant processing load effect (FS2 > FS4 detection rates) and the schizophrenic patients' detection rates were significantly impaired relative to the controls, especially at the higher processing load (FS4). These findings suggest deficient utilization of resource-dependent controlled serial processing in schizophrenics. In contrast, at the end of 320 trials of practice (block 5), the initial processing load effect was eliminated in the schizophrenics (FS2 = FS4 detection rates) and the detection rates of the two groups no longer differ significantly. These findings suggest that the schizophrenics were able to develop automatic detection responses after practice. Taken together, these MFST results are consistent with theories postulating resource limitations (Nuechterlein & Dawson, 1984) and greater deficiencies with controlled processing than with automatic processing (Neale & Oltmanns, 1980; Callaway & Naghdi, 1982) in schizophrenia.

Following the fifth block of MFST practice (Figure 3), subjects were required to simultaneously perform on the MFST and an auditory shadowing task (dual-task condition), where they repeated random letters presented at the rate of one per two seconds. In the dual-task condition, although the MFST accuracy of the schizophrenics deteriorated somewhat relative to their single-task (block 5) level of performance, this decline was not statistically significant. In contrast, the controls' MFST accuracy remained much more stable. Thus, although neither group's MFST performance was *significantly* affected by the additional resource demands of the dual-task condition, the patients' performance was

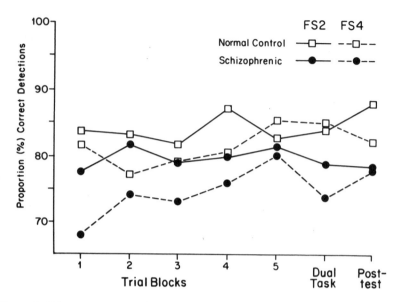

Figure 3. Mean percentage of correct target detections by schizophrenic patients and normal controls on a multiple-frame search task for frame sizes 2 and 4 (FS2, FS4) in five blocks of practice and during (Dual Task) and after (Posttest) simultaneous performance of an auditory shadowing task. (Reproduced with permission from Granholm et al., *Journal of Abnormal Psychology*, Vol. 100, copyright 1991 by American Psychological Association, Inc.)

somewhat more adversely affected, suggesting that they may not have automated detection and, thus, freed resources as well as normals.

Despite normal shadowing accuracy during single-task (shadowing alone) performance, the dual-task shadowing accuracy of the patients was significantly impaired relative to that of the controls and relative to the schizophrenics' own single-task shadowing performance. This pattern of shadowing task results indicates that, unlike controls, the schizophrenics were left with insufficient resources to maintain shadowing (secondary) task performance during simultaneous (primary) MFST performance. A specific processing stage deficit cannot account for the finding that the patients' single-task shadowing accuracy did not differ significantly from that of controls. Performance decrements were only observed during the increased processing load of the dual-task condition, where the patients' resource availability was exceeded.

To further investigate the automation of processing skills in schizophrenia, the relationships between motor procedural learning, tardive dyskinesia (TD), and MRI T_2 measures of basal ganglia structures were examined in schizophrenics (Granholm et al., 1993). A series of studies in the Butters lab (Butters et al., 1985; Martone et al., 1984; Heindel et al., 1989) suggested that the basal ganglia (especially the neostriatum) are involved in the acquisition of motor skills. In these studies, the performance of HD, but not amnesic or AD, patients was impaired on a variety of procedural learning tasks, including the pursuit rotor, the Tower of Hanoi, and a mirror-reading task. These findings suggested that patients with dementia due to pathology in the caudate (e.g., HD) have deficits in the automation of procedural skills. Based on these findings, and because pathology in the caudate produces movement disorders similar to TD, it was postulated that schizophrenics with TD would have caudate abnormalities and deficient automation of motor skills.

T_2 relaxation times calculated using high field MRI instruments was used as a measure of pathophysiology in basal ganglia structures. T_2 may provide an in vivo index of iron concentrations in brain tissue, with shortened T_2 (hypointensity) indicating increased iron deposition (Drayer, 1989). Increased deposition of iron in basal ganglia structures may indicate tissue abnormalities and has been reported in patients with degenerative basal ganglia diseases, such as HD (Drayer et al., 1986). If high caudate iron levels and caudate pathophysiology contributes to TD, then increased severity of abnormal involuntary movements should be associated with both decreased motor learning on the pursuit rotor and caudate T_2 shortening. In addition, if the caudate is involved in the automation of motor procedural skills (Heindel et al., 1989), the amount of motor learning on the pursuit rotor should be associated with caudate T_2.

In a preliminary study (Granholm et al., 1993), 11 patients with chronic schizophrenia (4 non-TD; 7 TD) and 11 normal controls practiced on the pursuit rotor for 6 trial blocks of 4 20-second trials each. The patients with TD showed significantly less motor learning (block 6-block 1 difference scores) than did the non-TD patients, but the motor learning of the TD and non-TD groups did not differ significantly from that of the normal controls (Figure 4). This finding of normal motor learning is consistent with several previous reports that schizophrenics can automate processing on other procedural learning tasks, such as the MFST described above, the Tower of Hanoi task (Goldberg et al., 1990) and other versions of the pursuit rotor (Huston & Shakow, 1949).

Table 1 summarizes the associations between the MRI and behavioral measures. Motor learning ability and caudate T_2 were both strongly associated with the severity of abnormal involuntary movements (AIMS ratings) in patients with schizophrenia. Motor learning ability was also strongly associated with bilateral caudate T_2. Both the motor learning and AIMS scores were

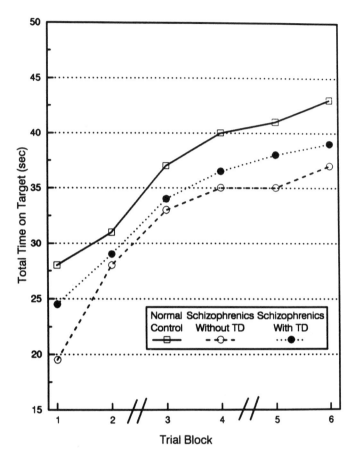

Figure 4. Performance of normal control subjects and schizophrenic patients with and without tardive dyskinesia (TD) on the pursuit rotor task. (Reproduced with permission from Granholm et al., *Psychiatry Research: Neuroimaging,* Vol. 50, copyright 1993 Elsevier Scientific Publishers Ireland Ltd.)

specifically associated with caudate T_2 and not with putamen or globus pallidus T_2, and caudate T_2 and motor learning were not associated with gross motor output (finger tapping). This pattern of associations supports the hypothesis that neostriatal abnormalities are associated with decreased motor procedural learning and provides converging evidence from neuropsychological and neuroimaging measures to suggest caudate nucleus abnormalities in schizophrenics with TD.

TABLE 1

Correlations Between Basal Ganglia T_2 Relaxation Times and
Behavioral Measures in 11 Schizophrenic Patients

	Motor Learning (Block 6 - 1)	AIMS	Finger Tapping
L-Caudate	.79**	-.71*	-.20
R-Caudate	.82**	-.53	.07
L-Putamen	-.06	-.01	-.66*
R-Putamen	.03	.04	-.71*
L-Pallidus	.20	-.39	-.49
R-Pallidus	.38	-.53	-.20

Notes: L = left; R = right;
AIMS = Abnormal Involuntary Movement Scale.
* $p < .05$; ** $p < .01$ (two-tailed).

CONCLUSIONS

Through the example of his work and his professional activities, Nelson Butters has significantly advanced the field of neuropsychology by promoting a symbiotic relationship between clinical and cognitive approaches to neuropsychology. This brief review attempts to illustrate how the application of theoretical concepts and paradigms from cognitive psychology to neuropsychology studies can provide a better understanding of the specific nature of impaired memory and attention. I am extremely fortunate to have learned this valuable lesson, firsthand, from one of the preeminent teachers and leaders of the field of neuropsychology.

ACKNOWLEDGEMENTS. Work on this manuscript was supported by the Scottish Rite Benevolent Foundation's Schizophrenia Research Program, N.M.J., U.S.A.

REFERENCES

Asarnow, R. F., Granholm, E. & Sherman, T. (1991). Span of apprehension in schizophrenia. In S. Steinhauer, J. H. Gruzelier, J. Zubin (Eds), *Handbook of Schizophrenia, Vol. 4, Neuropsychology, psychophysiology, and information processing.* Amsterdam: Elsevier, pp. 335-370.

Butters, N. (1984). The clinical aspects of memory disorders: Contributions from experimental studies of amnesia and dementia. *Journal of Clinical Neuropsychology, 6*(1), 17-36.

Butters, N. (1993). Editorial: Some comments on the goals and Directions of Neuropsychology. *Neuropsychology, 7*(1), 3-4.

Butters, N., Wolfe, J, Granholm, E., & Martone, M. (1986). An assessment of verbal recall, recognition and fluency abilities in patients with Huntington's Disease. *Cortex, 22*, 11-32.

Butters, N., Wolfe, Martone, M., Granholm, E. & Cermak, L. S. (1985). Memory disorders associated with Huntington's Disease: Verbal recall, verbal recognition and procedural memory. *Neuropsychologia, 6*, 729-744.

Butters, N., Granholm, E., Salmon, D.P. & Grant, I. (1987). Episodic and semantic memory: A comparison of amnesic and demented patients. *Journal of Clinical and Experimental Neuropsychology, 9*(5), 479-497.

Callaway, E. & Naghdi, S. (1982). An information processing model for schizophrenia. *Archives of General Psychiatry, 39*, 339-347.

Cermak, L.S., Uhly, B. & Reale, L. (1980). Encoding specificity in the alcoholic Korsakoff patient. *Brain and Language, 11*, 119-127.

Fuld, P.A. (1983). Psychometric differentiation of the dementias: An overview. In B. Reisberg (Ed.), *Alzheimer's Disease: The Standard Reference.* New York: Free Press.

Drayer, B.P. (1989). Basal ganglia: Significance of signal hypointensity on T2-weighted images. *Radiology, 173*, 311-312.

Drayer, B.P., Burger, P., Darwin, R., Reider, S., Herfkens, R. & Johnson, A.G. (1986). MRI of brain iron. *American Journal of Radiology, 147*, 103-110.

Gjerde, P. F. (1983). Attentional capacity dysfunction and arousal in schizophrenia. *Psychological Bulletin, 93*, 57-72.

Goldberg, T.E., Saint-Cyr, J.A. & Weinberger, D.R. (1990). Assessment of procedural learning and problem solving in schizophrenic patients by Tower of Hanoi type tasks. *Journal of Neuropsychiatry, 2*, 165-173.

Gophor, D. & Donchin, E. (1986). Workload -- examination of the concept. In K. R. Boff, L. Kaufman and J. P. Thomas (Eds.), *Handbook of Perception and Human Performance, Vol. 2, Cognitive Processes and Performance.* New York: Wiley and Sons, pp. 41-1 to 41-49.

Granholm, E. (1992). Processing resource limitations in schizophrenia: Implications for predicting medication response and planning attentional training. In D. I. Margolin (Ed.), *Cognitive Neuropsychology in Clinical Practice*. New York: Oxford University Press, pp. 43-69.

Granholm, E. & Butters, N. (1988). Associative encoding and retrieval in Alzheimer's and Huntington's disease. *Brain and Cognition, 7*, 335-347.

Granholm, E., Asarnow, R. F. & Marder, S. R. (1991). Controlled information processing resources and the development of automatic detection responses in schizophrenia. *Journal of Abnormal Psychology, 100*(1).

Granholm, E., Bartzokis, G., Asarnow, R. F. & Marder, S. R. (1993). Preliminary associations between motor procedural learning, basal ganglia T2 relaxation times, and tardive dyskinesia in schizophrenia. *Psychiatry Research: Neuroimaging, 50*, 33-44.

Hasher, L. & Zacks, R. T. (1979). Automatic and effortful processes in memory. *Journal of Experimental Psychology: General, 108*, 356-388.

Heindel, W.C., Salmon, D.P., Shults, C.W., Walicke, P.A. & Butters, N. (1989). Neuropsychological evidence for multiple implicit memory systems: A comparison of Alzheimer's, Huntington's, and Parkinson's disease patients. *Journal of Neuroscience, 9*, 582-587.

Hirst, W. & Kalmar, D. (1987). Characterizing attentional resources. *Journal of Experimental Psychology: General, 116*, 68-81.

Huston, P.E. & Shakow, D. (1949). Studies of motor function in   schizophrenia: I. Pursuit of learning. *Journal of Personality, 17*, 52-74.

Kahneman, D. (1973). *Attention and effort*. Englewood Cliffs, NJ: Prentice-Hall.

Martin, A. & Fedio, P. (1983). Word production and comprehension in Alzheimer's disease: The breakdown of semantic knowledge. *Brain and Language, 19*, 124-141.

Martone, M., Butters N., Payne, M., Becker, J. & Sax, D.S. (1984). Dissociations between skill learning and verbal recognition in amnesia and dementia. *Archives of Neurology, 41*, 965-970.

Neale, J. M. & Oltmanns, T. F. (1980). *Schizophrenia* (Chapter 3). New York: John Wiley and Sons, pp. 102-161.

Norman, D. A. & Bobrow, D. G. (1975). On data-limited and resource-limited processes. *Cognitive Psychology, 7*, 44-64.

Nuechterlein, K. H. & Dawson, M. E. (1984). Information processing and attentional functioning in the course of schizophrenic disorder. *Schizophrenia Bulletin, 10*, 160-203.

Ober, B.A., Dronkers, N.F., Koss, E., Delis, D.C. & Friedland, R.P. (1986). Retrieval from semantic memory in Alzheimer-type dementia. *Journal of Clinical and Experimental Neuropsychology, 8*, 75-92.

Posner, M.I. & Snyder, C. R. P. (1975). Attention and cognitive control. In R. L. Solso (Ed.), *Information Processing and Cognition: The Loyola Symposium*. Hillsdale, NJ: Lawrence Erlbaum Associates, pp. 55-85.

Schneider, W., Dumais, S. T. & Shiffrin, R. M. (1984). Automatic and controlled processing and attention. In R. Parasuraman, J. Beatty and J. Davies (Eds.), *Varieties of Attention*. New York: Academic Press, pp. 1-27.

Schneider, W. & Shiffrin, R. M. (1977). Controlled and automatic human information processing: I. Detection, search and attention. *Psychological Review, 84*, 1-66.

Squire, L.R. (1986). Mechanisms of memory. *Science, 232*, 1612-1619.

Thomson, D.M. & Tulving, E. (1970). Associative encoding and retrieval: Weak and strong cues. *Journal of Experimental Psychology, 86*, 255-262.

Tulving, E. & Thomson, D.M. (1973). Encoding specificity and retrieval processes in episodic memory. *Psychological Review, 80*, 352-373.

Tulving, E. (1983). *Elements of Episodic Memory.* New York: Oxford Univ. Press.

10

Cognitive Investigations in Huntington's Disease

JASON BRANDT[1]

As a graduate student in experimental and physiological psychology in the late 1970's, I was taught that the basal ganglia constituted a component of the "extrapyramidal motor system," a relatively undifferentiated set of nuclei which were responsible for the fine-tuning of movements. Even the major textbooks of the day rarely mentioned the contribution of the striatum to cognition. During this same period, Nelson Butters began publishing the first of his many papers on the cognitive impairments of patients with Huntington's disease (HD) (Butters, Tarlow, Cermak & Sax, 1976; Butters & Grady, 1977). The body of research on this topic by Nelson and his students over the past 17 years has been a major force in the re-conceptualization of the basal ganglia as a set of functionally discrete cortico-striato-thalamic loops regulating specific aspects of both motor programming and higher-order cognition (Alexander, DeLong & Strick, 1986; Crosson, 1992; Stern, 1983).

The origin of Nelson's interest in HD can probably be traced to his earlier work on the effects of caudate nucleus lesions on learning and memory in non-human primates. As a postdoctoral research fellow at the National Institute of Mental Health in the 1960's, Nelson found that lesions of the ventrolateral head of the caudate in rhesus monkeys resulted in excessive bar-press responding during experimental extinction and impaired performance on the delayed-alternation task (Butters & Rosvold, 1968). The similarity of these effects to those of prefrontal cortical lesions was noted, and the hypothesis was formulated that the orbital frontal cortex, along with its anatomically-related subcortical

[1] JASON BRANDT, Ph.D., • Department of Psychiatry, The John Hopkins University School of Medicine

Neuropsychological Explorations of Memory and Cognition: Essays in Honor of Nelson Butters, edited by Laird S. Cermak, Ph.D. Plenum Press, New York, 1994

structures (septal nuclei, caudate nucleus), formed a functional system related to perseveration.

In many ways, patients with Huntington's disease were ideally suited for addressing the questions in human neuropsychology of interest to Nelson. First, the disease is associated with a clear dementia syndrome, but one that is somewhat more selective than that in other dementias (Alzheimer's disease, for example). Second, the dementia of HD has its onset in middle age; thus, it does not confound cognitive changes of disease state with those associated with normal aging. Third, the neuropathology of HD is relatively well characterized and uniform across patients, at least at the macroscopic level. Finally, HD is a genetic disorder that is inherited as a dominant trait. This allows us to study the unfolding of the neuropsychological syndrome, from its presymptomatic state to full-blown dementia.

Reflection on Nelson's early studies of HD reveals three clear themes that have run throughout his human neuropsychological research. The first is that patients whose cognitive syndromes appear on the surface to be similar, but who have different underlying pathophysiology, will be found on more careful analysis to be quite dissimilar in their cognitive syndromes. This clearly calls for a *comparative approach* to clinical neuropsychological research (Butters, 1984; Butters, Granholm, Salmon *et al.*, 1987; Heindel, Salmon, Shults *et al.*, 1989). The second theme is that, within a given cognitive domain (be it spatial orientation, remote memory, implicit memory, or any other), distinct *varieties and subprocesses* can be discerned. Brain pathology can selectively impair some of these varieties and subprocesses while leaving others relatively unscathed. The third theme is the *developmental* one, no doubt influenced by Nelson's graduate education at Clark University. Much of Nelson's research has examined qualitative changes in behavior and cognition with disease progression, and the effects of neurologic disease on younger and older patients (*e.g.*, Albert, Butters & Brandt, 1981; Butters & Brandt, 1985; Ryan & Butters, 1980). His 1978 paper on the cognitive differences in early-stage and advanced HD (Butters, Sax, Montgomery & Tarlow, 1978), for example, has become a classic in the field. It has had a significant influence on my own efforts to detect cognitive alterations in the offspring of HD patients who remain asymptomatic but who carry the HD gene mutation (Brandt, Quaid, Folstein *et al.*, 1989; Strauss & Brandt, 1986, 1990; Rothlind, Brandt, Zee *et al.*, 1993).

COMPARATIVE NEUROPSYCHOLOGY OF HUNTINGTON'S DISEASE

The cognitive syndrome of HD has been shown by several laboratories to be distinct from that in Alzheimer's disease (AD), the most common cause of dementia in the elderly. In 1988, Brandt, Folstein and Folstein compared the performance profiles on the Mini-Mental State Exam (MMSE) of 84 HD patients and 145 AD patients. The patients in each group were stratified by severity of dementia (*i.e.*, total score on the MMSE). Relatively consistent differences were found. The HD patients performed more poorly on the "attention" item (*i.e.*, serial subtractions from 100), while the AD patients were more often disoriented to date and performed more poorly on the memory item (*i.e.*, recall of three items after a single intervening task). The profile differences, even on this very brief mental status exam, were sufficiently robust to correctly classify 84 percent of the subjects using discriminant function analysis. Subsequently, Salmon, Kwo-on-Yuen, Heindel, *et al.* (1989) essentially replicated this finding using a different, somewhat longer cognitive exam, the Dementia Rating Scale.

Patterns of verbal memory have also been described as being distinctly different in AD and HD. Butters and his collaborators have shown that HD patients can be as impaired as AD patients or patients with alcoholic Korsakoff's syndrome (KS) on measures of free recall, selective reminding, and paired-associate learning (Butters, 1984; Granholm & Butters, 1988). However, they have maintained that HD patients typically display much more normal performance on recognition memory tests (Butters, Wolfe, Granholm *et al.*, 1986; Butters, Wolfe, Martone *et al.*, 1985). This, it has been argued, supports the hypothesis that memory search and retrieval mechanisms are the major source of verbal learning impairment in HD, whereas encoding and storage are defective in AD and KS (Butters, 1984; Butters, Albert, Sax *et al.*, 1983; Brandt & Butters, 1986). As a result, when HD patients are tested with recognition memory procedures, they can perform relatively normally.

Recently, this hypothesis was tested explicitly by Brandt, Corwin & Krafft (1992) using the Hopkins Verbal Learning Test (HVLT; Brandt, 1991). In groups of HD and AD patients matched for MMSE score and first trial free recall, the learning curves of the AD and HD groups were essentially equivalent. However, in contrast to the usual findings with the California Verbal Learning Test (CVLT; Delis, Kramer, Kaplan & Ober, 1987) (Delis, Massman, Butters *et al.*, 1991; but *cf.* Kramer, Delis, Blusewicz *et al.*, 1988), Brandt *et al.* did not find that recognition accuracy was greater in the HD than in the AD group. In fact, the HD group had slightly (though insignificantly) *lower* recognition accuracy. However, the AD patients had a more distorted (liberal) response bias; that is, they tended more often to say "yes" to distractor items (especially those that were semantically related to the targets) than did the HD patients. The source of the differences in findings between studies using the CVLT and the HVLT remains unclear, but the nature of the recognition task (*e.g.*, number of distractors per target) and the statistical model used in evaluating recognition accuracy and response bias may be important (Snodgrass & Corwin, 1988).

VARIETIES AND SUBPROCESSES OF IMPLICIT MEMORY

Butters and his collaborators were the first to demonstrate a double dissociation between explicit recollection and skill learning. In 1984, Martone, Butters, Payne *et al.* found that KS patients had a normal rate of improvement in reading mirror-inverted word triads, but poor subsequent recognition of those words. HD patients displayed essentially the opposite deficits: their ability to acquire the mirror-reading skill was poor, while their subsequent recognition for those words was relatively normal. The HD patients did display a greater reduction in reading latency for repeated triads than for unique triads, suggesting that repetition priming of individual items is much less impaired than skill acquisition. This study and others like it from the Butters laboratory have inspired a great many studies of skill learning, many of which focus on motor skill acquisition. For example, Heindel, Butters and Salmon (1988) reported that HD patients are severely impaired in their ability to learn the pursuit rotor task, even when the rotor was slowed to allow HD patients to have essentially the same initial time-on-target as the other patient groups. Thus, HD patients appear to be impaired in motor tracking that requires the integration of visual perception and motor behavior.

The work of Butters, Salmon and Heindel (1990) has suggested that whereas some aspects of motor skill acquisition are impaired in HD, verbal/conceptual tests of implicit memory, such as word stem completion, can be performed normally (Heindel, Salmon, Shults *et al.*, 1989; Shimamura, Salmon, Squire & Butters, 1987). Recently, Bylsma, Rebok & Brandt (1991) employed a semantic decision-making task to investigate components of the lexical priming effect in HD. We were also interested in the possibility that an implicitly learned word list would be less vulnerable to the progressive deterioration seen in HD than would explicit learning. Fifteen mildly demented HD patients and a like number of healthy control subjects were asked to make the same semantic decision (*i.e.*, "Is this a living thing?") about 20 words presented individually on a computer screen. Reaction times to yes/no button-press responses were recorded. This same list of 20 words was repeated for four blocks of trials. On the fifth block of trials, 20 new words were presented. The degree of improvement from Block 1 to Block 4 reflects both practice effect (*i.e.*, skill learning) and item-specific learning. The degree of rebound in reaction times from Block 4 to Block 5 reflects primarily item-specific learning. The difference in reaction time between Block 1 and Block 5 reflects pure practice, as in both instances a novel list of words is encountered. As seen in the left panel of Figure 1, the HD patients had a slightly less steep learning curve from Block 1 to Block 4. However, the groups did not differ in the degree of RT rebound from Block 4 to Block 5, indicating that the HD patients learned the list-specific words as well as the normal subjects. On the other hand, the normal control group had a quicker reaction time on Block 5 than on Block 1, whereas this was

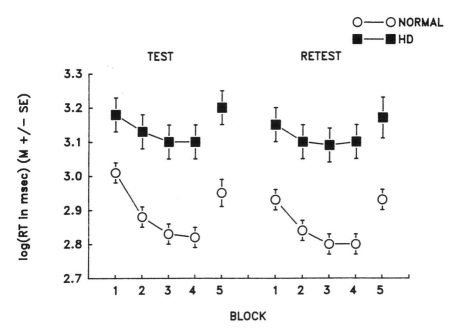

Figure 1. Initial performance (*left*) and 6-month re-test performance (*right*) of Huntington's disease patients and healthy control subjects on semantic decision priming test. In each session, the same set of 20 words is repeated in the first four blocks; a different set of 20 words is presented in the fifth block. [From, F.W. Bylsma, G. W. Rebok & J. Brandt (1991). Long-term retention of implicit learning in Huntington's disease. *Neuropsychologia, 12*, 1213-1221.]

not the case in the HD patients. This indicates a defect in perceptual-motor skill learning in the HD group.

These same subjects performed precisely the same experiment six months later (see right panel of Figure 1). On re-testing, the healthy subjects and, to a lesser extent, the HD patients displayed shorter reaction times than on the initial testing. This suggests that both groups retained their primed memory for the specific words over the 6-month interval. This is particularly striking in the HD group, as they displayed a trend toward *poorer* performance on a test of explicit memory for the primed words at re-test than initially. This experiment clearly shows the dissociation of implicit learning and explicit recollection and, within the domain of implicit memory, between skill learning and item-priming.

One of the key features of the pursuit rotor task that may be responsible for the poor performance of HD patients is that it requires a repetitive pattern of movements. This raises the possibility that a fundamental cognitive defect in these patients is their inability to detect and benefit from the regularity in, or patterning of, to-be-acted-upon stimuli. To address this hypothesis, Bylsma, Brandt & Strauss (1990) administered a "stepping-stone" maze learning task to early-stage HD patients. Three different mazes were used, and subjects were given five trials to learn each one. In two of the mazes, the correct route was unpredictable. In the third maze, the correct route followed a predictable, repetitive pattern (*i.e.*, up, right, down, right, up, right, down, right, etc.). The learning curves of the HD patients for the two mazes with unpredictable routes were no different from those of normal control subjects. However, whereas the healthy subjects learned the maze with the predictable route in fewer trials than the mazes with unpredictable routes, the HD patients showed no such effect. Thus, HD patients appear to be less able than healthy individuals to "pick-up" on the patterning or regularity in a sequence of movements.

Recently, several investigators have used a serial response time (SRT) task to further address the ability of HD patients to benefit from repeated motor sequences. In this task, visual stimuli appear in various locations on a computer screen, and the subject's task is to press a corresponding key or button. Unbeknownst to the subject, the visual targets do not appear at random, but rather appear in a sequence of positions that repeats itself. Normal subjects typically respond more quickly with repetitions of the sequence. Again, they appear to "pick up" on the predictability of the targets although, on questioning them later, they are often unaware of the sequence. Knopman and Nissen (1991) reported that HD patients are impaired on this task. Although the patients displayed even greater reduction in reaction time with repeated presentations of the sequence than the normal control subjects, they displayed less rebound in reaction time than expected when a new sequence of moves was introduced. This was interpreted as reflecting a defect in sequence-specific learning. Recently, Brandt and Bylsma (1993) administered a modified serial response time task to 14 patients with early to mid-stage HD and 14 healthy subjects. A five position sequence was repeated nine times. On the tenth block of trials, a new five-position sequence was administered. The degree of improvement from Block 1 to Block 9 reflects both skill acquisition and sequence-specific learning. The degree of rebound from Block 9 to Block 10 reflects sequence-specific learning. The difference in reaction time between Block 1 and Block 10 reflects pure skill learning, as in both instances a novel sequence of positions is encountered. As can be seen from Figure 2 (top panel), the HD patients are slower than the healthy control subjects in performing this task, but the shape of their learning function is comparable. Analysis of variance revealed significant effects of both Block and Group, but no Group x Block interaction. In the bottom panel of Figure 2, the group means are adjusted for Block-1 reaction times. The Block-1 minus Block-10 difference (skill learning) and the Block-10 minus Block-9 difference (sequence learning) were both virtually identical in the two groups.

Apparently, the type of motor sequence learning required for our version of the SRT task is very different from that required for performance on the pursuit rotor task. Recently, Willingham and Koroshetz (1993) have drawn a distinction between tasks requiring the repeating sequence of movements (which they maintain is impaired in HD) and those requiring the learning of new stimulus-response mappings (which they maintain are intact). However, they base their conclusions in part on the performance of HD patients on an SRT task. Like Knopman and Nissen (1991), Willingham and Koroshetz obtained an equivocal difference between HD and healthy subjects on this task. The essence of those motor skills that can be acquired normally by HD patients and those that can not remains to be determined.

DEVELOPMENTAL ASPECTS

Notwithstanding the ability of the Mini-Mental State Exam to reveal qualitative differences between HD and AD (Brandt *et al.*, 1988), the test is

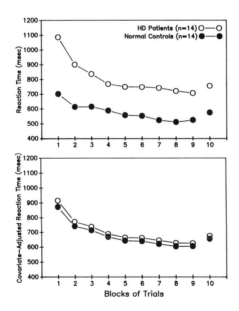

Figure 2. Performance of Huntington's disease patients and healthy control subjects on Serial Response Time task. The first 9 blocks consist of the same sequence of five responses; a different sequence appears on the 10th block. The figure depicts raw learning curves (*top*) and learning curves adjusted for overall speed by covarying for mean Block-1 reaction time (*bottom*).

relatively insensitive to the cognitive impairment of early-stage HD and probably other subcortical dementias as well (Rothlind & Brandt, 1993). Recently, Brandt, Bylsma & Gross (1993; Brandt & Butters, 1993) compared the neuropsychological test performance of a group of HD patients who performed perfectly on the Mini-Mental State Exam to an age- and education-matched group of persons at risk for the illness but who tested negative for the genetic mutation (Brandt, Quaid, Folstein *et al.*, 1989). Significant differences were found on many measures, with the largest effect sizes being on the Hopkins Verbal Learning Test and the Brief Test of Attention, an auditory working memory task (Schretlen & Bobholz, 1992).

In view of the fact that HD causes a progressive dementia, and given that Butters *et al.* (1978) found *qualitative* as well as *quantitative* differences between early-stage and later-stage patients, it is surprising that essentially no prospective, longitudinal studies of cognition in HD have ever been conducted. Brandt, Bylsma & Gross (1993) administered a set of nine neuropsychological tests to 52 HD patients on two occasions, separated by one year. The battery was reduced by principal components analysis to three cognitive factors: a "general" factor (WAIS-R Vocabulary, WAIS-R Block Design, Controlled Oral Word Association and Developmental Test of Visual-Motor Integration), a "memory and attention" factor (Hopkins Verbal Learning Test, Brief Test of Attention, Stroop Color-Word Test and Trail Making Test), and a "categorizing" factor (Wisconsin Card Sorting Test). Because patients with early-life onset of HD appear clinically to decline more rapidly than later-life onset cases, the cohort was divided into two groups: those with onset at or before age 40 (N=28) and those with onset after age 40 (N=24). The two groups did not differ in mean level of education, duration of illness, or MMSE score. Separate Group by Session analyses of variance failed to reveal a significant main effect of session for any of the three factors (sse Figure 3). Apparently, a one-year period is not sufficient to document decline on these cognitive factors. The Group effect was also not statistically significant for any of the factors. However, there was a significantly Group x Session interaction on Factor 2 (the memory and attention factor), such that early-onset patients declined over the one-year interval while later-onset patients actually improved. There was a nonsignificant trend in the same direction for Factor 3. These data suggest that early-onset HD results in a more rapid progression of dementia, but only for some aspects of cognition. Interestingly, those tests that load most highly on Factor 2 are also the one that are most sensitive to the presence of HD (Brandt *et al.*, 1993).

In an effort to determine whether there are any biological differences between the early- and later-onset groups, the length of the trinucleotide repeat that constitutes the genetic mutation responsible for HD was examined in all the patients from whom DNA was available (Huntington's Disease Collaborative Research Group, 1993; Duyao, Ambrose, Myers *et al.*, 1993). The early-onset patients had a significantly longer repeat length (mean=48.9 repeats) than the

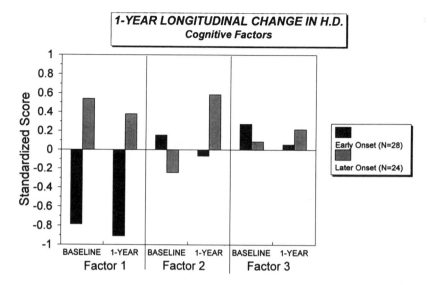

Figure 3. Standardized (Z) scores of early-onset and later-onset HD patients on three cognitive factors assessed at one-year intervals.

later-onset patients (mean=42.5 repeats) (p=.011). This appears to be the first demonstration that neuropsychological variability among HD patients is related to genotypic variability.

Over the past two decades, neuroscientists have learned a great deal about the role of the basal ganglia in memory and other cognitive domains. Without a doubt, the work of Nelson Butters on Huntington's disease has been a singular influence in shaping our thinking about the neuropsychology of the striatum. His ability to ferret out dissociations among cognitive subprocesses, and his keen appreciation of the developmental aspects of this neurodegenerative disease have been inspirational for the many students and fellows who have had the pleasure and honor of working with him.

ACKNOWLEDGEMENTS. Supported, in part, by NIH grants NS16375 and MH46034 to the Johns Hopkins University.

REFERENCES

Albert, M.S., Butters, N. & Brandt, J. (1981). Development of remote memory loss in patient with Huntington's disease. *Journal of Clinical Neuropsychology, 3,* 1-12.

Alexander, G.E., DeLong, M.R. & Strick, P.L. (1986). Parallel organization of functionally segregated circuits linking basal ganglia and cortex. *Annual Review of Neuroscience, 9*, 357-381.

Brandt, J. (1991). The Hopkins Verbal Learning Test: Development of a new memory test with six equivalent forms. *The Clinical Neuropsychologist, 5*, 125-142.

Brandt, J. & Butters, N. (1986). The neuropsychology of Huntington's disease. *Trends in Neuroscience, 93*, 118-120.

Brandt, J. & Butters, N. (1993). Neuropsychological characteristics of Huntington's disease. In, I. Grant & K. Adams (Ed.), *Neuropsychological Assessment of Neuropsychiatric Disorders, 2nd edition.* New York: Oxford University Press, in press.

Brandt, J. & Bylsma, F.W. (1993). Skill acquisition and sequence-specific learning of Huntington's disease patients on the serial response time task. Manuscript in preparation.

Brandt, J., Bylsma, F.W. & Gross, R. (1993). Selective cognitive decline in Huntington's disease. Manuscript in preparation.

Brandt, J., Corwin, J. & Krafft, L. (1992). Is verbal recognition memory really different in Huntington's and Alzheimer's disease? *Journal of Clinical and Experimental Neuropsychology, 14*, 773-784.

Brandt, J., Folstein, S.E. & Folstein, M.F. (1988). Differential cognitive impairment in Alzheimer's disease and Huntington's disease. *Annals of Neurology, 23*, 555-561.

Brandt, J., Quaid, K.A., Folstein, S.E., Gabber, P., Maestri, N.E., Abbot, M.H., Slavney, P.R., Franz, M.L., Kasch, L. & Kazazian, H.H. (1989). Presymptomatic diagnosis of delayed-onset disease with linked DNA markers: The experience in Huntington's disease. *Journal of the American Medical Association, 26*, 3108-3114.

Butters, N. (1984). The clinical aspects of memory disorders: Contributions from experimental studies of amnesia and dementia. *Journal of Clinical Neuropsychology, 6*, 17-36.

Butters, N., Albert, M.S., Sax, D.S., Miliotis, P., Nagode, J. & Sterste, A. (1983). The effect of verbal mediators on pictorial memory in brain-damaged patients. *Neuropsychologia, 21*, 307-323.

Butters, N. & Brandt, J. The continuity hypothesis: The relationship of long-term alcoholism to the Wernicke-Korsakoff syndrome. In M. Galanter (Ed.), *Recent Advances in Alcoholism, Vol. 2.* New York: Plenum Press.

Butters, N. & Grady, M. (1977). Effect of predistractor delays on short-term memory performance of patients with Korsakoff's and Huntington's disease. *Neuropsychologia, 15*, 701-706.

Butters, N. & Rosvold, H.E. (1968). The effect of caudate and septal nuclei lesions on resistance to extinction and delayed-alternation performance in monkeys. *Journal of Comparative and Physiological Psychology, 65, 397-403.*

Butters, N., Salmon, D.P. & Heindel, W.C. (1990). Dissociation of implicit memory in dementia: Neurological implications. *Bulletin of the Psychonomic Society, 28*, 359-366.

Butters, N., Sax, D.S., Montgomery, K., & Tarlow, S. (1978). Comparison of neuropsychological deficits associated with early and advanced Huntington's disease. *Archives of Neurology, 35*, 585-589.

Butters, N., Tarlow, S., Cermak, L. & Sax, D. (1976). A comparison of the information processing deficits of patients with Huntington's chorea and Korsakoff's syndrome. *Cortex, 12*, 134-144.

Butters, N., Wolfe, J., Martone, M., Granholm, E. & Cermak, L.S. (1985). Memory disorders associated with Huntington's disease: Verbal recall, verbal recognition, and procedural memory. *Neuropsychologia, 23*, 729-743.

Butters, N., Wolfe, J., Granholm, E. & Martone, M. (1986). An assessment of verbal recall, recognition and fluency abilities in patients with Huntington's disease. *Cortex, 22*, 11-32.

Bylsma, F.W., Brandt, J. & Strauss, M.E. (1990). Aspects of procedural memory are differentially impaired in Huntington's disease. *Archives of Clinical Neuropsychology, 5*, 287-297.

Bylsma, F.W., Rebok, G. & Brandt, J. (1992). Long-term retention of implicit learning in Huntington's disease. *Neuropsychologia, 29*, 1213-1221.

Crosson, B. (1992). *Subcortical Functions in Language and Memory*. New York: Guilford Press.

Delis, D.C., Kramer, J.H., Kaplan, E. & Ober, B.A. (1987). *The California Verbal Learning Test*. San Antonio, TX: The Psychological Corporation.

Delis, D.C., Massman, P.J., Butters, N., Salmon, D.P. Cermak, L.S. & Kramer, J.H. (1991). Profiles of demented and amnesic patients on the California Verbal Learning Test: Implications for the assessment of memory disorders. *Psychological Assessment: A Journal of Consulting and Clinical Psychology, 3*, 19-26.

Duyao, M., Ambrose, C., Myers, R. et al., (1993). Trinucleotide repeat length instability and age of onset in Huntington's disease. *Nature Genetics, 4*, 387-392.

Granholm, E. & Butters, N. (1988). Associative encoding and retrieval in Alzheimer's and Huntington's disease. *Brain and Cognition, 7*, 335-347.

Heindel, W.C., Butters, N. & Salmon, D.P. (1988). Impaired learning of motor skill in patients with Huntington's disease. *Behavioral Neuroscience, 102*, 141-147.

Heindel, W.C., Salmon, D.P., Shults, C.W., Walicke, P.A. & Butters, N. (1989). Neuropsychological evidence for multiple implicit memory systems: A comparison of Alzheimer's, Huntington's, and Parkinson's disease patients. *Journal of Neuroscience, 9*, 582-587.

Huntington's Disease Collaborative Research Group (1993). A novel gene containing a trinucleotide repeat that is expanded and unstable on Huntington's disease chromosomes. *Cell, 72*, 971-983.

Knopman, D.S. & Nissen, M.J. (1991). Procedural learning is impaired in Huntington's disease: Evidence from the serial reaction time task. *Neuropsychologia, 29*, 245-254.

Kramer, J.H., Delis, D.C., Blusewicz, M.J., Brandt, J., Ober, B.A. & Strauss, M. (1988). Verbal memory errors in Huntington's and Alzheimer's dementias. *Developmental Neuropsychology, 4*, 1-15.

Martone, M., Butters, N., Payne, M., Becker, J. & Sax, D.S. (1984). Dissociations between skill learning and verbal recognition in amnesia and dementia. *Archives of Neurology, 41*, 965-970.

Rothlind, J. & Brandt, J. (1993). Validation of a brief assessment of frontal and subcortical functions in dementia. *Journal of Neuropsychiatry and Clinical Neurosciences, 5*, 73-77.

Rothlind, J., Brandt, J., Zee, D., Codori, A.M. & Folstein, S.E. (1993). Unimpaired verbal memory and oculomotor control in asymptomatic adults with the genetic marker for Huntington's disease. *Archives of Neurology, 50*, 799-802.

Ryan, C. & Butters, N. (1980). Learning and memory impairments in young and old alcoholics: Evidence for the premature aging hypothesis. *Alcoholism: Clinical and Experimental Research, 4*, 288-293.

Salmon, D.P., Kwo-on-Yuen, P.F., Heindel, W.C., Butters, N. & Thal, L.J. (1989). Differentiation of Alzheimer's disease and Huntington's disease with the Dementia Rating Scale. *Archives of Neurology, 46*, 1204-1208.

Schretlen, D.J. & Bobholz, J.H. (1992). Standardization and initial validation of a brief test of executive attentional ability [Abstract]. *Journal of Clinical and Experimental Neuropsychology, 14*, 65.

Shimamura, A.P., Salmon, D.P., Squire, L.R. & Butters, N. (1987). Memory dysfunction and word priming in dementia and amnesia. *Behavioral Neuroscience, 101*, 347-351.

Snodgrass, J.G. & Corwin, J. (1988). Pragmatics of measuring recognition memory: Applications to dementia and amnesia. *Journal of Experimental Psychology: General, 117*, 34-50.

Stern, Y. (1983). Behavior and the basal ganglia. In, R. Mayeux and W.G. Rosen (Ed.), *The Dementias*. New York: Raven Press.

Strauss, M.E. & Brandt, J. (1986). An attempt at presymptomatic identification of Huntington's disease with the WAIS. *Journal of Clinical and Experimental Neuropsychology, 8*, 210-218.

Strauss, M.E., & Brandt, J. (1990). Are there neuropsychological manifestations of the gene for Huntington's disease in asymptomatic, at-risk individuals? *Archives of Neurology, 47*, 905-908.

Willingham, D.B. & Koroshetz, W.J. (1993). Evidence for dissociable motor skills in Huntington's disease patients. *Psychobiology, 21*, 173-182.

11

Magnetic Resonance Imaging and Memory Disorders

TERRY JERNIGAN[1]

In our presentations many of us acknowledge the intellectual debt we owe to Nelson, but before I begin mine, I'd like to express my gratitude to Nelson on a more personal level. Some of you may have been present at a reunion of Nelson's students, during which Edith Kaplan described an extraordinary kindness Nelson had extended to her involving the sale of her inoperable, and as far as I can remember, unenterable automobile. I'm sure after hearing that story, most people thought no one could produce a more impressive example of Nelson's generosity to his friends. However, imagine my plight when eight years ago, having recently left all of my friends at Stanford to join the faculty at UCSD, I found myself a lonely spinster, not getting any younger, and in possession of only one prospect: an enthusiastic but inaccessible Danish pen pal who happened to live 6000 miles away in Oxfordshire, England. After a few months of moping around in a particularly dreary mood, I confided my situation to Nelson, who I was later to find out knew all about it anyway. How he knew I can't imagine, because as everyone knows, Nelson never indulges in idle gossip. At any rate, those of you who know Nelson will perhaps not be surprised to learn that within a few weeks my husband-to-be Arne had been comprehensively vetted by Nelson in a long phone call to Freda Newcombe, arrangements had been made with Lew for a visiting faculty position for his first year in San Diego, and he had been introduced to the American expression about it being

---

[1] TERRY JERNIGAN, Ph.D. • Department of Veterans Affairs Medical Center, San Diego, CA

Neuropsychological Explorations of Memory and Cognition: Essays in Honor of Nelson Butters, edited by Laird S. Cermak, Ph.D. Plenum Press, New York, 1994

time to "fish or cut bait", which made a great impression on him at the time. The day after Christmas, less than a year after my heart-to-heart with Nelson, Arne and I were married in Copenhagen - and I defy anyone to beat that story as an example of why all of us who know Nelson, and have the privilege to work with him, could never begin to express our gratitude to him. Well, perhaps I should let Arne speak for himself...

Little more than a decade ago, most of what was written in the neuropsychological literature betrayed the naive assumption that all interesting mental phenomena arose from nervous activity in the cerebral cortex. The possibility that the deeper structures within the cerebrum might play an important role in cognition, while perhaps acknowledged, was rarely considered in the various treatises attempting to assign functions to gyri. However, since that time, Nelson, assisted by various colleagues, has, through the experimental analysis of the behavior of patients, developed a model that differentiates those cognitive processes in which the function of the cerebral cortex plays a critical role, from those more heavily dependent on the function of deep subcortical structures. Not only has this work forced a reconsideration of theories about so-called higher cortical functions, but it has served to impart to Nelson's clinician followers (among whom I rank myself) a deeper, more clinically useful understanding of the mental sequelae of neurological syndromes such as Alzheimer's Disease, Huntington's Disease, Parkinson's Disease, and the amnestic syndrome.

Modern brain imaging methods have the potential to contribute important anatomical information relevant to neurobehavioral models such as Nelson's; and for the last few years it has been my pleasure to work with Nelson on a series of studies of gross brain morphology in memory-impaired patients. I'd like to start by summarizing the results of these studies, with particular emphasis on the effects of different diseases on the cortical vs. the subcortical structures, in living patients.

Since the memory-impaired subjects we've been studying are all suffering from acquired damage to the brain, we have measured the effects on different brain structures by estimating the loss of volume in the structures. This is done by first estimating the present volume of brain structures in normal subjects using MRI. Then the correlation between the volume of a brain structure and the volume of the cranial cavity is determined. Since the size of the cranial cavity is unaffected by brain volume loss, this value can subsequently be used to estimate the premorbid volumes of brain structures in patients. When the present volume of a patient's brain structure is below that predicted from his cranial volume, the discrepancy is taken to be the amount of loss that has occurred. This discrepancy can be further adjusted relative to the amount of age-related loss that occurs in normal subjects, and it can be expressed in terms of the amount of variability observed in the patient's normal age-peers. In other words, the volume of a particular brain structure in a particular patient can be expressed as a z-score that indicates how aberrant it is relative to those of normal subjects with similar age and cranium size. The results I will present now are expressed in this way, as indices of abnormality in the volumes of the structures we've examined.

Figure 1 summarizes our results in a group of 40 patients meeting research criteria for probable AD. Note that the mean values for these indices of abnormality are, by definition, 0 in normal subjects. I have included the results for five brain structures of particular interest, and have arranged them with the cortical structures on the left and subcortical structures on the right. Consistent with the pathology studies of this disorder, particularly severe losses are observed in the cerebral cortex and in the structures on the mesial surface of the temporal lobe. For both measures, the average volume in the AD patients was 1.7 standard deviations below the control mean. The subcortical structures: the diencephalon, the caudate nucleus, and the deep white matter, while by no means normal (all of these deviations from 0 are statistically significant), are all less severely affected than the cortical and limbic structures.

Nelson has on numerous occasions noted the similarities between performances of AD patients and patients with Korsakoff's amnesia, particularly on memory tests. Therefore its not surprising that the pattern of cerebral damage observed in these patients is very similar to that in AD. The data shown in Figure 2 are from 11 Korsakoff patients studied by Laird Cermak, Nelson, Kim Schafer and myself. Again, both cortical and mesial temporal losses are pronounced, while the caudate and deep white matter are less affected. The diencephalon is somewhat more dramatically affected in Korsakoff patients than in AD, both in absolute terms and relative to the amount of cortical damage.

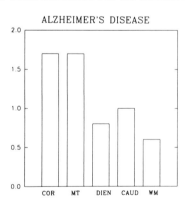

Figure 1. Bars show mean age- and cranium size-adjusted z-scores for gray matter volumes. COR = cerebral cortex, excluding mesial surface of the temporal lobe. MT = mesial temporal lobe. DIEN = diencephalon. CAUD = caudate nuclei. WM = cerebral white matter. Measures have been scaled so that higher values indicate increasing severity of volume loss.

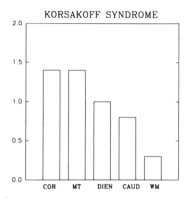

Figure 2. Bars show mean age- and cranium size-adjusted z-scores for gray matter volumes. COR = cerebral cortex, excluding mesial surface of the temporal lobe. MT = mesial temporal lobe. DIEN = diencephalon. CAUD = caudate nuclei. WM = cerebral white matter. Measures have been scaled so that higher values indicate increasing severity of volume loss.

This is especially true for the anterior diencephalic structures, which in our study included the hypothalamus, septal nuclei, and basal forebrain. I haven't shown this measure separately, but in our study it was affected as severely as the cortex and mesial temporal lobes. It was somewhat surprising to us that the volume losses were so pronounced in the mesial temporal lobe structures, given the traditional association of amnesia in this syndrome with diencephalic damage.

The volume losses in Korsakoff's Syndrome appear to be on a continuum with those observed in nonamnesic chronic alcoholics, but while significant caudate and thalamic losses were present in both amnesic and nonamnesic alcoholics, only the losses in the anterior diencephalon, the mesial temporal lobes, and orbitofrontal cortex were significantly more severe in the amnesic alcoholics.

Turning now to a putative subcortical dementia, Figure 3 shows the results for a group of 11 Huntington's Disease patients. What is most immediately apparent is the dramatic change in the gradient of abnormality from the cortical to the subcortical structures. As expected, the losses in caudate nucleus were very striking; putamen losses, though not shown here, were also quite severe. Somewhat more surprising was the degree of signal abnormality in the subcortical white matter. This finding, which has not received much attention in pathology studies, raises questions about the role of damaged fibers in the processing deficits of HD. Nevertheless, the pattern here is quite consistent with a description of this as a subcortical dementia. It should be

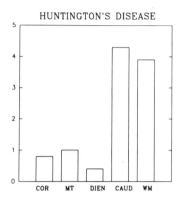

Figure 3. Bars show mean age- and cranium size-adjusted z-scores for gray matter volumes. COR = cerebral cortex, excluding mesial surface of the temporal lobe. MT = mesial temporal lobe. DIEN = diencephalon. CAUD = caudate nuclei. WM = cerebral white matter. Measures have been scaled so that higher values indicate increasing severity of volume loss.

noted though that the scale of this graph is different from the others. The degree of abnormality in mesial temporal lobe structures in HD patients is actually not much less than in Korsakoff patients.

Finally, we have studied a small group of 7 patients with Parkinson's Disease (Figure 4). While not frankly demented, these patients had mild deficits on psychomotor, attention, and fluency tasks. We found little evidence for any losses in gray matter structures, though we were unable to measure the substantia nigra. What we did observe, however, was a significant elevation of signal abnormality in the subcortical white matter. This was surprising, since it was substantially more white matter abnormality than we had observed in the AD patients, who in comparison had much more severe gray matter losses. Thus it seemed to us that, like in HD patients, there was some form of pathology in the white matter in these patients that was not likely to be Psecondary to the gray matter losses. It remains to be determined whether this pathology plays some specific role in the cognitive symptoms of HD and PD, and we are pursuing this question in our ongoing studies.

In summary, our brain imaging studies of these groups of patients largely confirm the expected patterns of damage to specific cortical and subcortical structures, but there were some surprises - such as the mesial temporal lobe losses in HD and Korsakoff patients, the white matter abnormality in the subcortical disorders, and the striatal losses in Alzheimer's disease and in alcoholic patients. Furthermore, we have been surprised by the within-group variability in each of our studies. We think that this heterogeneity underscores

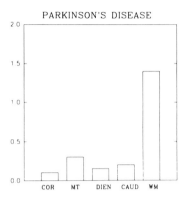

Figure 4. Bars show mean age- and cranium size-adjusted z-scores for gray matter volumes. COR = cerebral cortex, excluding mesial surface of the temporal lobe. MT = mesial temporal lobe. DIEN = diencephalon. CAUD = caudate nuclei. WM = cerebral white matter. Measures have been scaled so that higher values indicate increasing severity of volume loss.

both the need and the opportunity for examining directly the relationship between the amount of damage present in brain structures and the degree of impairment on specific cognitive tasks. However, in order to demonstrate correlation one has to examine subjects who are variable on the target measures. It is difficult, for example, to demonstrate an association between explicit memory scores and anatomical measures within groups of amnesics because on many explicit memory measures the amnesics are all essentially at chance performance. So with help from Nelson and Laird Cermak, Arne and I conducted a study of the relationship between anatomical measures and memory functions in a sample of subjects selected to exhibit a large degree of variability in the memory test scores and in the degree and regional distribution of anatomical changes.

The study that we did focussed on recognition memory and priming. To review very briefly for those who don't study memory, in recent years memory researchers have focussed increasing attention on dissociations between memory performances on traditional recall and recognition tasks requiring conscious recollection, and performances on tasks that assess memory more indirectly, and don't require conscious recollection - that is, between explicit and implicit memory tasks. A typical implicit memory task produces a measure of memory derived by contrasting a subject's performance when processing novel material to his or her performance when processing recently studied material. For example, naming speed for novel words may be compared to naming speed for words recently read. In most cases, subjects read studied words faster than unstudied words, whether they remember studying them or not. The increment in reading speed can therefore be taken as an indirect measure of the effect of study; that is, it can be treated as a memory measure. This kind of memory is referred to as priming.

There are several lines of evidence for a distinction between explicit memory performance and implicit memory such as priming. One that is particularly compelling is the repeated observation that some patients with severe impairments on explicit memory tasks seem to produce normal priming effects. This has led many to postulate that independent memory systems exist in the brain, one which depends upon the function of the mesial temporal lobe and related diencephalic structures, mediating explicit or conscious memory, and damaged in amnesic patients -- and a second, lying outside of the mesial temporal lobes, mediating priming effects, and spared in amnesia. So where is this memory that is measured with implicit memory tasks occurring? Well it depends to some extent on which implicit memory task. Nelson, Bill Heindel, and David Salmon have contrasted the performances of different patient groups on implicit memory tasks. They observed that while the learning of motor skills that occurs gradually over repeated trials is impaired in Huntington's Disease patients, such skill learning is normal in Alzheimer's Disease patients. In contrast, word priming effects were normal in Huntington's Disease patients but impaired in AD patients. From these results they hypothesized that skill learning may occur in the striatal structures (such as the caudate nucleus) so severely affected in HD patients, while word priming may occur in the neocortical association cortices, particularly temporo-parietal, affected early in AD. Keane, Gabrieli, Fennema, Growdon & Corkin (1991) and Schacter, Cooper, Tharan & Rubens (1991) have also hypothesized that priming may occur in posterior neocortical structures. So these are the hypotheses about the brain bases of explicit and implicit memory: the mesial temporal lobe is considered to mediate explicit memory; the striatum, skill learning; and posterior neocortical structures, priming. But note that these inferences, or, really, hypotheses, are based on comparisons of patient groups. Diagnosis is being used as a marker for a specific lesion. The diagnosis of amnesia is being used as a marker for damage to the mesial temporal lobe system, of Alzheimer's Disease as a marker for damage to temporo-parietal neocortex, Huntington's Disease as a marker for damage to the caudate nucleus. What Arne and I tried to do was to measure the amount of damage present in these different structures in the patients directly, with brain imaging, and examine the correspondence between the amount of damage present and the degree of impairment on recognition memory and priming.

The thirty subjects we studied were drawn from the subject samples I described earlier and had mixed diagnoses. We included subjects with memory impairments due to a variety of causes, including AD, HD, Korsakoff Syndrome, and anoxia.

Priming effects were measured in a tachistoscopic identification threshold task in which the subjects tried to identify words presented on a computer screen very briefly. Each word was initially presented for only 16 msec and immediately followed by a random pattern mask. Exposure duration was then gradually increased until the subject was able to identify the word. This exposure duration was the identification threshold. Repetition priming and recognition memory were measured with this task as follows: The subjects read aloud a list of words presented on a computer screen. After a delay, the identification threshold was measured for some of the words from the list and some new words. After each word identification, the subject was asked if the word was on the studied list. The measure of repetition priming was the difference between the mean identification threshold for all "old" word trials and the mean for all "new" word trials. The measure of recognition memory was the number of correct classifications of words as on or off the list (i.e., number of hits plus the number of correct rejections). In addition to these two measures, we examined the mean identification threshold for all of the "new" words, that is, the efficiency with which the subjects performed the baseline lexical identification task.

The three brain structures we examined were those I mentioned earlier, the caudate nucleus in the striatum; the posterolateral neocortex; and the mesial temporal lobe structures.

First we looked at the relationship between the performance measures. Consistent with many earlier studies, there was no simple correlation between the priming scores and the recognition memory scores, suggesting that they were measuring entirely independent processes. However, there was a significant correlation between performance on the baseline task (identification threshold for new words) and priming. The relationship at first seemed paradoxical, it was the subjects who had the largest thresholds, that is, who were most impaired on the baseline task, that had the highest priming scores. This finding is consistent, though, with results in normal subjects showing that if you degrade the stimuli in priming tasks, or use less familiar stimuli, the subjects have higher thresholds, but they also show larger priming effects for these stimuli. It appears from our study that when subjects have lexical or perceptual deficits, the stimuli are effectively degraded to them, and they show worse baseline performance and higher priming scores. We found it particularly interesting that when we predicted the priming scores in a multiple regression analysis with both the baseline and the recognition memory scores, the prediction was highly significant, and both measures contributed. In other words, when we controlled for the baseline deficits of the subjects, the residual variability in priming was correlated with recognition memory.

We next examined the relationships between the anatomical measures and the three performance measures. Each task measure was predicted by the three anatomical measures in a multiple regression analysis used to estimate the

BRAIN STRUCTURAL CORRELATES OF PRIMING TASK MEASURES

CRITERION VARIABLE

	RECOGNITION MEMORY		PRIMING		IDENTIFICATION THRESHOLD FOR NEW WORDS	
	r	β	r	β	r	β
Caudate	.49**	.17	-.35	-.54*	-.58***	-.38*
Posterolateral Neocortex	.50**	.16	-.09	-.08	-.48**	-.17
Temporal Limbic Cortex	66***	.49**	.17	.48*	-.53**	-.25
	R= .70***		R= .53*		R= .66**	

*	$p < .05$
**	$p < .01$
***	$p < .001$

r = Pearson correlation coefficient for simple correlation
β = Standardized regression coefficient from simultaneous multiple regression
R = Multiple R from simultaneous multiple regression

specific contributions to the different memory impairments made by damage to each of the target structures. The results are summarized in the table below.

Although all of the anatomical measures showed significant simple correlations with recognition memory; as expected, only the mesial temporal loss showed a significant specific association with poor recognition memory in the regression.

For the "new" word threshold, again, all simple correlations were significant; however, it appeared from the regression analysis that the caudate losses were most strongly related to inefficient lexical processing (as reflected in increased threshold).

Finally, none of the simple correlations of the anatomical measures with priming reached significance; however, the multiple regression analysis revealed significant contributions by both the caudate and the temporal limbic measures. However, the effects were in opposite directions: caudate volume loss was associated with increased priming, while temporal limbic loss was associated with decreased priming. At first this seems a very surprising result; however, remember that in normal subjects, several manipulations that make processing of lexical items more difficult result in increased priming for those items. We reasoned that perhaps impairment in the perceptual and lexical processing of the stimuli, associated with caudate damage, acted in a similar way to increase the priming effects of some of the subjects within the sample. If caudate losses result in poor lexical/perceptual processing, then such damage alone, like stimulus degradation, may actually increase priming effects. On the other hand, when temporal limbic losses occur in isolation, this might decrease priming effects. This would have resulted in the regression results we obtained for the priming measure. Also, if this explanation were correct, then a measure of priming which controlled for the subjects' performance on the "new" word (baseline) threshold should show a relationship to the temporal limbic measure. Such a residual priming score, removing variance associated with baseline threshold, was computed, and this score was correlated with each anatomical measure. The results suggested that, indeed, only temporal limbic losses were significantly correlated with this measure of priming.

As we expected, volume loss in the mesial temporal lobes was specifically related to poor recognition memory. Damage to the caudate, on the other hand, seemed particularly to affect lexical or perceptual processing of the words. This impairment of baseline performance was associated with larger priming effects; however, the magnitude of priming, holding baseline performance constant, was, like recognition memory, related to the integrity of the mesial temporal lobe structures. This means that what appears to be intact priming in memory-impaired subjects may in some cases be due to the contravening effects on priming of striatal and limbic damage.

These results may not generalize to other implicit memory tasks, although we think other tasks should be examined with these results in mind. Even if they do, other dissociations may not be attributable to the same factors that appeared to play a role here. The important point is that we believe it is necessary to examine each implicit memory task in the same way that we have traditionally examined explicit memory tasks. That is, we should try to identify each of the component processes required by the task, and then to understand how deficits in each of these processes affects the performance measure. In the past, we have tended to assume that nonmemory processing deficits, such as linguistic or attentional deficits, could act only to decrease memory scores. But now we should at least consider the possibility that deficits in nonmemory processing components of memory tasks can actually be associated with increased memory scores -- and in this case appeared to account for dissociations between priming and recognition memory.

In closing, I'd like to say that few in the neurosciences today would deny that the development of powerful new technologies, like the in vivo brain imaging modalities, opens up exciting new opportunities for revealing the structure of normal and disordered human cognition. But it is equally clear to all working in this field that the techniques have virtually no value unless they are married to the kind of careful experimental analysis of behavior that Nelson Butters' work exemplifies. Thanks to his extraordinary gifts as a teacher, and to his dedication to the nurturance of young psychologists, he has ensured that the best traditions of experimental psychology are well represented by his intellectual offspring, whether they call themselves neuropsychologists, cognitive scientists, cognitive neuroscientists, or whatever emerges as the next un-psychology science of behavior. Thank you very much, Nelson.

REFERENCES

Butters, N., Heindel, W.C., & Salmon, D.P. (1990). Dissociation of implicit memory in dementia: Neurological implications. *Bulletin of the Psychonomic Society, 28*(4), 359-366.

Jernigan, T.L., Archibald, S.L., Berhow, M.T., Sowell, E.R., Foster, D.S., Hesselink, J.R. (1991). Cerebral structure on MRI, Part I: Localization of age-related changes. *Biological Psychiatry, 29*(1), 55-67.

Jernigan, T.L., Schafer, K., Butters, N., & Cermak, L.S. (1991). Magnetic resonance imaging of alcoholic Korsakoff patients. *Neuropsychopharmacology, 4*(3), 175-186.

Jernigan, T.L., & Ostergaard, A.L. (1993). Word priming and recognition memory are both affected by mesial temporal lobe damage. *Neuropsychology, 7*(1), 14-26.

Jernigan, T.L., Salmon, D.P., Butters, N., & Hesselink, J.R. (1991). Cerebral structure on MRI, Part II: Specific changes in Alzheimer's and Huntington's Diseases. *Biological Psychiatry, 29*, 68 - 81.

Keane, M.M., Gabrieli, J.D.E., Fennema, A.C., Growdon, J.H., & Corkin, S. (1991). Evidence for a dissociation between perceptual and conceptual priming in Alzheimer's disease. *Behavioral Neuroscience, 105*(2), 326-342.

Norris, D. (1984). The effects of frequency, repetition and stimulus quality in visual word recognition. *Quarterly Journal of Experimental Psychology. A, Human Experimental Psychology, 36*, 507-518.

Schacter, D.L., Cooper, L.A., Tharan, M., & Rubens A.B. (1991). Preserved priming of novel objects in patients with memory disorders. *Journal of Cognitive Neuroscience, 3*, 117-130.

12

The Mammillary Bodies Revisited

Their Role in Human Memory Functioning

NARINDER KAPUR[1], KEITH SCHOLEY[1], ELIZABETH MOORE[2], SIMON BARKER[1], ANDREW MAYES[3], JASON BRICE[1], and JOHN FLEMING[2]

Of the many research studies carried out by Nelson Butters, that part of his work which embraced the relationship between the mammillary bodies and human memory developed from two separate directions, clinical neuropsychology and primate neuropsychology. From the direction of clinical neuropsychology, the oft-cited association between damage to the mammillary bodies and the memory disorder associated with Alcoholic Korsakoff's syndrome was noted by Butters & Cermak (1980) in their classic monograph on this condition. As pointed out by Butters and Cermak, this association dated back to the beginning of the century, yet it has remained controversial. Victor, Adams & Collins (1987) played down

[1] NARINDER KAPUR, Ph.D., KEITH SCHOLEY, SIMON BARKER, JASON BRICE • Wessex Neurological Centre, Southampton General Hospital, England
[2] ELIZABETH MOORE , JOHN FLEMING • Department of Medical Physics, Southampton General Hospital, England
[3] ANDREW MAYES, Ph.D. • Department of Neurology, University of Sheffield, England

Neuropsychological Explorations of Memory and Cognition: Essays in Honor of Nelson Butters, edited by Laird S. Cermak, Ph.D. Plenum Press, New York, 1994

the importance of mammillary body pathology in the memory disorder found in Alcoholic Korsakoff patients. By contrast, other authors (e.g. Torvik, 1987), proposed from a similar set of post-mortem material that mammillary body lesions were critical to the memory loss shown by Alcoholic Korsakoff patients.

In the case of primate neuropsychology, Holmes, Jacobson, Stein & Butters (1983) found that mammillary body lesions resulted in impaired performance on a new spatial memory task which the monkeys had never tried prior to surgery, but that pre-operatively acquired visuospatial discriminations were spared by such lesions. Across the range of non-human species, it is fair to say that the effects of mammillary body lesions on memory have at best been variable, with some researchers finding memory deficits, and others failing to observe any major memory loss (see Markowitsch, 1988 and Zola-Morgan & Squire, 1993 for summaries of some of this research).

The major causes of amnesia, such as Alcoholic Korsakoff's syndrome, Herpes Simplex Encephalitis and hypoxia may all result in mammillary body damage to a varying degree, but this is usually in the context of additional damage to other anatomical structures (Hierons, Janota & Corsellis, 1978; Squire, Amaral & Press, 1990). A major limitation to our understanding of the role of the mammillary bodies in human memory stems from the fact that few disease states actually result in focal mammillary body damage that is unaccompanied by damage to other memory-related structures in the brain. Such 'absence of evidence' has tempted many researchers to conclude that there is therefore 'evidence of absence' for the importance of the mammillary bodies in human memory. In recent years, some evidence has emerged that points to a significant role for the mammillary bodies in human memory. On the basis of a series of patients with penetrating missile injuries, Jarho (1973) concluded - "The present author's major finding is that the most severe and least recovering Korsakoff-like amnesic syndromes are associated with bilateral hypothalamic lesions, especially with lesions of the mammillary bodies or in their closest connections" (1973, p. 148). Squire, Amaral, Zola-Morgan, Kritchevsky & Press (1989) in a follow-up study of the noted case NA, who was originally thought to have a focal left thalamic lesion (Squire & Moore, 1979), found bilateral mammillary body damage and some additional right anterior temporal lobe pathology. In our initial report of a similar penetrating missile injury case (Dusoir, Kapur, Byrnes, McKinstry & Hoare, 1990), we found evidence for mammillary body damage as part of injury to adjacent structures, namely other parts of the hypothalamus and the pituitary gland.

A summary of the state of the field in relation to the mammillary bodies and memory was succinctly outlined by Amaral (1987, p. 236), when he noted - 'Whether the mammillary complex actually plays a role in memory processing, and what that role might be, remains controversial'. In an attempt to resolve at least some of this controversy, we therefore present some recent evidence relating to normal/damaged mammillary bodies and the presence of severe anterograde/retrograde amnesia. We sought to address four questions -

1.   Can one find severe anterograde amnesia in a patient with normal mammillary bodies?
2.   Can one find severe retrograde amnesia in a patient with normal mammillary bodies?
3.   Is mammillary body pathology associated with normal retrograde memory?
4.   Is mammillary body pathology associated with normal anterograde memory?

SEVERE ANTEROGRADE AMNESIA IN A PATIENT WITH NORMAL MAMMILLARY BODIES

In their series of Wernicke-Korsakoff cases, Victor *et al.* (1989) were unable to find any patients with normal mammillary bodies - "The medial mammillary nucleus was affected in every case in which it was available for study" (1989, p. 78). However, recent studies of non-alcoholic amnesic patients have reported cases with anterograde amnesia who have normal mammillary bodies. For example, in their post-mortem study, Zola-Morgan *et al.* (1986) found that their patient RB, who suffered amnesia following hypoxia, had normal mammillary bodies. In a further study of patients with amnesia following probable hypoxia, on this occasion using magnetic resonance imaging, Squire *et al.* (1990) found that two of their four patients had mammillary body volumes that were within normal limits. We present a case of amnesia following carbon monoxide poisoning where we also were able to gather evidence on the integrity of the mammillary bodies.

CASE REPORT

Clinical History

MM, a 49 yr old right-handed man (d.o.b. April 8, 1944), who had previously worked as an insurance salesman, suffered carbon monoxide poisoning in October 1992. He was left with marked memory impairment and no other sequelae of note.

On the WAIS-R, he had a Verbal IQ = 122, a Performance IQ = 105, and a Full Scale IQ = 115. He performed normally on a picture naming test (McKenna and Warrington, 1983) and on the 'F.A.S.' verbal fluency test (Lezak, 1983). On the Wechsler Memory Scale-Revised, he had a General Memory Quotient of 86 and a Delayed Memory Quotient of <50. He showed a mild impairment (41/50 - 25th percentile) in recognition memory for faces, and a marked impairment (34/50 - <5th percentile) in his recognition memory for words (Warrington, 1984). On the Autobiographical Memory Interview (Kopelman, Wilson and Baddeley, 1990), he had retrograde amnesia for events/incidents, with less impairment for semantic memory items.

MRI scanning showed discrete globus pallidus lesions and, more importantly from the point of view of his memory disorder, hippocampal atrophy - further localization of the lesion within the hippocampal formation was not possible. This atrophy can be clearly seen in Figure 1. Fluorodeoxyglucose (FDG) PET scanning at rest (Figure 2) showed bilateral medial temporal lobe hypometabolism.

A detailed analysis of his mammillary bodies and those of an age, sex and education-matched control subject showed that they were very similar in shape and size to those of the control subject. Figure 1a shows the patient's mammillary bodies and Figure 1b shows those of the control subject.

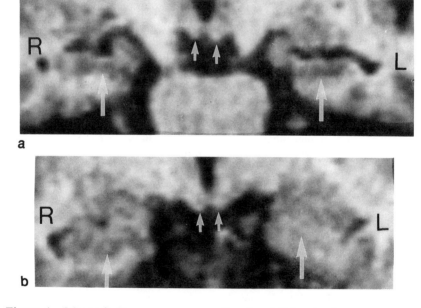

Figure 1. Magnetic Resonance scans of patient MM and of an age, sex and education-matched normal control subject. Enlarged coronal T_1 view (Figure 1a) shows mammillary bodies (small arrows) and hippocampal atrophy (large arrows). Analogous cuts through the brain of a matched control subject (Figure 1b) show mammillary bodies (small arrows) and normal hippocampi (large arrows).

AMNESIA FOLLOWING C.O. POISONING

BILATERAL HIPPOCAMPAL HYPOMETABOLISM

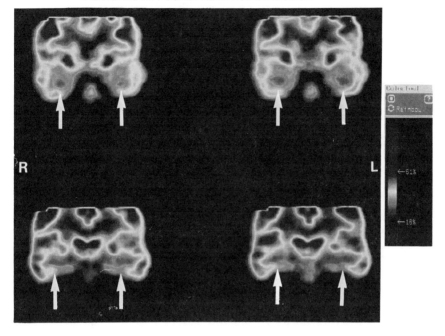

Figure 2. FDG resting PET scan in patient MM showing bilateral hippocampal hypometabolism in coronal section (arrowed). Level of metabolic activity is colour coded, with red and yellow representing high levels of activity and blue representing low or absent activity.

SEVERE RETROGRADE AMNESIA IN A PATIENT WITH NORMAL MAMMILLARY BODIES

In Alcoholic Korsakoff patients, who invariably display both anterograde and retrograde amnesia, the finding of shrunken mammillary bodies might lead one to conclude that mammillary body pathology plays a part in retrograde memory loss. Few studies of non-alcoholic patients with severe retrograde amnesia have attempted to examine their mammillary bodies in detail. We present a case of severe retrograde amnesia where we were able to carry out such an examination.

CASE REPORT

Clinical History

SP, a 46 yr old left-handed lady (dob July 7, 1948), who had previously worked as a marketing manager, suffered a severe closed head injury in February 1992, as a result of a road traffic accident. After the accident, she was unconscious for around five days, and appeared to be rather confused for a further six weeks after this. Early physical signs included a marked right hemiparesis, complete right third nerve palsy with an associated diplopia, and a right homonymous hemianopia. Her hemiparesis largely recovered, though her visual deficits have remained.

General cognitive testing in November/December 1992 yielded a WAIS-R Verbal IQ of 92, a Performance IQ of 88 and a Full Scale IQ of 89. On the Wechsler Memory Scale-Revised, she had a General Memory Quotient of 81 and a Delayed Quotient of 73. Both she and her husband considered her everyday memory to be minimally impaired, and her major memory loss to be for events that occurred prior to her head injury. They also observed that she appeared to have a very long-term (i.e. months) anterograde memory deficit, one that seemed to be similar to that reported by De Renzi and Lucchelli (1993) - at present, we are in the process of empirically assessing this symptom. There was, however, little doubt as to her retrograde memory loss which was apparent on the Autobiographical Memory Interview (Kopelman, Wilson & Baddeley, 1990), with marked impairment in her memory for specific incidents/events (Table 1).

TABLE 1

SP's Autobiographical Memory Performance

	PERSONAL SEMANTIC	INCIDENTS
Childhood	12.5/21(abnormal)	0/9 (abnormal)
Early Adult Life	13.5/21(abnormal)	0/9 (abnormal)
Recent Life	8/21(abnormal)	3/9 (abnormal)

Magnetic resonance imaging (Figure 3) showed significant pathology in the left temporal lobe, and a smaller lesion in the region of the right uncus and right anterior hippocampus. The left temporal lesion appeared to particularly involve the anterior portions of the inferior, middle and superior temporal lobe gyri. Figure 4 shows enlarged views of her mammillary bodies (Figure 4a),

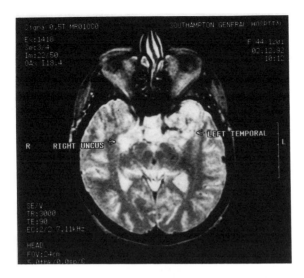

Figure 3. T$_2$ weighted axial MR scan showing left temporal lobe lesion, and right uncal and right anterior hippocampal lesion in patient SP.

and those of a control subject matched for age, sex and handedness (Figure 4b). Detailed analyses of these structures showed them to be of similar shape and size in SP and in the control subject.

MAMMILLARY BODY PATHOLOGY - RETROGRADE AND ANTEROGRADE MEMORY FUNCTIONING

For the remaining part of this chapter, we will ask whether mammillary body pathology may be associated with normal retrograde memory, and whether it can be found in association with normal anterograde memory. Retrograde memory functioning will be considered briefly. The patient NA (Squire *et al.*, 1989) was found to have virtually absent mammillary bodies on detailed MR imaging. His performance on retrograde memory tasks has been found to be largely intact (Cohen and Squire, 1981), though the nature of tests of this type is such that a short, mild retrograde amnesia of several weeks or months often cannot be excluded with certainty. Similarly, our report of patient BJ (Dusoir *et al.*, 1990), who also suffered mammillary body destruction, indicated the absence of any major retrograde memory loss. There would thus appear to be little support for any hypothesis that mammillary body damage results in significant retrograde memory deficits.

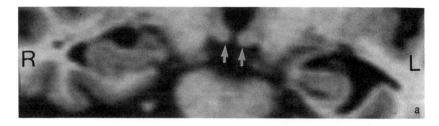

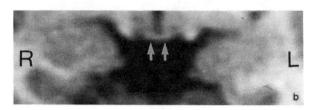

Figure 4. Enlarged coronal T$_1$ view of SP's MR scan (Figure 4a) shows mammillary bodies (arrowed). Analogous cuts through the brain of a matched control subject (Figure 4b) also show mammillary bodies (arrowed). An incidental finding is that the mammillary bodies appear to be 'fused' together in the control subject.

We shall now turn to the more controversial issue as to whether mammillary body pathology may result in impaired anterograde memory performance. We will return to the patient BJ whom we reported several years ago, and we shall present more recent brain imaging and memory test data.

CASE REPORT

Clinical History

Details of our patient's clinical history have been presented in our earlier report (Dusoir *et al.*, 1990). To summarize, our patient (dob January 3, 1959) suffered a penetrating paranasal snooker cue injury in October, 1986. In addition to his memory disorder, he suffered from hypopituitarism, some diabetes insipidus, and hypothalamic signs such as lack of normal sweat reaction, poor sleep control, voracious appetite and temper outbursts. Most of these signs have abated but remain to some extent. He continues to take cortisone replacement therapy.

Magnetic Resonance Imaging

Magnetic Resonance scanning on a 0.5 Tesla GE Signa Scanner comprised an initial sagittal T1W survey, followed by a 3D SPGR T_1 coronal scan of the whole brain (24 field of view. TR = 50, TE = 14. Matrix size = 256 x 192. Flip angle = 45 degrees). This was followed by a whole brain proton density and T_2 axial scan, with 'temporal lobe orientation', i.e. with cuts parallel to the temporal horn as seen on the sagittal scout view (5mm contiguous slices. TR = 3000, TE = 30/90). A final sequence was conducted, this consisting of whole brain, non-contiguous coronal Proton Density & T_2 weighted orthogonal scan (5mm slices, 1mm gap. TR = 3000, TE = 30/90). This sequence was formatted from a sagittal survey cut which showed the angle used for the T_2 axial sequence, and the angle of the coronal cut was at right-angles to the angle used in the axial sequence.

Quantitative analyses were carried using a SUN workstation and ANALYSE software. Purpose-built software routines were developed to enable the MR data to be transferred from the GE scanner in a form that can be readily analysed at the SUN workstation. We carried out volumetric analyses using a statistical random marking method (Bentley and Karwoski, 1988) that is incorporated within ANALYSE. We used a pre-defined anatomical protocol similar to those used by other researchers (e.g. Cook *et al.*, 1992; Watson *et al.*, 1992).

As can be seen in coronal (Figure 5a) and sagittal (Figure 5b,c) views from our patient and from an age-, sex- and education-matched normal control subject (Figure 5d, e, f), the mammillary bodies can be clearly demarcated in the normal control subject, but are not even visible in our patient.

The only other evidence of pathology related to an absent pituitary gland, hypothalamic damage, and a minor extrusion of orbital frontal tissue through the jugulum sphenoidale (Figure 5g), this presumably occurring at the time of surgery.

The results of volumetric analyses of left and right hippocampus are shown in Table 2. When defining the boundary of the hippocampus, we included the subiculum, dentate gyrus, alveus, and the fimbria as far as the crus of the fornix. BJ showed a mild (around 28%) reduction in the volume of the left hippocampus, compared to that of the matched control subject. His right hippocampus value was close to that for the control subject. The reduction in size of the left hippocampus cannot be explained by a general reduction in size of the left temporal lobe, since this volume was similar in BJ and the control subject. Our normal control values for the hippocampus were in fact close to those derived by other researchers using similar analytical procedures (e.g. Jack *et al.*, 1992).

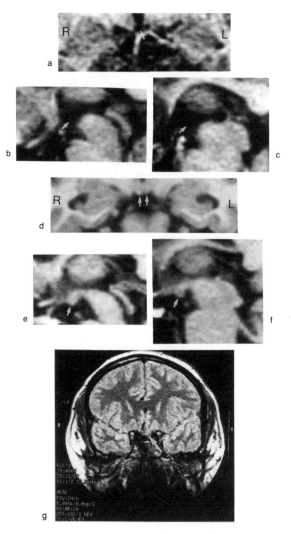

Figure 5. Enlarged coronal view of BJ's MR scan (Figure 5a) shows absence of mammillary bodies at bottom of third ventricle (arrowed). Analogous cuts through the brain of a matched control subject (Figure 5d) show mammillary bodies (arrowed). Left (Figure 5b) and right (Figure 5c) sagittal T_1 sections in patient BJ also show absence of mammillary bodies (arrowed area), whereas these are readily visible in the corresponding left sagittal (Figure 5e) and right sagittal (Figure 5f) T_1 sections of the control subject. Minor extrusion of left frontal lobe tissue (arrowed) through the jugulum sphenoidale is seen on the coronal proton density image (Figure 5g).

Positron Emission Tomography

The results of FDG PET scanning, which was carried out at St Thomas' Hospital, London, can be seen in Figure 6. There was evidence for a limited degree of focal, left hippocampal hypometabolism, this being evident on one axial (Figure 6a) and several coronal (Figure 6b) images. This hypometabolism was relatively mild, being 16-17% lower than the corresponding right hippocampal area. On the basis of experience in the PET scanning unit where the scan was carried out, a 10% difference is usually employed as a cut-off point to indicate some degree of abnormality. The abnormality appeared to primarily involve the mid and posterior portions of the left hippocampus. Both thalamic structures appeared quite normal, and quantitative analyses of anterior thalamic metabolic activity, when compared with the cerebellum, showed no significant asymmetry. There was no evidence of any hypometabolism in frontal lobe structures.

General Cognitive Functioning

On the basis of six subtests of the Wechsler Adult Intelligence Scale-Revised (Wechsler, 1981), BJ had a Verbal IQ of 103, a Performance IQ of 99 and a Full-Scale IQ of 101. These scores are in fact rather higher than IQ scores (estimated Full Scale IQ = 91) derived from his performance on an adult reading test (Nelson, 1982). BJ's educational and occupational achievements since leaving school suggest that his Full Scale IQ score probably represents a more reliable estimate of his premorbid cognitive functioning than his reading score alone.

TABLE 2

VOLUMETRIC VALUES, DERIVED FROM MAGNETIC RESONANCE IMAGES, FOR HIPPOCAMPUS AND LEFT TEMPORAL LOBE

STRUCTURE	VALUE FOR BJ	CONTROL VALUE
Left Hippocampus	$1.6cm^3$	$2.2cm^3$
Right Hippocampus	$2.8cm^3$	$2.6cm^3$
Left Temporal Lobe	$74.8cm^3$	$62.3cm^3$

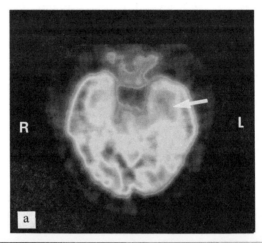

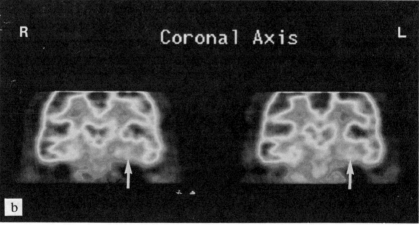

Figure 6. FDG resting PET scan in patient BJ showing left hippocampal hypometabolism in axial section (Figure 6a), and coronal section (Figure 6b). Level of metabolic activity is colour coded, with red and yellow representing high levels of activity and blue representing low or absent activity.

Standard Anterograde Memory Tasks

BJ was aware of everyday memory difficulties, mainly relating to situations such as remembering a message or remembering where he had put something. BJ's anterograde memory functioning was assessed over a range of tests. His performance on the Revised Wechsler Memory Scale (Wechsler, 1987) is outlined in Table 3.

Table 3
BJ's Memory Test Scores

TEST	RAW SCORE	STATISTIC SCORE
VERBAL MEMORY AND LEARNING		
Word recognition	46/50	9 (scaled-score)
Story recall (Immediate)	21/50	25th percentile
Story recall (Delayed)	6/50**	3rd percentile
Verbal Paired-associate learning (Immediate)	11/24**	
Verbal Paired-associate learning (Delayed)	3/8**	
VISUAL-NONVERBAL MEMORY AND LEARNING		
Faces recognition	45/50	11 (scaled-score)
Designs recall (Immediate)	36/41	74th percentile
Designs recall (Delayed)	15/41**	5th percentile
Pattern-Colour learning (Immediate)	9/18*	
Pattern-Colour learning (Delayed)	3/8*	
WMS-R GENERAL MEMORY QUOTIENT		85*
WMS-R DELAYED MEMORY QUOTIENT		56**

* *Mild Impairment*
** *Marked Impairment*

His Delayed Memory quotient of 56 indicated a marked degree of impairment. On closer scrutiny of individual subtests, he could not spontaneously recall any of the two stories presented 30m earlier, and only remembered a few further items after being provided with cues. It is of note that his delayed recall of visual designs also showed a marked drop from immediate to delayed retention testing. His scores on the Wechsler Memory Scale-Revised were similar to those that we obtained previously (Dusoir *et al.*, 1990). For example, his current Delayed Memory Quotient of 56 is similar to the score of 54 that was reported in the earlier paper. On a words and a faces recognition memory test (Warrington, 1984), he now performed normally for both faces and words subtests, this representing an improvement on the words subtest compared to the previous testing in 1988. BJ also performed normally on a visual pattern recognition memory test, which included continuous recognition memory and delayed retention after 20 minutes (Trahan and Larrabee, 1988). His scores on this test were - Total Score = 85, d-prime = 2.59, Delayed Retention = 4 / 7, Visual Discrimination = 7 / 7.

Nonverbal location memory

In order to further examine the extent to which BJ showed only verbal memory deficits, we assessed an aspect of nonverbal memory that has been found to be sensitive to right hippocampal damage, namely memory for spatial location of items. The pictures used for this test are shown in Figure 7. The subject is shown the top picture for 60s and then shown the bottom picture. The same items occur in both pictures, but ten items have been re-arranged, and the subject is asked to circle those items that have been moved. For example, the ghost has moved in the lower retention test picture. The pictures were identical, except for the ten items that were moved about. Three tests were admininistered, with a different picture set in each test. As can be seen in Figure 8, BJ's performance on this test is significantly impaired compared to that of three matched control subjects.

Rate of Forgetting

Four matched stories were used for this experiment. Free recall and four-choice recognition were separately tested at 20 seconds and at 10 minutes, with both intervals being filled with other activities. Thus, four story retention tests were administered. BJ was given three repetitions of the story to match his initial retention scores to those of control subjects, who received one repetition of the story (see Mayes, 1988 for further rationale relating to such matching procedures). Figure 9a shows the recall performance of BJ, nine Alcoholic Korsakoff patients, one patient with amnesia resulting from bilateral medial temporal lobe pathology following Herpes Simplex Encephalitis, and 18 control subjects. Figure 9b shows corresponding data relating to story recognition memory.

As can be seen, BJ showed an abnormally fast forgetting rate from 20s to 10 minutes, equivalent to that of Alcoholic Korsakoff patients. A further memory test was carried out after seven days, testing for retention of items in the 10-minutes recognition story. The order of items within each four-choice question was changed from that used seven days earlier. This assessment was

Presentation

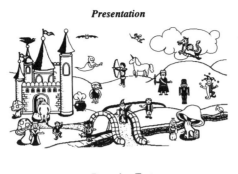

Retention Test

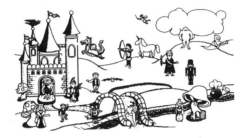

Figure 7. 'Spot-the-difference' memory test, where subject is shown upper picture for 60 seconds, and is then shown the lower picture. See text for further details.

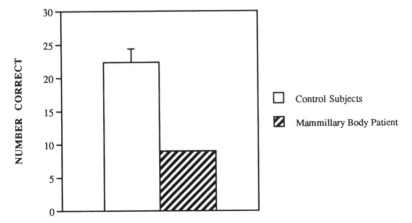

Figure 8. Performance of BJ and control subjects on 'Spot-the-difference' memory test. Score relates to number of items correctly identified as having moved (Maximum = 30). Error bar shows standard deviation value for control subjects.

carried out by post, with BJ completing the recognition memory test while instructions were given by one of the authors (NK) by phone. BJ scored 6/12, a drop of only two items over the seven days and well above chance level. For two of his erroneous responses, he in fact initially selected the correct item but then crossed this out to chose a distractor item instead. Thus, although we do not have control data for this delay interval, it seems very unlikely that BJ shows an abnormal rate of forgetting from ten minutes to seven days.

Contextual Memory

Memory for verbal context (indicating in which of two lists of sentences a target sentence was presented) was assessed using the materials and procedure described by Parkin and Hunkin (1993). Six sentences were presented, each for five seconds, and were read aloud by BJ. He was told that his memory

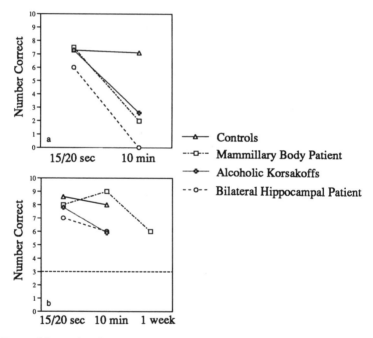

Figure 9. Rate of forgetting for recall of story material from 15-20 seconds post presentation to 10 minutes (Figure 9a). Rate of forgetting for recognition story material from 15-20 seconds post presentation to 10 minutes (Figure 9b). [Control subject data were initially only available for 15 seconds retention, but differed little from subsequent 20 seconds control data]. Further data are presented for BJ in respect of his performance one week later. Chance level of performance is indicated by the horizontal dotted line.

for the sentences would be tested later. The following three minutes were spent in conversation. A second matched list of sentences was presented in a similar fashion. Then BJ was shown 24 sentences, 12 of which had occurred previously and 12 of which were new. He was asked to indicate whether each sentence was in one of the two lists of sentences, and if so in which list it had been presented. BJ performed well on this task. He was able to correctly recognize 10/12 sentences as having occurred previously. He correctly apportioned 9/10 sentences that he correctly recognized. He also only made one false positive response to the distractor sentences. BJ's performance was similar to that of control subjects tested by Parkin and Hunkin (1993), and well above that of Alcoholic Korsakoff patients.

BJ was also tested on his temporal context memory for words. Using a similar presentation format to that of the Recognition Memory Test (Warrington, 1984), he was shown a list of 50 high frequency words, each for three seconds, after which he was shown 23 pairs of words. He had to indicate which of the two words appeared earlier in the list. The distribution of temporal distance between words in the 23 pairs was as follows - immediately adjacent (0 items in between) = 3 pairs; 10 items = 5 pairs; 20 items = 5 pairs; 30 items = 5 pairs; 40 items = 5 pairs. His performance, together with that of control subjects is shown in Figure 10. As can be seen, he performed well on the task.

'Fluency versus Recollection' Recognition Memory
        To explore whether BJ was similar to Alcoholic Korsakoff patients in showing an impaired ability to use recollective processes in order to exclude the interference effects of previous stimuli, we employed an experimental design and set of stimuli similar to those used by Cermak and Verfaellie (1992). BJ was

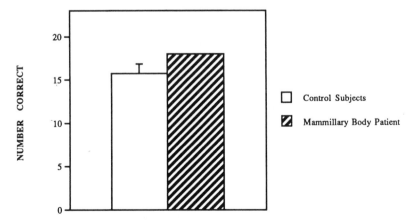

Figure 10. Performance of BJ and control subjects on the 50 words verbal temporal context memory task.

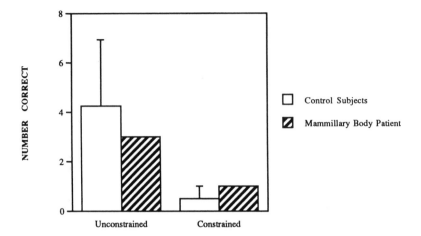

Figure 11. Performance of BJ and control subjects on 'stem fluency' test.

asked to read a list of ten words, and after a filled interval of 30 seconds, he was shown the first three-letter stems of the words in a different order. He was asked to indicate the first words that came to mind as a result of seeing the word stem. Several hours later, a similar experiment was carried out, with a matched list of words (but with different word stems). On this occasion, when he was asked to generate words from word stems, he was asked to specifically exclude words that he had read 30 seconds before. As can be seen in Figure 11, there was no evidence to indicate that, within the short-term temporal limits of this task, BJ showed impaired recollective ability, and thus increased 'fluency' effects, compared to control subjects.

Release from Proactive Interference
                    Patients with diencephalic pathology, such as Alcoholic Korsakoff patients, have been found to show significant intereference effects in certain short-term memory tasks. In view of the mammillary body damage and hypothalamic damage sustained by our patient, the links between the hypothalamus and the frontal lobes, and the minor extrusion of frontal lobe tissue seen on one of the MR images, we assessed his performance in a paradigm designed to assess release from proactive interference. We used an identical set of procedures to those used by Squire (1982). Essentially, five sets of word triads were presented. Words were selected from various semantic categories. The fifth set of words was either of the same category as the preceding four sets or was from a different semantic category (release condition). As can be seen from Figure 12, BJ showed normal release from proactive interference, and he performed similar to NA and to the control subjects in the Squire (1982) study.

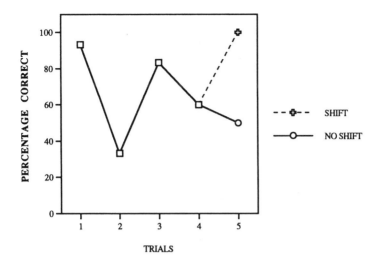

Figure 12. Performance of BJ on release from proactive interference task.

Autobiographical Memory

BJ's retrograde memory for autobiographical material had been previously shown to be relatively intact, with only relatively patchy memory loss for a six month period prior to his injury (Dusoir et al., 1990). On this examination, BJ's pre-traumatic amnesia had now shrunk to around several days. His last clear memory is of returning to England from Ireland three to four days before the injury. He does not, however, have any clear memory for attending his brother's wedding a week before his injury, though he does clearly remember journeys by car and by plane to and from the wedding. He appears to have clear and continuous memory for events prior to this wedding. Other aspects of his pre-injury autobiographical memory are discussed in the previous report of this case (Dusoir et al., 1990).

BJ's autobiographical memory for events *after* his head injury was assessed by means of a structured interview covering personal events, and we used similar procedures to those described elsewhere (Kapur et al., 1992). In addition to the structured interview, we also administered a short questionnaire, the Shared Experiences Test, which is described below. The structured interview with BJ and his parents resulted in the following observations -

1. HOLIDAYS/TRIPS - He could remember going to Butlins' holiday camp in Scotland three years earlier, and he could recount some entertainment events at the camp. He came to London in September 1992 for his compensation hearing, and could recall items such as the layout of the room, where the hearing took place, and some of the points raised at the hearing.

2. HOSPITAL TREATMENT - He did not spontaneously recall being in hospital the year before, but when cued about this he did remember it, and could offer items such as the names of some of his visitors. He could recall phoning his wife at one point during his stay.

3. BIRTHS - He could indicate that three of his nephews had been born in the past few years, and he could name them. However, he did forget that he visited one of his nephews in hospital at the time of the child's birth.

Shared Experiences Test.
      In this test, BJ and his parents independently filled in a check-list of 66 items. This mostly covered towns in his home country of N Ireland, but also included parts of London (e.g. Buckingham Palace) and situations such as being on an aeroplane, at a circus, in a restaurant, etc. BJ had to indicate those places where he had been with his parents in the past six years since the injury, and his parents similarly but independently completed the checklist. BJ correctly indicated seven of the eight places/situations marked by his parents, the one omission being a circus. When cued about this, he indicated that he did recall going to the circus, could recollect where it was, and the fact that he went with his nephew. It is worth noting that BJ in fact marked two events (attending his brother's wedding and attending the funeral of his father-in-law) which his parents forgot that BJ had attended along with them!
      It would appear on the basis of the structured interview and also the Shared Experiences Test that BJ has minimal memory loss for personal events that have occurred in the past six years since his injury. Two provisos need to be borne in mind. Firstly, he admits that his memory for the first year after his injury is poor, and this is understandable in view of his post-traumatic confusional state. Secondly, when specifically asked to compare the clarity in his mind of the five subsequent years after this year and the five years immediately preceding his injury, BJ is confident that the pre-injury years are significantly clearer in his mind than the post-injury years. It would, therefore, be fair to classify his memory for post-injury experiences as being impaired, but to a relatively mild degree.

Post-Injury Knowledge Acquisition
      Aspects of his pre-injury knowledge of items such as public events is given in our earlier paper (Dusoir et al., 1990). In this investigation, we concentrated on his long-term acquisition of knowledge. Due to the restricted time period of items/events that were assessed, it was not feasible to collect temporal dating information from subjects. BJ and four age, sex and education-matched control subjects (mean age = 36 yrs) were administered several general knowledge tests -

(1) *Famous Names Identification Test.* This test assesses memory for personalities who have been in the public eye over the previous six years since his injury. We included names that had recently become famous (e.g. Bill Clinton), or people who had died or taken part in a major event in this period. Forty-four names were chosen. BJ and control subjects were required to indicate if the name was familiar to them, whether it was that of a British or a Foreign citizen, what the occupation of the person was (recall followed by forced-choice recognition if incorrect), which of three events was associated with the person, whether he/she was dead or alive, and if dead - the manner of death (from four choices - natural causes, suicide, murdered or accident).

(2) *Real-Fictitious News Events Test.* This test is similar to the test devised by Kapur (1991). Twenty-five news events that had occurred in the past six years since BJ's injury were inter-mingled with 25 fictitious but plausible events. Subjects had to indicate those events they thought had actually occurred.

(3) *Newsreaders Test.* This test comprised 20 names of TV personalities who had become prominent in the past six years, ten of whom read daily news bulletins on one of the major TV channels and ten of whom were involved in reporting news events or similar political programmes but who did not actually read the news bulletins. Subjects had to indicate which of the personalities actually read news bulletins.

(1) *Famous Names Identification Test.* Figure 13 provides scores on various components of this task as they relate to BJ's post-injury knowledge of these names. Thus, he could identify as familiar most names that had come into prominence since his injury, but his score was still somewhat lower than that of control subjects. Such a test inevitably has slight ceiling effects, with two of our control subjects obtaining perfect performance, so that BJ's score probably represents a mild impairment. From the set of items for this test, those names that did not appear or sound foreign were considered for nationality rating (British or Foreign), and BJ was also mildly impaired on this part of the test. His ability to identify the occupation of the person, either by recall or by recognition, was mildly impaired. When one considers those names who were involved in a major news event since 1987, BJ's ability to choose the correct event in association with such names also showed a mild impairment. For those personalities who had died since 1987, his knowledge of such deaths was moderately impaired, as was his ability to choose the correct manner of death.

(2) *Real-Fictitious News Events Test.* BJ could correctly identify almost as many items as control subjects (Figure 14), and made a similarly small number of false positive responses.

(3) *Newsreaders Test.* BJ scored as well as control subjects on this task (Figure 15).

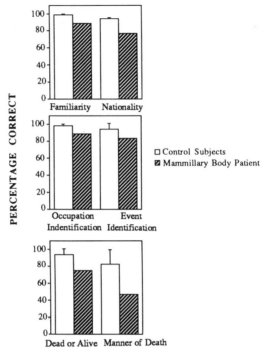

Figure 13. Performance of BJ and control subjects on various components of famous names memory test - indicating familiarity of name, nationality of personality, occupation and event associated with the personality, whether the person is dead or alive and manner of death (see text for more details).

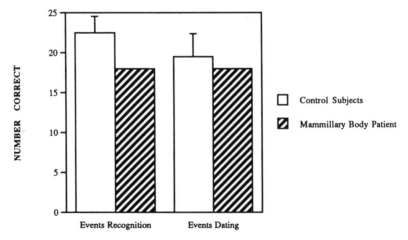

Figure 14. Performance of BJ and control subjects on real-fictitious news events test.

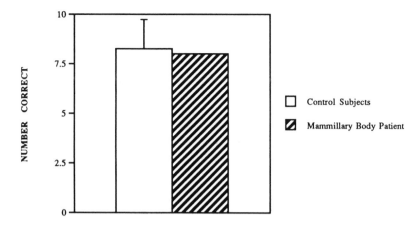

Figure 15. Performance of BJ and control subjects on newsreaders test.

This test was in fact designed as a simple screening test, and the similar scores of BJ and control subjects suggests that they all had equivalent amounts of exposure to news items through the TV media.

DISCUSSION

Our patient BJ, who suffered destruction of the mammillary bodies following a penetrating head injury, continued to show marked memory impairment on delayed recall components of standard memory tests. Recollective ability, especially on verbal recall tests over short-term intervals, is relatively normal - this finding suggests that his recall deficit may only become striking after a delay or where his immediate memory span is significantly over-stretched. There was a relative sparing of recognition memory functioning. His improvement in recognition memory since our previous assessment five years earlier suggests that the critical lesion produced a transient effect on some aspects of recognition memory but a permanent effect on recall. He showed an abnormally fast rate of forgetting on a story recall task, but normal short-term and long-term rate of forgetting for recognition of similar material. There was no evidence of any contextual memory deficit. BJ's post-injury autobiographical memory appeared to be only mildly impaired. His post-injury knowledge acquisition did show a limited deficit, especially where he had to indicate specific information that was associated with a famous personality. While dedicated MRI scanning protocols confirmed that major structural damage in memory-related structures was limited to the mammillary bodies, volumetric MRI analyses and PET scanning revealed a mild degree of left hippocampal abnormality.

There are several possible factors that may explain the partial hippocampal abnormality found in our patient. Firstly, it is possible that it represents retrograde degeneration via the fornix. However, this is unlikely in view of primate evidence that transection of the fornix does not lead to retrograde degeneration in the hippocampus (Clark & Meyer, 1950). In addition, it is uncertain why such degeneration would be restricted to the left hippocampus and not extend to both hippocampi, since mammillary body damage in our patient was bilateral in extent. Secondly, if - as seems possible - the supramammillary area was lesioned at the time of the injury, secondary damage via efferent connections from this area to the hippocampus (Veazey, Amaral & Cowan, 1982) may have resulted in hippocampal dysfunction (cf. Kirk and McNaughton, 1991). However, there is no hard evidence to support such transneuronal degeneration, and the current resolution of MR imaging is such that it is not possible to say for certain if supramammillary damage in fact occurred, and if it was unilateral or bilateral. In partial support of the first and second possibilities, several studies of alcoholic Korsakoff patients have pointed to the presence of hippocampal abnormality in addition to the well-established mammillary body and thalamic damage, either at the neuropathological level (Mayes, Meudell, Mann & Pickering, 1987) or at the level of metabolic activity/cerebral blood flow (e.g. Hata, Meyer, Tanahashi, Ishikawa, Imai, Shinohara, Velez, Fann, Kandula & Saki, 1987; Fazio, Perani, Gilardi, Colombo, Cappa, Vallar, Bettinardi, Paulesu, Alberoni, Bressi, Franceschi & Lenzi, 1992). A third possibility revolves around the vascular supply of the mammillary bodies and the hippocampus. Both of these structures receive their blood supply from branches of the posterior cerebral artery (Haymaker, 1969; Marinkovic, Milisavljevic & Puskas, 1992). This particular area in the base of the brain is perhaps more susceptible than most other areas to arterial disruption, simply due to the extensive network of major and perforating arteries that are present - e.g. Holmes et al. (1983) found that most of their mammillary body lesioned and sham-operated monkeys suffered temporal lobe infarction as a result of surgery in this region. Since it is well known that disruption of blood supply in the area of the posterior cerebral artery may result in memory impairment (Cramon, Hebel & Schuri, 1988), this may have caused both the initial period of retrograde amnesia (which covered a period of several years), and the anterograde memory impairment. However, if such arterial disruption did in fact occur, one might have expected to find evidence of infarction in the left hippocampus. Although this was not present, the possibility of mild ischaemia remains open.

While there have been a number of clinical descriptions of memory-disordered patients with well documented mammillary body damage (e.g. Kahn and Crosby, 1972), and observations relating to memory and mammillary body integrity in Alcoholic Korsakoff patients (Bigler, Nelson & Schmidt, 1989), the only published case of non-alcoholic bilateral mammillary body damage where memory functioning was studied in detail relates to the patient NA. (Squire *et al.*, 1989). However, this patient also suffered left thalamic damage, together with damage to the right anterior temporal lobe. Damage as a result of the injury/surgery was also considered by Squire *et al.* to have included the fornix and amygdala to some extent. The patient's hypothalamic damage was evident on T_2 weighted images, whereas this was not seen in corresponding images of our case. Two further cases of possible mammillary body damage are worthy of brief mention. One is a case of a hypothalamic glioma reported by Parkin & Hunkin (1993). Unfortunately, no imaging data were reported on this patient, but his Wechlser Memory Scale-Revised scores were very similar to those of our patient, showing a marked drop from General to Delayed Memory Quotients. It is of note that he also showed a similar sparing of recognition memory to the one displayed by BJ. The second case is also a patient with a hypothalamic lesion which appeared to involve the mammillary bodies (Cohen and Albers, 1991), though the authors did not specifically discuss this possibility. Their patient showed significant impairment on a number of memory tests. The patient also displayed changes in circadian rhythm, and it is possible that this may have exacerbated her memory impairment.

The pattern of memory impairment shown by BJ - impaired recall with relatively intact recognition memory - is partly similar to that which has sometimes been reported for patients with frontal lobe damage (Shimamura, Janowsky and Squire, 1991). However, our patient's delayed recall deficits were particularly severe. In addition, we found no brain imaging or functional evidence of significant frontal lobe pathology, and it would therefore seem that the two sets of recall impairments are due to the involvment of different brain circuits.

Could the left hippocampal abnormality alone, that was seen on BJ's PET scan and on volumetric MR analysis, have resulted in his memory impairment? This seems unlikely for a number of reasons. Firstly, BJ showed impairments in both verbal and nonverbal retention testing, as indicated by his delayed visual design recall deficits and spatial item location impairment. Secondly, while discrete left hippocampal vascular pathology is rare, those cases that have been reported have been associated with minimal residual memory impairment (Landi, Giusti & Guidotti, 1982; Tanabe, Haskikawa, Nakagawa, Yamamoto, Harada, Tsumoto, Nishimura, Shiraishi & Kimura, 1991). The case reported by Tanabe *et al.* (1991) is particularly revealing, since MRI showed a residual discrete left hippocampal lesion in the CA1 region of the hippocampus, yet the patient had a WMS-R Delayed Memory Quotient of 108, compared to the markedly impaired score of 56 obtained by BJ. Thirdly, Goldstein and Polkey (1992, 1993) found that patients who had left amygdalo-hippocampectomy showed a mild impairment on story recall, with only a slightly lower drop from immediate to delayed (one hour) recall of stories compared to control subjects. This contrasted with the very poor delayed story recall by our patient, and a rapid rate of forgetting over a ten minute period. In addition, their left amygdalo-hippocampectomy patients' mean screening score of 7.57 on the Rivermead

Behavioural Memory Test was much higher than the score of 2 obtained by BJ (Dusoir *et al.*, 1990). The study by Frisk & Milner (1990), which reported significant decline in forgetting rate for story recall after major hippocampal ablation, found much less drop in recall levels over a 20-minute period than was shown by BJ over ten minutes. The major hippocampal ablation group in the Frisk and Milner study probably sustained a lesion that was greater in extent than that indicated by BJ's PET scan - the Frisk and Milner patient group that sustained more limited anterior left hippocampal ablation (which included the uncus and the amygdala) showed little drop in story recall over a 20-minute period. In considering such data and the data gathered in this investigation, it is important to allow for some differences in test procedures between studies, and to allow for the fact that epilepsy patients who have undergone ablation may be rather unique in the combination of beneficial and deleterious effects of surgery on brain functioning (cf. Solomon, Solomon, Schaaf & Perry, 1983). Fourthly, in volumetric studies of patients with temporal lobe epilepsy, most patients with significant pathology in the hippocampus have volumes lower than the value of $1.6cm^3$ that we found in our patient (Cascino, Jack, Parisi, Sharbrough, Hirschorn, Meyer, Marsh & O'Brein, 1991). These four sets of data, when taken together, render unlikely the possibility that our patient's focal left hippocampal abnormality would by itself have resulted in his particular profile of memory disorder. However, we should stress that it remains possible that mammillary body lesions alone do not result in the pattern of memory deficits which we found, and that deficits such as accelerated rate of forgetting only arise when mammillary body lesions are accompanied by a second lesion, however minor, elsewhere in the limbic circuit.

In many respects, our patient's memory disorder was similar to that shown by patients with damage to the fornix (Hodges and Carpenter, 1991). A recently reported case of presumed fornix damage, from a paranasal injury which had a more anterior trajectory compared to the snooker cue injury sustained by our patient, also found significant memory disorder to be present (Botez-Marquard & Botez, 1992). In our patient, we could not find any firm evidence to suggest damage to the fornix, though the convoluted shape of this structure render it difficult to discern minor degrees of damage. It would be reasonable to expect that bilateral mammillary body damage would be similar in its effects to bilateral damage of the anterior columns of the fornix, such as that sustained by one of the two patients reported by Hodges and Carpenter. In both their patients and in our patient, there was an anterograde memory loss that was particularly marked for delayed recall and for paired-associate learning, with relative sparing of recognition memory, and also with minimal retrograde memory impairment. In spite of their memory difficulties, both our patient and the two patients reported by Hodges and Carpenter had everyday memory symptoms that were not as severely disabling as those seen in Alcoholic Korsakoff or Herpes Encephalitic amnesics.

The rate of forgetting shown by our patient on a story recall task was as steep as that shown by Alcoholic Korsakoff patients and a little less severe than that shown by an amnesic patient with medial temporal lobe damage following Herpes Simplex Encephalitis. This finding suggests that the rapid forgetting shown by Alcoholic Korsakoff patients in delayed recall paradigms may well be due to the mammillary body component of their pathology. By contrast, BJ's recognition memory for similar material did not show such a rapid decline. Our findings demonstrate that damage to the limbic-diencephalic circuit leads to rapid loss of information over a ten minute period. It also confirms other findings (e.g. McKee & Squire, 1992) that longer term retention over a period of days is associated with normal rates of forgetting in amnesia, at least where recognition memory is concerned.

In other research studies, there has been little documentation of post-injury knowledge acquisition, and so our own report of a relatively consistent, though mild, impairment in this domain of memory functioning cannot be easily compared with published evidence. In the case of the patient HM, who probably sustained both hippocampal damage and also damage to adjacent limbic system and white matter structures, Gabrielli, Cohen & Corkin (1988) noted impaired 'semantic learning' for new knowledge such as vocabulary terms. In a study of a patient with amnesia following Herpes Simplex Encephalitis, Warrington and McCarthy (1988) and McCarthy and Warrington (1992) reported sparing of memory for definition of new terms, but impaired knowledge of events associated with famous personalities. The data from HM and the Herpes Encephalitic patient partly paralleled what we found in our patient, though the deficits shown by BJ in the area of knowledge acquisition appeared to be much milder than those found in the other two published cases. His impairment was particularly evident in respect of deaths of famous personalities - such events tend by their very nature to occur and to be reported as discrete events, rather than extend over a prolonged period as is the case for some news events. It is, therefore, not surprising that this proved to be the most sensitive measure of his limited impairment in knowledge acquisition.

In summary, it would appear that human mammillary body damage results in impaired anterograde memory. This is particularly evident where retention testing of items is - (i) Delayed; (ii) Tested by recall; (iii) Subject to interference from other items; (iv) Requires the retrieval of associations with other specific items, associations which normal subjects can typically exploit at retention test. Mammillary body damage does not result in permanent impairment of retrograde memory functioning. Mammillary body damage only affects recognition memory to a mild degree. The rapid forgetting shown by alcoholic Korsakoff patients in delayed recall settings may be due to the mammillary body component of their pathology. The syndrome found in Alcoholic Korsakoff patients is probably due to a combination of mammillary body damage, thalamic damage and neocortical damage. Mammillary body damage appears similar in its effects on memory to that of bilateral fornix or bilateral discrete hippocampal lesions. In itself, it is not a prerequisite for the presence of anterograde amnesia, but it appears to contribute as part of the limbic/Papez circuit. Finally, it remains possible that mammillary body lesions alone do not result in marked memory impairment, but that this impairment only arises when mammillary body lesions are accompanied by a second lesion, however minor, elsewhere in the limbic circuit.

ACKNOWLEDGEMENTS. The Wellcome Trust kindly provided financial support for this research. We thank Pamela Kimber and Rebecca Lund for their assistance. We are grateful to Alan Parkin for use of the sentence context memory task. We thank Dr John Aggleton, Professor L McLellan and Dr C Ward for helpful discussions about these cases. We also thank Dr S McKinstry and Dr J Winder of the Royal Victoria Hospital, Belfast for their cooperation with MR scanning. We are grateful to Dr P Lewis for assistance with the analyses of BJ's PET scan.

REFERENCES

Amaral DG. (1987). Memory: anatomical organization of candidate brain, In: J M Brookhard, VB Mountcastle (Eds) *Handbook of Physiology. The Nervous System, Volume V, Higher Functions of the Nervous System*. Bethesda. American Physiological Society: 211-293.

Bentley MD, Karwoski RA (1988) Estimation of tissue volume from serial radiographic sections: a statistical random marking method. *Investigative Radiology*, 23: 742-747.

Bigler ED, Nelson JE, Schmidt RD (1989) Mammillary body atrophy identified by magnetic resonance imaging in alcoholic amnestic (Korsakoff's) syndrome. Neuropsychological correlates. *Neuropsychiatry, Neuropsychology and Behavioural Neurology*, 3: 189-201.

Botez-Marquard T, Botez MI (1992) Visual memory deficits after damage to the anterior commissure and right fornix. *Archives of Neurology*, 49: 321-324.

Butters N, Cermak LS (1980) *Alcoholic Korsakoff's Syndrome: An Information Processing Approach*. New York: Academic Press.

Cascino GD, Jack CR, Parisi JE, Sharbrough FW, Hirschorn KA, Meyer FB, Marsh WR & O'Brein PC (1991) Magnetic resonance imaging-based volume studies in temporal lobe epilepsy: pathological correlations. *Annals of Neurology*, 30: 31-36.

Cermak LS, Verfaellie M (1992) The role of fluency in the implicit and explicit task performance of amnesic patients. In: Squire LS, Butters N (Eds) *The Neuropsychology of Memory, Second Edition*. New York: Guilford Press, 36-45.

Clark WE, Meyer M (1950) Anatomical relationships between the cerebral cortex and the hypothalamus *British Medical Bulletin*, 6: 341-345.

Cohen NJ, Squire LR (1981) Retrograde amnesia and remote memory impairment. *Neuropsychologia*, 19: 337-356.

Cohen AR & Albers HH. (1991) Disruption of human circadian and cognitive regulation following a discrete hypothalamic lesion.: A case study. *Neurology*, 41: 726-729.

Cook MJ, Fish DR, Shorvon SD, Straughan K, Stevens JM (1992) Hippocampal and morphometric studies in frontal and temporal lobe epilepsy. *Brain*, 115: 1001-1015.

Cramon Von DY, Hebel N, Schuri U (1988) Verbal memory and learning in unilateral posterior cerebral infarction. A report of 30 cases. *Brain*, 111: 1061-1077.

De Renzi, E., & Lucchelli, P. (1993). Dense retrograde amnesia, intact learning capability and abnormal forgetting rate: A consolidation deficit? *Cortex*, 29: 449-466.

Dusoir, H. Kapur, N. Byrnes, D. McKinstry S. & Hoare, R.D. (1990). The role of diencephalic pathology in human memory disorder: evidence from a penetrating paranasal brain injury. *Brain*, 113, 1695-1706.

Fazio F, Perani D, Gilardi MC, Colombo F, Cappa SF, Vallar G, Bettinardi V, Paulesu E, Alberoni M, Bressi S, Franceschi M & Lenzi GL. (1992) Metabolic impairments in human amnesia: A PET study of memory networks. *Journal of Cerebral Blood Flow and Metabolism*, 12, 353-358.

Frisk V, Milner B. (1990) The role of the left hippocampal region in the acquisition and retention of story content. *Neuropsychologia*, 28: 349-359.

Gabrieli, J. D. E., Cohen, N. J., & Corkin, S. (1988). The impaired learning of semantic knowledge following bilateral medial temporal lobe resection. *Brain and Cognition*, 7: 157-177.

Goldstein, LH, Polkey CE (1992) Behavioural memory after temporal lobectomy or amygdalo-hippocampectomy. *British Journal of Clinical Psychology*, 31: 75-81.

Goldstein, LH, Polkey CE (1993) Short-term cognitive changes after unilateral temporal lobectomy or unilateral amygdalo-hippocampectomy for the relief of temporal lobe epilepsy. *Journal of Neurology, Neurosurgery and Psychiatry*, 56: 135-140.

Hata T, Meyer JS, Tanahashi N, Ishikawa Y, Imai A, Shinohara T, Velez M, Fann WE, Kandula P & Sakai F. (1987) Three-dimensional mapping of local cerebral perfusion in alcoholic encephalopathy with and without Wernicke-Korsakoff syndrome. *Journal of Cerebral Blood Flow and Metabolism*, 7: 35-44.

Haymaker W. (1969) Blood supply of the human hypothalamus. In: Hayamker W, Anderson E, Nauta W (Eds) *The Hypothalamus*. Springfield, Ill.: Charles Thomas: 210-218.

Hierons R, Janota I, Corsellis JAN (1978) The late effects of necrotising encephalitis of the temporal lobes and limbic areas: a clinico-pathological study of ten cases. *Psychological Medicine*, 8: 21-42.

Hodges JH, Carpenter K. (1991) Anterograde amnesia with fornix damage following removal of IIIrd ventricle cyst. *Journal of Neurology, Neurosurgery & Psychiatry*, 54: 633-638.

Holmes EJ, Jacobson S, Stein BM, Butters N. (1983) Ablations of the mammillary nuclei in monkeys: Effects on post-operative memory. *Experimental Neurology*, 81: 97-113.

Jack CR, Sharborough FW, Cascino GD, Hirschorn KA, O'Brien PC, Marsh WR (1992) Magnetic resonance image-based hippocampal volumetry: correlation with outcome after temporal lobectomy. *Annals of Neurology*, 31: 138-146.

Jarho L (1973) Korsakoff-like amnesic syndrome in penetrating brain injury. *Acta Neurologica Scandinavica*, 49 (Supplementum 54): 1-156.

Kahn EA, Crosby EC (1972) Korsakoff's syndrome associated with surgical lesions involving the mammillary bodies. *Neurology*, 22: 117-125.

Kapur, N., Ellison, D., Smith, M., McLellan, D. L., & Burrows, E. H. (1992). Focal retrograde amnesia: a neuropsychological and magnetic resonance study. *Brain*, 115: 73-85.

Kapur N (1991) Amnesia in relation to fugue states - distinguishing a neurological from a psychogenic basis. *British Journal of Psychiatry*, 159: 872-877.

Kirk IJ, McNaughton N (1991) Supramammillary cell firing and hippocampal slow activity. *NeuroReport*, 2: 723-725.

Kopelman, M. D., Wilson, B., & Baddeley, A.D. (1990). *The Autobiographical Memory Interview*. Bury St Edmonds: Thames Valley Test Company.

Landi G, Giusti MC, & Guidotti M. (1982) Transient global amnesia due to left temporal lobe haemorrhage. *Journal of Neurology, Neurosurgery and Psychiatry*, 45: 1062-1063.

Lezak M (1983) *Neuropsychological Assessment. Second Edition*. New York: Oxford University Press.

Marinkovic S, Milisavljevic M, Puskas L. (1992) Microvascular anatomy of the hippocampal formation. *Surgical Neurology*, 37: 339-349.

Markowitsch, HJ (1988). Diencephalic amnesia: A reorientation towards tracts. *Brain Research Reviews*, 13: 351-370.

Mayes AR, Meudell R, Mann D, Pickering A (1987) Location of lesions in Korsakoff's syndrome: Neuropsychological and neuropathological data on two patients. *Cortex*, 24: 367-388.

Mayes, AR (1988). *Hunan Organic Memory Disorders*. New York: Cambridge University Press.

McCarthy RA, Warrington EK (1992) Actors but not scripts: The dissociation of people and events in retrograde amnesia. *Neuropsychologia*, 30: 633-644.

McKee RD, Squire LR (1992) Equivalent forgetting rates in long-term memory for diencephalic and medial temporal lobe amnesia. *The Journal of Neuroscience*, 12: 3765-3772.

McKenna, P., & Warrington, E. K., (1983). *Graded Naming Test*. Windsor: NFER-Nelson.

Nelson, H. E. (1982). *National Adult Reading Test*. Windsor: NFER-Nelson.

Parkin AJ, Hunkin NM (1993) Impaired temporal context memory on anterograde but not retrograde tests in the absence of frontal pathology. *Cortex*, 29: 267-280.

Shimamura AP, Janowsky JS, Squire LR (1991) What is the role of frontal lobe damage in memory disorders? In: HS Levin, HM Eisenberg , AL Benton (Eds), *Frontal Lobe Function and Dysfunction*. New York: Oxford University Press, pp. 173-198.

Solomon PR, Solomon SD, Schaaf EV & Perry HE (1983) Altered activity in the hippocampus is more detrimental to classical conditioning than removing the structure. *Science*, 220: 329-331.

Squire LR, Amaral DG, Zola-Morgan S, Kritchevsky M, Press G. (1989) Description of brain injury in the amnesic patient N.A. based on magnetic resonance imaging. *Experimental Neurology*, 105: 23-35.

Squire LR, Moore RY (1979) Dorsal thalamic lesion in a noted case of human memory dysfunction. *Annals of Neurology*, 6: 503-506.

Squire LR, Amaral DG, Press GA. (1990) Magnetic resonance imaging of the hippocampal formation and mammillary nuclei distinguish medial temporal lobe and diencephalic amnesia. *The Journal of Neuroscience*, 10: 3016-3117.

Squire LR   (1982) Comparisons between forms of amnesia: Some deficits are unique to Korsakoff's syndrome. *Journal of Experimental Psychology: Learning, Memory and Cognition*, 8: 560-571.

Tanabe H, Haskikawa K, Nakagawa Y, Yamamoto H, Harada K, Tsumoto T, Nishimura N, Shiraishi H & Kimura K (1991). Memory loss due to transient hypoperfusion in the medial temporal lobes including hippocampus. *Acta Neurologica Scandinavica*, 84: 22-27 & 463.

Torvik A. (1987) Topographic distribution and severity of brain lesions in Wernicke's encephalopathy. *Clinical Neuropathology*, 6: 25-29.

Trahan DE, Larrabee GJ. (1988) *Continuous Visual Memory Test*. Odessa, Florida: Psychological Assessment Resources.

Veazey RB, Amaral DG, Cowan WM (1982) The morphology and connections of the posterior hypothalamus in the cynomolgus monkey. II. Efferent connections. *Journal of Comparative Neurology*, 207: 135-156.

Victor M, Adams RD, Collins GH (1989) *The Wernicke-Korsakoff Syndrome and related neurologic disorders due to alcoholism and malnutrition. Second Edition.* Philadelphia: Davis.

Warrington, E. K. (1984). *Recognition Memory Test*. Windsor: NFER-Nelson.

Warrington, E. K., & McCarthy, R. (1988). The fractionation of retrograde amnesia. *Brain and Cognition*, 7: 184-200.

Watson C, Andermann F, Gloor P, Jones-Gotman M, Peters T, Evans A, Olivier A, Melanson D, Leroux G (1992) Anatomic basis of amygdaloid and hippocampal volume measurement by magnetic resonance imaging. *Neurology*, 42: 1743-1750.

Wechsler, D. (1981). *Wechsler Adult Intelligence Scale-Revised*. The Psychological Corporation: San Antonio.

Wechsler, D. (1987). *Wechsler Memory Scale- Revised*. San Antonio: Psychological Corporation.

Zola-Morgan S, Squire LR. (1993). Neuroanatomy of memory. *Annual Review of Neuroscience*, 16: 547-563.

Zola Morgan, S., Squire, L., & Amaral, D. (1986). Human amnesia and the medial temporal lobe region: Enduring memory impairment following a bilateral lesion limited to field CA1 of the Hippocampus. *The Journal of Neuroscience*, 6: 2950-2967.

13

Functional and Anatomical Specificity of Frontal Lobe Functions

DONALD T. STUSS[1] and MICHAEL P. ALEXANDER[2]

We both started our professional academic careers as fellows at the Boston Veterans Administration Medical Centre, one in psychology research and the other in behavioural neurology. It was a time of intellectual ferment and excitement, a period that has significantly influenced our subsequent academic endeavours. During that time there were at least four major areas of active neurobehavioural research at the V.A. - in neurology (Geschwind, Benson and Albert), in psycholinguistics and neuropsychology (Goodglass, Kaplan, Blumstein and Zurif), in right hemisphere cognition (Gardner) and in memory (Butters, Cermak and Oscar-Berman). Those of us lucky enough to work in that setting learned many important rules for our subsequent careers. It is difficult, looking back, to identify any one person as the creator or embodiment of any one rule, but Nelson Butters certainly was a critical teacher and example of them all.

First, collaborate. No one can know or do everything. Find people who complement your skills. Second, always remember the 'neuro' when doing neurobehavioural or neuropsychological research. There is, and must be, a

[1] DONALD T. STUSS, Ph.D. • Rotman Research Institute of Bayrest Centre, Departments of Psychology and Medicine (Neurology), University of Toronto

[2] MICHAEL P. ALEXANDER, M.D. • Braintree Hospital, Department of Neurology, Boston University

Neuropsychological Explorations of Memory and Cognition: Essays in Honor of Nelson Butters, edited by Laird S. Cermak, Ph.D. Plenum Press, New York, 1994

neural basis for the behaviours we study. In research grounded in lesion studies of animals the relationship is clear. In human lesion research this neural basis can be quite difficult to establish, but it should always be sought (Butters & Stuss, 1989). Third, a well-studied single case can illuminate cerebral function as well as any standard group experiment, but the case should motivate a particular neurobehavioural theory, not just report a "look-what-we-found" event. Fourth, test material must be able to answer the question. If it does, it doesn't matter if it is subverted from unrelated uses, applied exactly as its creator intended, or designed de novo for the specific question.

We would like to review some old and recent research that we hope demonstrate that we have been true to the lessons we learned from Nelson and his VA colleagues twenty years ago in Boston.

CLARIFICATION OF BRAIN - BEHAVIOR RELATIONS IN A GROUP STUDY

We had the opportunity to study five patients with spontaneous persistent confabulation (Stuss, Alexander, Lieberman, & Levine, 1978). At that time, several mechanisms of confabulation had been proposed, but none was satisfactory. The hypothesized causes ranged from a direct consequence of memory loss to psychological defense mechanisms. Our patients were all amnesic - although not all terribly severe - but they had different aetiologies. Thorough neuropsychological, neurological and CT imaging assessments pointed to a common biological factor in all five of our patients: each had documented frontal lobe pathology.

The frontal lobe pathology was, in turn, the key to illuminating the neuropsychological mechanism of confabulation. All five patients had substantiated deficits in higher level executive functions. In particular, all five had grossly deficient capacity to monitor their on-going performance, whether on neuropsychological tasks (i.e. card sorting) or in conversation (i.e., confabulations that defied elementary real world semantic knowledge). Even when constrained to generate a correct response, in testing by providing feedback or in conversation by providing cueing, the patients would not self correct their responses. The failure in attention and monitoring of immediate experience combined with defective access to accurate memories produced confabulations. The frontal lobe pathology was the neural basis for the monitoring deficits, a conclusion entirely compatible with then current (and still accepted) notions of prefrontal procedural function.

The simultaneous explanation at the levels of both anatomy and behaviour enabled us to present a unified theory about the mechanism of confabulation. These hypotheses have subsequently been supported and enlarged

at the levels of psychological theory (Johnson, 1991; Moscovitch, 1989) and
anatomy (Fischer et al., in press).

CASE STUDY

While group studies of well defined patients were a hallmark of the
Butters approach, investigation of the unique individual patient was always an
important methodology used by Butters and colleagues. A particular valuable
insight on the mechanisms of autobiographical memories was obtained by the
study of one patient, a university professor. This individual had written multiple
research papers, books and chapters, including an extensive autobiography
published two years prior to the acute onset of an amnesic condition secondary to
alcoholic Korsakoff Syndrome (Butters & Cermak, 1986). This detailed case
study provided convincing evidence for a two factor model of alcoholic retrograde
amnesia (Butters, 1984).

We had the opportunity to study a patient with a prolonged Capgras
Syndrome in which the patient was convinced that a new family (wife and five
children), almost identical to his "first family", had taken the place of the
original family (Alexander, Stuss, & Benson, 1979). Ten months after suffering
a serious traumatic brain injury and after a long difficult recovery, the patient
returned home for a weekend pass. There had been unusual circumstances
associated with the wife taking him home for that weekend. His wife had not
forewarned him of her arrival, her usual custom. She was driving a new car.
The teenage children were close to a year older and had physically changed. On
his return from the weekend, the patient demonstrated a focal problem of
disorientation.

In this family, the wife and all five children had the same names and
general appearances as the wife and children of his "first" family. He
acknowledged that they looked a great deal alike but that he could - through some
intuition that he could not explain - tell them apart, i.e., tell the "first" (real)
from the "second" (imposter) families. This delusion of imposters, known as
Capgras Syndrome in psychiatry, had been described in schizophrenia, psychotic
depression and dementia. We suggested that there was a significant parallel
between the Capgras Syndrome and a neurologic disorder labelled reduplicative
paramnesia. Following the hierarchal theory -anatomy into psychology - that
we developed for the confabulation group, we proposed a similar theory for
Capgras Syndrome and reduplicative paramnesia. All three - confabulation,
reduplication and Capgras delusions - seem to require a disturbance in higher
order executive functions as described above. Furthermore, confabulation and
reduplication seem invariably to have these executive deficits due to structural
frontal lesions. The neural lesion in schizophrenia is, of course, different, but
the functional effects are still profound. The relevance of frontal system

dysfunction in the emergence of Capgras delusions in schizophrenia has recently been confirmed in psychiatric patients without acute acquired brain pathology. Two groups of schizophrenic patients matched in most regards except for the presence or absence of the Capgras Syndrome were compared. There was significant pathology in the anterior brain regions of those patients who exhibited the Capgras Syndrome (Joseph, O'Leary, & Wheeler, 1990).

Additional observations in this case provided closure with other disparate clinical observations. One observation has great relevance for our subsequent research in frontal functions which has always proposed specific regional and lateral frontal lesion effects. Our patient had predominantly right hemispheric pathology. The importance of the right hemisphere in the patients with reduplicative paramnesia, particularly the right frontal region (perhaps in combination with other brain lesions), had been emphasized earlier (Benson, Gardiner, & Meadows, 1976). A more recent publication also emphasized that the right frontal lobe plays a significant role in the disorder of personal recollections such as the Capgras Syndrome (Malloy, Cimino, & Westlake, 1991).

Pick, in his description of reduplicative paramnesia, emphasized the importance of intuitive familiarity for a sense of conscious continuity of experience. The possibility that the right hemisphere's limbic circuitry had particular importance for generating familiarity judgements came from the epilepsy literature (Mullan & Penfield, 1959). That our patient could not maintain a sense of familiarity across time, or had two separate but similar familiarity judgements which he could not reconcile, seemed to be critical to his reduplication. We concluded that one role of higher order frontal functioning might be monitoring familiarity and that disturbed monitoring was related to disturbed thinking and problem solving. One of us have subsequently expanded these observations (Benson & Stuss, 1990; Stuss, 1991 a,b) to a general theory for the psychological mechanism of delusions in both psychiatric and neurologic diseases.

THE COGNITIVE APPROACH

Nelson Butters always emphasized detection of specifically disturbed cognitive processes. Butters and his colleagues used tests devised by other theoreticians as they might be applicable to the population being studied (Brown, 1958; Peterson & Peterson, 1959), or developed their own tests (Albert, Butters, & Brandt, 1980). The value of this approach was clear; consequently, we in turn were ready to borrow from Butters and Cermak. In an early study of the effects of frontal lobe damage on memory, we examined patients who had undergone prefrontal leucotomy 25 years earlier for treatment of schizophrenia (Stuss, Kaplan, Benson, Weir, Chiulli, & Sarazin, 1982). A large series of clinical neuropsychological memory tests were administered. Cognitive tests were borrowed from other published work, particularly that of Butters and Cermak (Butters & Cermak, 1974; Cermak & Butters, 1972), based on the Brown-Peterson paradigm.

The Brown-Peterson test that we used required the subject to recall three consonants after varying delays filled by interference by the subject counting backwards by threes. The results were striking. The patients with leucotomy who had achieved good recovery, and who also had the largest frontal brain lesions (Naeser, Levine, Benson, Stuss, & Weir, 1981), were equivalent to a matched control group on standard memory tasks, including the Wechsler Memory Scale. In contrast, their performance on the Brown-Peterson was significantly impaired. Even though there was no amnesia defined operationally by an IQ minus MQ difference, it was clear that the leucotomized patients were significantly impaired in recalling the information after having created interference by counting backwards. This important difference between performance on a clinical test of memory and the Brown-Peterson test, derived from the theoretical cognitive processing literature, is illustrated in Figure 1.

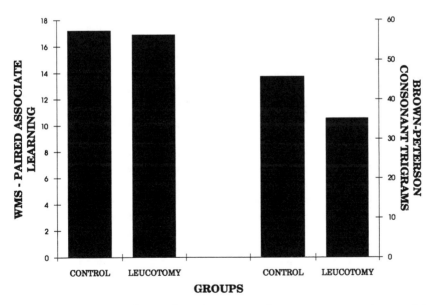

Figure 1.   A comparison of performance of two groups, patients with orbitofrontal leucotomies and matched controls, on two "memory tests".

The discrepancy between the results on the paired associate and Brown-Peterson tests conformed to contemporary theories of frontal function (Fuster, 1980; Moscovitch, 1981). We suggested that the impairment on the Brown-Peterson reflected deficient performance in supervisory executive function, essentially a working memory deficit due to poor control of attention. Furthermore, we proposed that prefrontal structures (right and left) were critical to maintain this control. Modern theories of the attentional responsibilities of the frontal lobes (Shallice, 1988; Stuss, Eskes, & Foster, in press) support our findings. The particular sensitivity of the Brown-Peterson test to damage in the frontal region (although localization is yet to be clearly specified) has also been confirmed (Parkin, Leng, Stanhope, & Smith, 1988).

Focus on Specific Processes and Patient Groups

All amnesics are not the same. Considerable disagreement in initial research on amnesia arose from different laboratories studying different amnesic populations. The controversy about the appropriate grouping of amnesics - by deficit profile or by lesion or by aetiology - has influenced our research strategies. In our current research on frontal deficits we have attempted to use the most appropriate elements of grouping by lesions and by comparable aetiology to be certain that different behaviours were not uninteresting artifacts of neurology as opposed to principled regional differences. We can illustrate this operational lesson from ongoing work (Stuss, Alexander, Palumbo, Buckle, Sayer, & Pogue, in press).

In our attempts to understand the memory deficits reported in patients with frontal lobe damage, we began with our conclusion: frontal lobe functions cannot be reduced to a single process. To ensure that we could generalize our behavioural conclusions to specific frontal regions, we used the two selection criteria, focused lesions and comparable aetiologies: 1) all patients had lesions restricted to frontal structures and grouped by regional involvement, and 2) all patients had damage of acute onset - haemorrhage, infarction, trauma or surgical complication.

In addition to characterizing the patient lesion as specifically as possible, we hypothesized particular deficit profiles and selected tests that would assess and measure these domains unambiguously. The dependent measure came from psychology - word list learning. The independent measures came from experimental psychology. Manipulations in the dependent measures were informed by extensive observations in cognitive science. Standard clinical neuropsychological tests provided a descriptive measure of baseline functioning. CT and MR imaging created independent variables of regional frontal lesion location and of lesion site.

The results were clear: performance on the word list learning task was determined by many factors and there was not a single 'frontal' factor. A certain number of patients were actually impaired on delayed recognition memory, unanticipated from available research, but the reasons were clear from imaging studies and from clinical neuropsychological findings. The presence of any pathology in the relatively small frontal limbic structures - septum, basal forebrain or posterior part of the anterior cingulate - even without clinical significant amnesia was associated with significant recognition impairment (see Figure 2). Second, the presence of even the mildest naming deficits on neuropsychological testing uniformly predicted impaired recognition memory, even though the anomic patients had unilateral left dorsolateral - not limbic - lesions. Thus, a quantitatively similar level of performance on a recognition test could be due one of two entirely different factors.

Many patients had impaired secondary memory, defined by the number of items that intervened between encoding and recall. These patients were characterized by the size of the lesion in the left frontal region, and by a correlation with language performance. Another group of patients were not significantly impaired on free recall, but had a significant deficit in their ability to monitor their performance, as though they could not recognise previously recalled words. These patients tended to have damage in the right frontal region. In addition to these highly regionally specific causes of impaired memory after

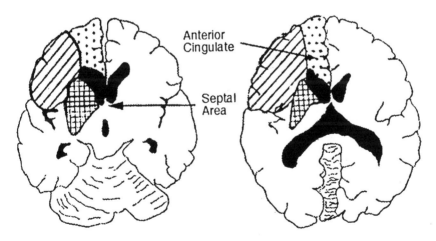

Figure 2. A depiction of the brain region related to a deficit in performance on a one hour delayed recognition performance.

frontal lesion, there was one general deficit of all frontal lesions: organization of recall. Thus, a single task -list learning - revealed four different region-specific processes affecting learning and recall and one general process that seems related to supervisory control.

AN OVERVIEW

We have reviewed how our own research has attempted to incorporate the lessons learned from Nelson Butters' and his colleagues at the Boston V.A. Nelson, however, has had more impact than that based on his research, important as that is. A word of encouragement, a letter of recommendation, a suggestion of important areas to research - through these and other means he has fostered many careers. Nelson Butters has provided us with many examples to emulate.

All great teachers do more than provide rules for careers. They provide examples and support. Never one to suffer fools gladly or blandly encourage the unacceptable, Nelson's advice to us on all professional matters was direct and critical - critical in the good sense of considered not rash, rooted in data and experience, and detailed and correct even when we were not.

ACKNOWLEDGEMENTS. Research presented in this chapter has been assisted by grants funds to the first author from the Ontario Mental Health Foundation and the Medical Research Council of Canada. We are grateful to our collaborators noted in the original publications. P. Mathews typed the manuscript.

REFERENCES

Albert, M.S., Butters, N., & Brandt, J. (1980). Memory for remote events in alcoholics. *Journal of Studies in Alcohol, 41*, 1071-1081.

Alexander, M.P., Stuss, D.T., & Benson, D.F. (1979). Capgras syndrome: a reduplicative phenomenon. *Neurology, 29*, 334-339.

Benson, D.F., Gardner, H., & Meadows, J.C. (1976). Reduplicative paramnesia. *Neurology, 26*, 147-151.

Benson, D.F., & Stuss, D.T. (1990). Frontal lobe influences on delusions: A clinical perspective. *Schizophrenia Bulletin, 16*, 403-411.

Brown, J. (1958). Some tests of the decay theory of immediate memory. *Quarterly Journal of Experimental Psychology, 10*, 12-21.

Butters, N. (1984). Alcoholic Korsakoff's Syndrome: An update. *Seminars in Neurology, 4*, 229-247.

Butters, N., & Cermak, L. (1974). Some comments on Warrington and Baddeley's report of normal short-term memory in amnesic patients. *Neuropsychologia, 12*, 283-285.

Butters, N., & Cermak, L.S. (1986). A case study of the forgetting of autobiographical knowledge: Implications for the study of retrograde amnesia. In D.C. Rubin (Ed.), *Autobiographical memory*. Cambridge: Cambridge University Press, pp. 253-272.

Butters, N. & Stuss, D.T. (1989). Diencephalic amnesia. In F. Boller & J. Grafman (Eds.), *Handbook of neuropsychology, Vol. 3*. Amsterdam: Elsevier, pp. 107-148.

Cermak, L.S., & Butters, N. (1972). The role of interference and encoding in the short-term memory deficits of Korsakoff patients. *Neuropsychologia 10*, 89-95.

Fischer, R.S., Alexander, M.P., D'Espesito, M., & Otto, R. (in press). Neuropsychological and neuroanatomical correlates of confabulation. *Journal of Clinical and Experimental Neuropsychology*.

Fuster, J.M. (1980). *The prefrontal cortex. Anatomy, physiology and neuropsychology of the frontal lobe*. New York: Raven Press.

Johnson, M.K. (1991). Reality monitoring: Evidence from confabulation in organic brain disease patients. In G.P. Prigatano & D.L. Schacter (Eds.), *Awareness of deficit after brain injury: Clinical and theoretical issues*. New York: Oxford University Press, pp. 176-197.

Joseph, A.B., O'Leary, D.H., & Wheeler, H.G. (1990). Bilateral atrophy of the frontal and temporal lobes in schizophrenic patients with Capgras Syndrome: A case-control study using computed tomography. *Journal of Clinical Psychiatry, 51*, 332-325.

Malloy, P., Cimino, C., & Westlake, R. (1991). Differential diagnosis of primary and secondary Capgras delusions. *Neuropsychiatry, Neuropsychology, and Behavioral Neurology, 4*, 90-108.

Moscovitch, M. (1981). Multiple dissociations of function in the amnesic syndrome. In L.S. Cermak (Ed.), *Human memory and amnesia*. Hillsdale, N.J.: Lawrence Erlbaum Associates.

Moscovitch, M. (1989). Confabulation and the frontal systems: Strategic versus associative retrieval in neuropsychological theories of memory. In H.L. Roediger III & F.I.M. Craik (Eds.), *Varieties of memory and consciousness: Essays in honour of Endel Tulving*. Hillsdale, N.J.: Lawrence Erlbaum Associates, pp. 133-160.

Mullan, S., & Penfield, W. Illusions of comparative interpretation and emotion. *Archives of Neurology and Psychiatry, 81*, 269-289.

Naeser, M.A., Levine, H.L., Benson, D.F., Stuss, D.T., & Weir, W.S. (1981). Frontal leukotomy size and hemispheric asymmetries on computerized tomographic scans of schizophrenics with variable recovery. *Archives of Neurology, 38*, 30-37.

Parkin, A.J., Leng, N.R.C., Stanhope, N., & Smith, A.P. (1988). Memory impairment following ruptured aneurysm of the anterior communicating artery. *Brain and Cognition, 7*, 231-243.

Peterson, L. & Peterson, M.J. (1959). Short-term retention of individual verbal items. *Journal of Experimental Psychology, 58*, 193-198.

Shallice, T. (1988). *From neuropsychology to mental structure*. Cambridge: Cambridge University Press.

Stuss, D.T. (1991a). Self, awareness, and the frontal lobes: A neuropsychological perspective. In J. Strauss & G.R. Goethals (Eds.), *The self: Interdisciplinary approaches*. New York: Springer-Verlag, pp. 255-278.

Stuss, D.T. (1991b). Disturbance of self-awareness after frontal system damage. In G. Prigatano & D. Schacter (Eds.), *Awareness of deficit after brain injury. Clinical and theoretical issues*. New York: Oxford University Press, pp. 63-83.

Stuss, D.T., Alexander, M.P., Lieberman, A. & Levine, H. (1978). An extraordinary form of confabulation. *Neurology, 28*, 1166-1172.

Stuss, D.T., Alexander, M.P., Palumbo, C.L., Buckle, L., Sayer, L. & Pogue, J. (in press). Organizational strategies of patients with unilateral or bilateral frontal lobe injury in word list learning tasks. *Neuropsychology*.

Stuss, D.T., Eskes, G.A., & Foster, J.K. (in press). Experimental neuropsychological studies of frontal lobe functions. In F. Boller & J. Grafman (Eds.), *Handbook of Neuropsychology, Vol. 9*. Elsevier, Amsterdam.

Stuss, D.T., Kaplan, E.F., Benson, D.F., Weir, W.S., Chiulli, S. & Sarazin, F.F. (1982). Evidence for the involvement of orbitofrontal cortex in memory functions: An interference effect. *Journal of Comparative and Physiological Psychology, 6*, 913-925.

14

Recovery of Function after Focal Cerebral Insult

A Pet Activation Study

MURRAY GROSSMAN[1], LETICIA PELTZER[1], MARK D'ESPOSITO[1], ABASS ALAVI[2], and MARTIN REIVICH[1]

Nelson Butters is world-renowned for his investigations of human cognitive disorders. Butters' seminal explorations of subhuman primate cognition with his collaborators Donald G. Stein and Jeffrey J. Rosen, while not as well-known, have been equally influential in directing another important area of research. These investigators were pathbreaking in their examinations of the mechanisms underlying recovery of function following lesions of dorsolateral frontal cortex in monkeys. Butters and his colleagues [e.g. 1973, 1974; Rosen et al, 1971] hypothesized that cortex immediately adjacent to a cortical lesion, as well as more distant association cortices, play a critical role in recovery and reorganization of function following cortical ablation in the adult. This work anticipated more recent investigations of CNS plasticity and reorganization following insult in subhuman primates [e.g. Kaas, 1992]. As we suggest below, the lessons derived from Butters' prescient observations of primates may also provide powerful constraints on modeling in human cognitive neuroscience.

---

[1] MURRAY GROSSMAN, M.D., LETICIA PELTZER, MARK D'ESPOSITO, M.D., MARTIN REIVICH • Department of Neurology, University of Pennsylvania School of Medicine
[2] ABASS ALAVI • Department of Radiology, University of Pennsylvania School of Medicine

Neuropsychological Explorations of Memory and Cognition: Essays in Honor of Nelson Butters, edited by Laird S. Cermak, Ph.D. Plenum Press, New York, 1994

Cognitive neuroscientists have typically assumed that the residual cognitive architecture following a lesion is the normal system minus the lesioned component. This view has been articulated most elegantly by Caramazza [1986] as his "transparency assumption". Briefly, Caramazza stated that the effects of brain damage on a cognitive system must leave the remaining components undamaged, and that new processing structures must not be created as a consequence of brain damage. Indeed, he felt that normal cognitive processes could not be informed by neuropsychological investigations unless the neural network remaining after insult reflected the normal state except for the ablated element. The conservation of function inherent in the "transparency assumption" has been adopted without challenge by several different theoretical approaches within cognitive neuroscience. For example, flow diagrams often characterize information processing models of neurologically impaired performance simply by deleting the abnormal process or connection from the model [McCarthy & Warrington, 1991]. Similarly, parallel distributed processing models of cognitive functioning attempt to replicate abnormal behavior by "lesioning" a trained system, that is, by removing some proportion of the units from a fully functional model [Hinton & Shallice, 1991; Patterson et al, 1989b].

Counter-examples to the "transparency assumption" have been suggested from time to time. For example, deep dyslexia is said to follow a large lesion in the left hemisphere, and the peculiar pattern of reading errors associated with this syndrome has been attributed to the intact right hemisphere or to non-lesioned regions within the left hemisphere [e.g. Coltheart, 1980; Landis et al, 1983; Patterson et al, 1989a]. Explanations for deep dyslexia such as these imply that the remaining brain regions supporting reading do not reflect only the normal reading system, but the unusual errors may mirror the contribution of brain regions that do not ordinarily participate in reading. The reading process thus may have been reorganized in an attempt to compensate in part for the impairment. Examples such as these are potentially important since they may provide important neurophysiological constraints on the nature of modeling in cognitive neuroscience. In the context of observations such as these, investigators such as Kosslyn and van Kleek [1990] have called to question Caramazza's "transparency assumption", and have emphasized the importance of understanding the cerebral basis for neuropsychological functioning. *In vivo* neurophysiological monitoring of cerebral functioning during the performance of a cognitive task in a brain-damaged state has been rare [e.g. Grady et al, 1990; Weiller et al, 1992], however, so it has been difficult to marshall support for this alternative. We present preliminary evidence from a PET activation study of a stroke patient that challenges the "transparency assumption". If accurate, our preliminary observations begin to suggest that additional components must be incorporated in models of cognitive functioning to make them biologically more plausible.

RC is a 64-year-old, right-handed salesman with an unremarkable past medical history who suffered an acute hemorrhagic stroke in the posterior aspects of the left temporal convexity (Figure 1). His recovery during the subsequent 24 months prior to the PET study was unremarkable but incomplete. Clinical examination at the time of the PET study revealed the patient to have fluent spontaneous speech with frequent word-finding pauses and semantic paraphasic errors. He misnamed knife "nail", a safety pin was "stick", a padlock was "keys", and a spoon was "...a dish, no a cup, no a drink", for example. His comprehension of single words and simple sentences was impaired, although his repetition was relatively preserved. He found it difficult to understand or execute sequential commands such as "Point to the pen after the book", although he could repeat these sentences. RC's clinical examination thus was consistent with a so-called transcortical sensory aphasia, as confirmed by his performance on the Western Aphasia Battery [Kertesz, 1979] (Table 1).

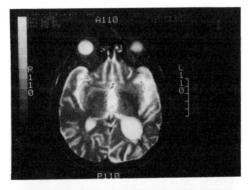

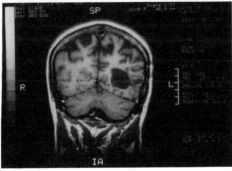

Figure 1. MRI of RC showing infarction in the postero-lateral aspects of the left temporal lobe. The left hemisphere is displayed on the right of each image. The upper panel shows a transaxial view at a mid-temporal level; the lower panel shows a coronal view at a posterior temporal level.

TABLE 1

PERFORMANCE OF RC ON THE WESTERN APHASIA BATTERY

TASK	SCORE
Spontaneous speech	14/20
Comprehension	6/10
Repetition	8/10
Naming	6/10

Additional studies documenting the nature of RC's cognitive impairment are provided in Table 2. These observations confirmed the difficulty experienced by RC in manipulating semantic information. He often erred in his category membership decisions of pictures and words, accepting semantically-related foils (e.g. "lemon") as instances of a target superordinate (e.g. "vegetable") although not confusing these with semantically unrelated superordinates (e.g. "furniture"). On a multiple choice recognition picture naming task, all of his errors were semantically related to the target name.

TABLE 2

PERFORMANCE OF RC ON ADDITIONAL COMPREHENSION MEASURES

TASK	SCORE
Semantic judgments (pictures)[1]	
-targets	22/29 (75.9% correct)
-semantic foils	12/24 (50.0% correct)
Multiple choice recognition picture naming[2]	80% correct - 100% errors semantic foils
Quantifier-picture match[3]	18/30 (60% correct)
-semantic errors	8/12 (67%)
-grammatical errors	4/12 (33%)
Semantic anomaly sentence judgments[4]	145/196 (74.0% correct)
New word learning[5]	
-semantic characteristics	10/20 (50.0% correct)
Triadic comparison judgments[6]	51% category violations

NOTES

1. RC was asked to evaluate color pictures according to the probe: "Is this a vegetable?" There were equal numbers of targets and foils, and some foils violated semantic attributes of the target category [Grossman & Mickanin, submitted].

2. RC was asked to match an orally-presented word with one of four line drawings. Foils included semantic, perceptual and unrelated alternatives to the target picture's name.

3. RC matched quantifiers such as "much" and "few" used in simple sentences ("Show me the container with many") to one of four pictures depicting (large/small) amounts of (mass/count) types of material [Grossman et al, 1993 c].

4. RC judged the anomaly of simple subject-predicate sentences such as "The cow is hungry" and *"The door is hungry". There were equal numbers of coherent and anomalous sentences [Grossman et al, in preparation b].

5. RC was exposed to a new verb in a naturalistic setting, and 10 minutes later we probed his recall of semantic and grammatical attributes of the new word. Semantic knowledge was assessed with a picture judgment task, where half of the pictures violated a specific attribute associated with the word's meaning [Grossman et al, in press].

6. RC chose the pair of three available verbs that went best together. The set of words consisted of 5 motion verbs (e.g. "crawl", "jump") and 5 cognition verbs ("think", "suggest") [Grossman et al, in preparation c].

He made semantic errors on a sentence-picture matching task (e.g. matching "the jar contains many" with a picture of a small number of grapes). RC also encountered difficulty detecting semantic anomalies on a sentence judgment task (e.g. he was as likely to accept "the plate is thirsty" as "the boy is thirsty"). In his acquisition of a new word, he performed randomly in his judgments of pictures that depicted the new word's meaning. On a triadic comparison task involving similarity judgments of a set of 5 cognition verbs and 5 motion verbs, his judgments violated the semantic distinction between motion and cognition as often as he respected this distinction.

PET scanning of RC used an equilibrium technique [Jones et al, 1985] described in greater detail elsewhere [Grossman et al, 1992]. Briefly, the equilibrium CBF technique involves the administration of ^{15}O-H_2O through an antecubital vein while arterial samples are obtained every 3 minutes from the opposite radial artery at the wrist. ^{15}O-H_2O is infused for 8 minutes at a constant rate at the beginning of each study to attain a steady state. The ^{15}O-H_2O infusion is then continued at the same rate while positron emission data are then collected for PET scans during ten minute segments, allowing us to capture enough counts at a favorable signal-to-noise ratio to produce an easily interpretable image for each individual. Eight minute gaps separate successive PET scans. rCBF is calculated from the equation [Subramanyam et al, 1978]:

$$rCBF = \frac{1}{C_a/C_T - 1/p}.$$

where l is the decay constant of ^{15}O (0.335/min), C_a is the arterial concentration of ^{15}O-H_2O obtained from arterial blood samples drawn during the equilibrium phase, C_T is the tissue concentration of ^{15}O obtained from the PET scan, and p is the brain-blood partition coefficient for water (0.98ml/g in gray matter).

CBF was assessed in RC and 6 age- and education-matched control subjects. The room had subdued lighting and a white noise background was heard. A foam head restraint was used to position a subject's head during the scan, and head position was continuously monitored with a laser alignment system. The PET images were obtained by a scanner (UGM, Philadelphia PA) that acquires 64 transverse slices simultaneously as a volume with a voxel size of 2 x 2 x 2 mm^3. The spatial resolution of the device is 5.5 mm in X, Y, and Z axes [Karp et al, 1990]. The attenuation correction method assumed an average attenuation coefficient for each image [Bergstrom et al, 1982]. The images were analyzed using a semi-automated region of interest (ROI) template system based on the Talairach and Tournoux [1988] atlas. Thus, each patient's MRI was sliced in the anterior commissure-posterior commissure (AC-PC) plane. The computerized atlas was then applied to each patient's MRI in order to create an individualized anatomic atlas. The PET images, 8 mm thick and overlapping 4 mm, were sliced in the same AC-PC plane as the MRI according to a reliable procedure used in our laboratory. The individualized anatomic template was then applied to every other transaxial slice of each subject's PET image in a user-independent fashion.

We report the results of an "activation baseline" and two "cognitive challenges". During the activation baseline, the subject responds simply to the presentation of each successive stimulus by alternately dorsiflexing and plantarflexing the great toes. One cognitive challenge was a letter judgment task, where the patient was asked to decide whether a word contains the letter "r". The second cognitive challenge was a semantic category judgment task, where the patient was asked to decide whether the stimulus word is a vegetable. Subjects responded to the cognitive challenge by dorsiflexing ("yes") or plantarflexing ("no") their toes. Subjects were trained on each task during a portion of the 8 minute break between scans. The stimulus material for each PET scan was the same set of 80 single familiar words printed in lower case white block letters on a black background. There were equal numbers of positive and negative stimuli associated with each cognitive challenge. Thus, half of the stimuli did not contain the target letter, and half of the words were non-target foils (e.g. fruit or furniture). Across each dimension of interest, the words were matched for frequency of occurrence, word length, and grammatical form class.

During the PET protocol, RC and the control subjects were accurate at identifying target letters in words (99% correct). Control subjects were 96.5% correct in their category membership judgments, but RC was correct only in 82% of his category membership judgments. He was random in his judgments of semantically related foils, accepting fruit names as vegetables, and he also erred on some judgments of less representative exemplars of the target category.

Table 3 presents rCBF during the activation baseline in control subjects, and ratio data for letter judgments and category membership judgments. In order to account for individual differences in overall brain activity, the activation data were normalized to whole brain CBF under each condition. These ratios were then normalized to the activation baseline region:whole brain ratios for each region in order to account for non-specific task demands. Analyses of variance (ANOVAs) for PET activation effects in each brain region of control subjects revealed a significant difference between conditions in left angular gyrus [F(2,12)=3.17; p<.05]. Figure 2 summarizes the differences in normalized rCBF between the letter judgments and the category membership judgments. Since these tasks were identical in every way except for the cognitive probe, we could subtract rCBF during the letter judgment condition from rCBF during the category membership judgment condition in order to identify the critical brain regions contributing to category membership judgments. Figure 2 thus reveals that the significant condition effect was due to the increased CBF in left angular gyrus under the category membership condition. This increase, averaging 13%, was seen in each of the 6 control subjects.

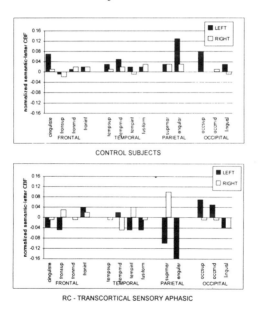

Figure 2. Differences between normalized regional cerebral blood flows (rCBFs) during the category membership judgment condition and the letter judgment condition. The upper panel shows rCBF differences in control subjects; the lower panel shows rCBF differences in RC.

TABLE 3

MEAN (S.E.M.) REGIONAL CEREBRAL BLOOD FLOW (rCBF) DURING
   BASELINE,
AND NORMALIZED CBF RATIOS DURING LETTER JUDGMENTS
AND CATEGORY MEMBERSHIP JUDGMENTS

REGION	WNL baseline[1]	letter[2]	category [2]	RC - TCS APHASIC baseline[1]	letter[2]	category [2]
FRONTAL						
lcingant	45.8 (9.2)	1.47	1.41	25	1.33	1.27
rcingant	42.9 (7.4)	1.46	1.47	25	1.24	1.23
lfronsup	29.4 (3.5)	0.98	0.97	21	0.95	0.90
rfronsup	27.9 (4.2)	1.01	0.99	21	0.99	1.03
lfronmid	29.4 (3.8)	1.05	1.06	19	1.00	1.00
rfronmid	26.8 (3.4)	0.94	0.95	23	1.24	1.23
lfroninf	35.1 (5.1)	1.19	1.18	20	1.05	1.09
rfroninf	30.3 (3.7)	1.07	1.09	26	1.38	1.41
TEMPORAL						
ltempsup	30.8 (4.3)	1.02	1.03	18	0.95	0.95
rtempsup	30.0 (4.4)	1.02	1.00	25	1.33	1.32
ltempmid	27.3 (3.1)	0.93	0.98	14	0.71	0.73
rtempmid	28.0 (3.3)	0.98	0.99	24	1.33	1.27
ltempinf	28.2 (3.1)	0.98	1.01	11	0.57	0.55
rtempinf	28.3 (3.3)	0.96	0.98	23	1.14	1.18
lfusiform	41.5 (6.4)	1.43	1.39	19	1.10	1.05
rfusiform	45.0 (7.3)	1.37	1.36	25	1.38	1.36
PARIETAL						
lsuprmar	24.5 (8.6)	0.83	0.89	18	1.00	0.91
rsuprmar	24.6 (3.3)	0.84	0.88	25	1.10	1.23
langular[3]	23.5 (3.7)	0.80	0.88	15	0.95	0.82
rangular	23.6 (3.5)	0.82	0.85	20	1.14	1.13
OCCIPITAL						
loccsup	41.5 (5.9)	1.35	1.46	22	1.19	1.27
roccsup	37.9 (5.8)	1.24	1.22	24	1.33	1.32
loccmid	34.1 (4.1)	1.17	1.19	18	0.95	1.00
roccmid	31.4 (4.2)	1.09	1.09	23	1.19·	1.18
llingual	42.3 (7.1)	1.31	1.30	19	0.95	0.91
rlingual	39.8 (6.2)	1.30	1.25	24	1.24	1.18
whole brain	29.3 (3.6)	-	-	19.3	-	-

Notes
   1. Baseline data are cerebral blood flow (CBF) in ml/100cc/min.

2. Letter and category membership data are rCBF normalized to whole brain CBF during each activation, and this ratio is normalized to region:whole brain CBF obtained at baseline.

3. A significant condition effect was seen in left angular gyrus, where an F-ratio exceeded p<.05. T-tests comparing normalized CBF during activations found a significant difference between category membership judgments and letter judgments.

Table 3 also reveals the baseline rCBF and the normalized rCBF under letter judgment and category membership judgment conditions for RC. It can be seen that there was a mild reduction in CBF in many left hemisphere regions when compared to the homologous right hemisphere regions. The largest deviation from right hemisphere rCBF was evident in left posterior temporal regions where RC's stroke was located. Figure 2 summarizes differences in the rCBF recruitment patterns of RC during the letter judgment condition and category membership judgment condition. As can be seen, increases in rCBF were seen in the right inferior parietal lobule rather than the left, and in left occipital association regions adjacent to the stroke. When contrasted with the recruitment pattern seen during his letter judgments, the single brain region exhibiting the greatest rCBF increase during category membership judgments was the right supramarginal gyrus (10%).

In summary, these preliminary findings indicate that RC has a characteristic semantic impairment. He apparently confuses exemplars of a concept with related items that are not exemplars, and has semantic paraphasic errors in his naming and spontaneous expression. Since parallel deficits were seen in comprehension and expression, his problem could not be easily attributed to the modality of assessment. His deficit is unlikely to be due to the material used to present the stimuli since the impairment involves both pictures and words. This pattern of findings has been documented previously in other patients clinically resembling RC [Grossman and Wilson, 1986; Grossman and Carey, 1987; Hillis et al, 1989]. Moreover, investigators such as Bouchard et al [1979], Hart and Gordon [1989], and Rubens and Kertesz [1983] have demonstrated semantic impairments following lesions to similar, posterior temporal and inferior parietal areas of the left hemisphere. PET studies of neurologically intact subjects have also emphasized the critical nature of this brain region in the processing of single words for meaning [Demonet et al, 1992; Wise et al, 1991].

Importantly, insult to this region has not completely devastated semantic processing in RC since he appeared to be able to make some, albeit crude, semantic decisions. While unable to determine reliably whether a lemon is a vegetable, for example, RC was accurate in deciding that a chair is not a vegetable. Investigators such as Zaidel [1978] have claimed that the right hemisphere is capable of appreciating some semantic distinctions, and speculation has been that this is due to a disinhibition of right hemisphere functioning following an interruption of left hemisphere control. Investigators such as Patterson et al [1989a] and Landis et al [1983] have invoked observations such as these in their explanation for the semantic paralexias and other errors seen in deep dyslexia. Others have noted that residual left hemisphere functioning may contribute to the reading errors seen in deep dyslexia [e.g. Besner, 1983; Marshall & Patterson, 1983; Roeltgen, 1987], possibly associated with collateral sprouting of axons from partially damaged neurons into adjacent cortical fields that are intact. Regardless of the specific neurophysiologic mechanism that underlies the apparent plasticity of the adult central nervous system, it is evident that considerable recovery of function can be attained following insult to the mature brain [St. James-Roberts, 1981; Teuber, 1975]. We hypothesize that the pattern of performance in RC may not be associated simply with a lesion that interrupts the cognitive architecture supporting the manipulation of semantic information. Instead, our preliminary PET activation findings in RC suggest that his pattern of cognitive performance may also associated with the recruitment of brain structures that are not ordinarily activated in controls. These observations support Butters' [e.g. 1973, 1974] primate work, and specifically suggest that alternative brain structures adjacent to the lesion or related association cortex structures at some distance from the lesion may compensate in part for the consequences of insult that interferes with cognitive performance.

Most approaches to the modeling of cognition in neuropsychology have accepted without challenge that the residual cognitive system following a lesion is a straightforward reflection of the native cognitive apparatus that supported the task prior to the lesion. If our preliminary observations are correct, recovery of function data suggest that additional components must be incorporated into these cognitive models. These components may not have participated in the task prior to a lesion, as suggested by observations of control subjects during PET activation procedures [also cf. Demonet et al, 1992; Wise et al, 1991], but it may be possible to recruit components such as these to bootstrap a compromised cognitive architecture after a lesion has removed a critical element. Clearly additional work is needed to help characterize the nature of these compensatory mechanisms. *In vivo* neurophysiological observations such as these nevertheless help constrain future modeling in cognitive neuroscience, and specifically guide these models in a biologically plausible fashion. Butters' prescient observations of cortical reorganization in primates thus may provide important lessons for current approaches to cognitive neuroscience.

Several caveats must be kept in mind when interpreting these data. A variety of materials and modalities were sampled in an attempt to define the impairment in RC, but additional studies should be performed to confirm the semantic nature of his cognitive difficulty. We have identified the same cortical reorganization phenomenon for semantic aspects of lexical and picture processing

·in other populations such as Alzheimer's disease [Grossman et al, 1993 a] and for other types of cognitive impairments such as object recognition difficulty [Grossman et al, 1993 b], but RC represents only one case. Clearly additional studies of this sort are needed in order to confirm our observations. Because of limitations associated with the patient's maximum allowable radiation exposure, we were unable to determine whether the pattern of cortical recruitment seen during word judgments was also evident during RC's category membership judgments of pictures. We can only assume on the basis of his cognitive assessment that RC's rCBF pattern during category membership judgments of words reflects his apparently supramodal semantic difficulty. With these caveats in mind, we tentatively conclude that modeling in cognitive neuroscience has failed to take into account alternative cerebral structures that appear to be recruited *de novo* by the human brain in an attempt to compensate for an interruption of a cerebral network subserving a cognitive process.

ACKNOWLEDGEMENTS. This work was supported in part by grants from the US Public Health Service (AG09399, DC00039, and NS14867). We express our appreciation to Dr. Guila Glosser for her helpful comments on an earlier version of this report. Trish Giampapa provided valuable assistance in preparing the manuscript.

REFERENCES

Bergstrom M, Litton J, & Eriksson K. (1982). Determination of object contour from projections for attentuation correction in cranial positron emission tomography. *J Comput Assist Tomog, 6*, 365-372.

Besner, D. (1983). Deep dyslexia and the right hemisphere hypothesis.: Evidence from the USA and the USSR. *Can J Psychol, 37*, 565-571.

Bouchard, R., Lecours, A.R., & Lhermitte, F. (1979). Physiopathologie et localisation des lesions cerebrales responsables de l'aphasie. In A.R. Lecours & F. Lhermitte (Eds.), *L'aphasie* (pp. 269-276). Paris: Flammarion.

Butters, N., Butter, C., Rosen, J.J., & Stein, D.G. (1973). Behavioral of sequential and one-stage ablations of orbital prefrontal cortex in the monkey. *Exp Neurol, 39*, 204-214.

Butters, N., Rosen, J.J., & Stein, D.G. (1974). Recovery of behavioral functions after sequential ablation of the frontal lobes of monkeys. In D.G. Stein, J.J. Rosen, & N. Butters (Eds.), *Plasticity and recovery of function in the central nervous system* (pp. 429-508). New York: Academic Press.

Caramazza, A. (1986). On drawing inferences about the structure of normal cognitive systems from the analysis of patterns of impaired performance: The case for single-patient studies. *Cognition, 5*, 41-66.

Coltheart, M. (1980). Deep dyslexia: A right hemisphere hypothesis. In M. Coltheart, K. Patterson, & J.C. Marshall (Eds.), *Deep dyslexia* (pp. 326-380). London: Routledge and Kegan Paul.

Demonet, J.-F., Chollet, F., Ramsay, S., Cardebat, D., Nespoulos, J.-L., Wise, R., Rascol, A., & Frackowiak, R.S.J. (1992). The anatomy of phonological and semantic processing in normal sujects. *Brain, 115*, 1753-1768.

Grady, C.L., Haxby, J.V., Horwitz, B., Schapiro, M., Carson, R., Herscovitch, P., & Rapoport, S.I. (1990). Activation of regional cerebral blood flow (rCBF) in extrastriate cortex during a face matching task in patients with dementia of the Alzheimer type (AD). *Society for Neuroscience Abstracts, 16*, 149.

Grossman, M., & Carey, S. (1987). Selective word-learning deficits in aphasia. *Brain Lang, 32*, 306-324.

Grossman, M., Carvell, S., & Peltzer, L. (1993). The sum and substance of it: The appreciation of mass and count adjective-noun pairs in Parkinson's disease. *Brain Lang, 44*, 351-384.

Grossman, M., Crino, P., Stern, M.B., Hurtig, H.I., & Reivich, M. (1992). Attention and sentence comprehension in Parkinson's disease: The role of anterior cingulate cortex. *Cerebral Cortex, 2*, 513-525.

Grossman, M., D'Esposito, M., Mickanin, J., & Hughes, E. (in preparation b). Anomaly judgments of simple sentences in probable Alzheimer's disease.

Grossman, M., Galetta, S., Mickanin, J., Alavi, A., & Reivich, M. (1993b). Visual comprehension in agnosia: Cognitive and PET studies in two patients. *Neurology, 43*, A275.

Grossman, M., Hughes, E., Mickanin, J., Carvell, S., D'Esposito, M. (in preparation c). Grammatical and semantic judgments of verbs in probable Alzheimer's disease and Parkinson's disease.

Grossman, M., Hughes, E., Mickanin, J., Ding, X.-S., Alavi, A., & Reivich, M. (1993a). Selective defect in a neural network subserving semantic judgments in Alzheimer's disease: A PET activation study. *Ann Neurol, 34*, 256.

Grossman, M., & Mickanin, J. (submitted). Picture comprehension in probable Alzheimer's disease.

Grossman, M., Stern, M.B., Gollomp, S., Vernon, G., & Hurtig, H.I. (in press). Verb learning in Parkinson's disease. *Neuropsychology.*

Grossman, M., & Wilson, M. (1986). Stimulus categorization by brain-damaged patients. *Brain Cognit, 6*, 55-71.

Hart, J., & Gordon, B. (1990). Delineation of single word semantic comprehension deficits in aphasia, with anatomical correlation. *Ann Neurol, 27*, 226-231.

Hillis, A.E., Rapp, B.C., Romani, C., & Caramazza, A. (1989). Selective impairment of semantics in lexical processing. *Cognit Neuropsychol, 7*, 191-243.

Hinton, G.E., & Shallice, T. (1991). Lesioning an attractor network: Investigations of acquired dyslexia. *Psych Review, 98*, 74-95.

Jones, S.C., Greenberg, J.H., Dann, R., Robinson, G.D., Kushner, M., Alavi, A., & Reivich, M. (1985). Cerebral blood flow with the continuous infusion of oxygen-15 labelled water. *J Cereb Blood Flow Metab, 5*, 565-575.

Karp, J.S., Muehllehner, G., Mankoff, D.A., Ordonez, C.E., Ollinger, J.M., Daube-Witherspoon, M.E., Haigh, A.T., & Beerbohm, D.J. (1990). Continuous slice Penn-PET: A volume tomograph with volume imaging capability. *J Nucl Med, 31*, 617-627.

Kertesz, A. (1979). *Aphsia and associated disorders*. New York: Grune & Stratton.

Kosslyn, S.M., & van Kleek, M. (1990). Broken brains and normal minds: Why humpty dumpty needs a skeleton. In E.L. Schwartz (Ed.), *Computational neuroscience* (pp. 390-402). Cambridge: MIT Press.

Landis, T., Regard, M., Graves, R., & Goodglass, H. (1983). Semantic paralexias: A release of right hemispheric function from left hemispheric control. *Neuropsychologia, 21*, 359-364.

Marshall, J.C., & Patterson, K.E. (1983). Semantic paralexia and the wrong hemisphere: A note on Landis, Regard, Graves, and Goodglass. *Neuropsychologia, 21*, 425-427.

McCarthy, R.A., & Warrington, E.K. (1991). *Cognitive neuropsychology: A clinical introduction*. New York: Academic Press.

Patterson, K., Vargha-Khadem, F., & Polkey, C.E. (1989a). Reading with one hemisphere. *Brain, 112*, 39-63.

Patterson, K., Seidenberg, M.S., & McClelland, J.L. (1989b). Connections and disconnections: Acquired dyslexia in a computational model of reading. In R.G.M. Morris (Ed.), *Parallel distributed processing: Implications for psychology and neurobiology* (pp. 523-568). Oxford: Oxford University Press.

Roeltgen, D.P. (1987). Loss of deep dyslexic reading ability from a second left-hemispheric lesion. *Arch Neurol, 44*, 346-348.

Rosen, J.J., Stein, D.G., & Butters, N. (1971). Recovery of function after serial ablation of prefrontal cortex in the rhesus monkey. *Science, 173*, 353-356.

Rubens, A.B., & Kertesz, A. (1983). The localization of lesions in transcortical aphasias. In A. Kertesz (Ed), *Localization in neuropsychology* (pp 245-268). NY: Academic Press, 1983.

St. James-Roberts, I. (1981). A reinterpretation of hemispherectomy data without functional plasticity of the brain. *Brain Lang, 13*, 31-53.

Subramanyam, R., Alpert, N.M., & Hoop, B. (1978). A model for regional cerebral oxygen distribution during continuous inhalation of 15O2, C15O, and C15O2. *J Nucl Med, 19*, 48-63.

Talairach, J., & Tournoux, P. (1988). *Co-planar stereotaxic atlas of the human brain*. NY: Thieme Med Pub Inc.

Teuber, H.-L. (1975). Recovery of function after brain injury in man. R. Perter & D.W. Fitzsimons (Eds.), *Outcome of severe damage to the nervous system* (pp. 159-190). Ciba Foundation Symposium 34. Amsterdam: Elsevier.

Weiller, C., Chollet, F., Friston, K.J., Wise, R.J.S., & Frackowiak, R.S.J. (1992). Functional reorganization of the brain in recovery from striatocapsular infarction in man. *Ann Neurol, 31*, 463-472.

Wise, R., Chollet, F., Hadar, U., Friston, K., Hoffner, E., & Frackowiak, R.S.J. (1991). Distribution of cortical neural networks in word comprehension and word retrieval. *Brain, 114*, 1803-1817.

Zaidel, E. (1978). Lexical organization in the right hemisphere. In Buser, P.A. & Rougeul-Buser, A. (Eds.), *Cerebral correlates of conscious experience* (pp 177-197). Amsterdam: North Holland Press.

15

Remote Memory in Retrospect

WILLIAM W. BEATTY[1]

I first encountered the phenomenon of remote memory early in my sabbatical leave in San Diego in 1984. Nelson was preparing a lecture on the neuropsychology of alcoholic Korsakoff's (AK) syndrome, and as was his habit, he practiced the talk at a meeting of the Psychology Service. His delight when he showed the slide of Charlie Chaplin to introduce the segment on remote memory was unmistakable. No less interesting to me was the clear temporally graded retrograde amnesia (RA) function for the group of AK patients reported by Albert, Butters and Levin (1979). Of even greater importance were the then unpublished findings on patient PZ. PZ, as you will recall, was a famous research psychologist who developed AK a few years after publishing his autobiography. Nelson and his colleagues (Butters & Cermak, 1986) were able to show that PZ exhibited the usual temporally graded RA for Famous Faces and Public Events. Furthermore, PZ showed an entirely comparable pattern of loss of memory for details of his professional life (as reported in his autobiography) and even for the facts and theories of experimental psychology. For example, PZ could describe the trichnomatic theory of color vision in precise detail, but appeared completely unfamiliar with the ideas of the opponent process theory, which was not widely known until the late 1950s.

For a person just entering human neuropsychology after 15 postdoctoral years in animal psychobiology, the case of PZ was an important lesson in the power of the single case method. Because PZ had published his autobiography before he developed AK, there was available a rich store of information from

---

[1] WILLIAM W. BEATTY, Ph.D. • Department of Psychiatry and Behavioral Sciences, University of Oklahoma Health Sciences Center

Neuropsychological Explorations of Memory and Cognition: Essays in Honor of Nelson Butters, edited by Laird S. Cermak, Ph.D. Plenum Press, New York, 1994

various past decades that PZ must have once known. The striking similarity of the functions describing PZ's loss of remote memories for autobiographical details, professional knowledge and of Famous Faces and Public Events enhanced the validity of the latter measures. PZ's apparent loss of information about past public persons and events (information that he might never have known or particularly cared about) followed exactly the same time course as his loss of personal and professional knowledge that he certainly once knew and clearly was important since it comprised the history of his own professional career.

The opportunity to apply these lessons was not long in coming. A patient (identified as MRL or LM in the literature) was admitted to the San Diego VA Hospital following an episode of hypoxia. After he recovered from a confusional state, a neuropsychological workup revealed a moderate and global anterograde amnesia, mild anomia (which subsequently cleared) and the hint of temporally graded RA. Using the standard and revised Albert remote memory batteries, David Salmon and I (Beatty, Salmon, Bernstein & Butters, 1987) confirmed a steeply sloping temporal gradient of RA extending back about 15 years and also documented the patient's loss of knowledge of his own profession (surveying). While in the hospital, MRL complained of inability to find his way from his room to the smoking room (a distance of about 30 feet), and he was quite unable to draw an accurate floor plan of the hospital room in which he had lived for five weeks. I wondered if his clear anterograde amnesia for spatial information might be paralleled by some sort of spatial RA. Examination of floor plans of homes in which MRL had resided throughout his life indicated that MRL's drawings were almost identical to those provided by his relatives for the period from birth until about 15 years before his hypoxic episode. Thus, the gradients of RA for famous faces, public events and drawings of former residences were highly similar. Subsequently, Squire and his colleagues (Squire, Haist & Shimamura, 1989) confirmed our observations and extended them to several other patients who had suffered hypoxicischemic episodes. They also demonstrated that all of these patients exhibited bilateral hippocampal atrophy with varying damage to overlying cortical regions (Press, Amaral & Squire, 1989).

Although the strategy of having MRL draw floor plans of residences he had occupied at various times in his life worked well in describing his spatial retrograde amnesia, its success depended on the availability of knowledgeable and cooperative family members. An attempt to replicate the procedure with an AK patient convinced me that a standardized test which did not depend on family members to determine the accuracy of performance was needed. Geographical knowledge or, more precisely, knowledge of the location of cities in regions of the country in which a person had lived seemed an appropriate knowledge base, so I constructed what came to be the standard version of the Fargo Map Test (Beatty, 1988) and administered it to everyone at the San Diego VA I could persuade to take it. Fearful that Nelson might regard this attempt to create a new neuropsychological test by an unschooled rookie as the height of folly, I did not tell him of my project. Eventually, he found out and asked me "What's this I hear about your map test?" Caught red-handed, I could only stammer, "Do you want to take it?" Much to my surprise, Nelson agreed to take the test; his data are included among the controls for patient SS in a paper describing geographical knowledge in amnesia and following right temporal lobectomy (Beatty, MacInnes, Porphyris, Tröster & Cermak, 1988).

The Alzheimer's Research Center at UCSD was just beginning operation during my sabbatical year of 1984-85. Sparked by a clinical observation by Marilyn Albert that AD patients always showed relatively better remote memories for the distant than for the recent past, I decided to study remote memory in these patients. If true, this observation would have indicated that the pattern of remote memory loss in AD was different from that in the subcortical dementias such as Huntington's disease (HD; Albert, Butters & Brandt, 1981), Parkinson's disease (PD; Freedman, Rivoira, Butters, Sax & Feldman, 1984; Huber, Shuttleworth & Paulson, 1986) and, as we eventually showed, multiple sclerosis (MS; Beatty, Goodkin, Monson, Beatty & Hertsgaard, 1988). There was just one problem. At the time, the only published study of remote memory (Wilson, Kaszniak & Fox, 1981) indicated that in AD, RA was not temporally graded, but equivalent across all past decades. This suggested that in dementia, regardless of its cause, the temporal pattern of RA was fundamentally different than in amnesia.

Our study (Beatty, Salmon, Butters, Heindel & Granholm, 1988), using a revised version of the Famous Faces and Public Events tests developed by Albert et al. (1979), showed that in mildly to moderately demented AD patients, there was a slight but significant temporal gradient of RA, superimposed upon a massive loss of the ability to remember information from all past decades. HD patients tested on the same battery, exhibited the expected "flat" temporal gradient of RA (i.e., equivalent lossacross decades). At about the same time, Sagar and colleagues (Sagar, Cohen, Sullivan, Corkin & Growdon, 1988) and Kopelman (1989) reported similar findings using different instruments that tapped essentially the same knowledge domain (i.e., public persons and events).

Salmon and I wanted to test the generality of the finding that RA in AD is temporally graded in a completely different knowledge domain. We exploited a useful property of geographical knowledge as measured by the Fargo Map Test -- namely, that if an individual has resided in a particular area of the country for a number of years, his memory for that region remains quite good even if he does not return to the region for extended periods (Beatty, 1988; Beatty & Spangenberger, 1988). By comparing the accuracy of knowledge of the geography of the region in which a person was born and raised with that of the region in which she currently resided, we could measure the temporal gradient of RA for spatial information.

Obviously this technique depends upon recruiting patients and controls who have resided in more than one region of the country during their lives. By the time this project got started, my sabbatical had ended and I had returned to North Dakota. Since almost no one (voluntarily) moves to North Dakota to retire, the project had to be conducted in a more appealing venue. With Nelson's assistance and David Salmon's skill at identifying appropriate patients and persuading technicians to "slip" just one more test into the battery, we were able to gather enough AD patients and controls to complete the study. As predicted, the AD patients' overall accuracy on tests of geographical knowledge was lower than that of controls. However, they were able to locate significantly more places on maps of the region in which they were born and raised than on the map of California where they currently lived. Controls were equally able to locate place on both maps (Beatty & Salmon, 1991). This tendency for "old" spatial knowledge to be relatively better preserved than more recently acquired spatial memories is seen in AD but not in HD. In an earlier study (Beatty, 1989a), using the same strategy, I found that HD patients showed equivalent deficits in locating places on maps of regions in which they were born and raised and in the region (California) in which they lived at the time of testing. These findings indicate that, regardless of the method of assessment, differing patterns of RA are observed in HD and AD. Although patients with MS and PD show impairments in geographical knowledge (Beatty, Goodkin et al., 1988; Beatty & Monson, 1989), the temporal pattern of RA for this form of spatial knowledge has not been studied.

For studies of remote memory in middle aged and elderly adults, tests such as the Remote Memory Battery and its numerous revisions and the Fargo Map Test provide useful assessments. For younger subjects, however, I have found them to be rather inadequate. This point was driven home several years ago when I attempted to devise a way of studying remote memory in outpatient depressed patients (mostly younger women). My initial idea was simply to create an age-appropriate battery of famous faces and public events questions. Since I had access to a large population of undergraduate students, I elected to do the initial normative work on them. Unfortunately, even after discarding the most difficult items (fully 50% of the test), the accuracy of the "normal" controls ranged from 15% to 98%. Obviously, a battery with such variability in controls can't be of much use for studying patients.

The remarkable ignorance of geography of modern college students has been reported so often in the popular media that I hardly need to document the existence of the phenomenon. It is sufficient to note that the performance of subjects between 18 and 29 years of age is substantially inferior to that of older subjects on all of the subtests of the Fargo Map Test, except for locating very gross geographical features (Beatty, 1989b).

After several months of doubting whether modern college students knew anything (more precisely, anything that could be used as the basis of a remote memory test), I hit upon a knowledge base that should have been obvious all along -- popular music. Over a period of several years, we have been developing the Famous Tunes Test which requires recalling and recognizing the titles, artists and year of initial popularity of 50 songs that were popular from 1955-1986. Although our results are still preliminary, the performance of controls from North Dakota and Oklahoma was remarkably similar and head-injured patients from both regions exhibited marked impairments which were evident long after they had emerged from post-traumatic amnesia (Beatty, Scott & Moreland, submitted).

The discussion so far has been focused along lines that are traditional in neuropsychology -- the description and analysis of deficits in remote memory exhibited by various patient groups. It seems appropriate, especially in a volume of this sort, to end with a new direction. Recently, we have begun to study patients with AD and other dementias who retain certain cognitive skills like playing bridge or canasta or playing musical instruments. To date, we have published descriptions of six patients: one pianist, one trombonist, one bridge player, one canasta player, one domino player and one patient who solved jigsaw puzzles (Beatty, Zavadil, Bailly, Rixen, Zavadil, Farnham & Fisher, 1988; Beatty, Winn, Adams, Allen, Wilson, Prince, Olson, Dean & Littleford, in press). At this point, we know little about the prevalence of preserved cognitive skills in dementia or what skills may be preserved. It is tempting to explain this phenomenon away as the unusual manifestation of remote procedural memory, but I believe that it is more than that. The first patient we studied retained considerable skill at playing the piano, and could transfer her skill to an unfamiliar instrument, the xylophone. Yet she could not learn the pursuit rotor task and showed no evidence of pictorial priming on the Gollin figures task. Another patient took up solving jigsaw puzzles after he demented.

At this point, my hypothesis is that the display of these skills by the demented patients arises because access to the memories that guide the skilled behaviors is somehow enhanced relative to the access available to neural systems controlling behaviors that are no longer displayed. To test this idea and, more generally, to study the phenomenon of preserved cognitive skills in dementia, we in Oklahoma have joined forces with the Alzheimer Research Centers at UC San Diego and UC Irvine. Best of all, Nelson is a Co-Investigator on the project. I am deeply grateful.

REFERENCES

Albert, M.S., Butters, N., & Brandt, J. (1981). Patterns of remote memory in amnesic and demented patients. *Archives of Neurology, 38*, 495-500.

Albert, M.S., Butters, N., & Levin, J. (1979). Temporal gradients in the retrograde amnesia of patients with alcoholic Korsakoff's disease. *Archives of Neurology, 36*, 211-216.

Beatty, W.W. (1988). The Fargo Map Test: A standardized method for assessing remote memory for visuospatial information. *Journal of Clinical Psychology, 44*, 61-67.

Beatty, W.W. (1989a). Remote memory for visuospatial information in patients with Huntington's disease. *Psychobiology, 7*, 431-435.

Beatty, W.W. (1989b). Geographical knowledge throughout the lifespan. *Bulletin of the Psychonomic Society, 27*, 379-381.

Beatty, W.W., Goodkin, D.E., Monson, N., Beatty, P.A., & Hertsgaard, D. (1988). Anterograde and retrograde amnesia in patients with chronic progressive multiple sclerosis. *Archives of Neurology, 45*, 611-619.

Beatty, W.W., MacInnes, W.D., Porphyris, H.S., Tröster, A.I., & Cermak, L.S. (1988). Topographical memory following right temporal lobectomy. Brain and Cognition, 8, 67-76.

Beatty, W.W. & Monson, N. (1989). Geographical knowledge in patients with Parkinson's disease. *Bulletin of the Psychonomic Society, 27*, 473-475.

Beatty, W.W. & Salmon, D.P. (1991). Remote memory for visuospatial information in patients with Alzheimer's disease. *Journal of Geriatric Psychiatry and Neurology, 4*, 14-17.

Beatty, W.W., Salmon, D.P., Bernstein, N., & Butters, N. (1987). Remote memory in a patient with amnesia due to hypoxia. *Psychological Medicine, 17*, 657-665.

Beatty, W.W., Salmon, D.P., Butters, N., Heindel, W.C., & Granholm, E.L. (1988). Retrograde amnesia in patients with Alzheimer's disease or Huntington's disease. *Neurobiology of Aging, 9*, 181-186.

Beatty, W.W. & Spangenberger, M. (1988). Persistence of geographical memories in adults. *Bulletin of the Psychonomic Society, 26*, 104-105.

Beatty, W.W., Scott, J.G., & Moreland, V.J. Head injury effects on a new measure of remote memory: The Famous Tunes Test. Submitted.

Beatty, W.W., Winn, P., Adams, R.L., Allen, E.W., Wilson, D.A., Prince, J.R., Olson, K.A., Dean, K., & Littleford, D. (in press). Preserved cognitive skills in dementia of the Alzheimer type. *Archives of Neurology.*

Beatty, W.W., Zavadil, K.D., Bailly, R.C., Rixen, G.J., Zavadil, L.E., Farnham, N., & Fisher, L. (1988). Preserved musical skill in a severely demented patient. *International Journal of Clinical Neuropsychology, 10*, 158-164.

Butters, N. & Cermak, L.S. (1986). A case study of forgetting of autobiographical knowledge: Implications for the study of retrograde amnesia. In D. Rubin (Ed.). Autobiographical Memory. Cambridge: Cambridge University Press.

Freedman, M., Rivoira, P., Butters, N., Sax, D.S., & Feldman, R.S. (1984). Retrograde amnesia in Parkinson's disease. *Canadian Journal of the Neurological Sciences, 11*, 297-301.

Huber, S.J., Shuttleworth, E.C., & Paulson, G.W. (1986). Dementia in Parkinson's disease. *Archives of Neurology, 43*, 987-990.

Kopelman, M.D. (1989). Remote and autobiographical memory, temporal context memory and frontal atrophy in Korsakoff and Alzheimer patients. *Neuropsychologia, 27*, 437-460.

Press, G.H., Amaral, D.G., & Squire, L.R. (1989). Hippocampal abnormalities in amnesic patients revealed by high-resolution magnetic resonance imaging. *Nature, 341,* 54-56.

Sagar, H.J., Cohen, N.J., Sullivan, E.V., Corkin, S., & Growdon, J.H. (1988). Remote memory function in Alzheimer's disease and Parkinson's disease. *Brain, 111,* 185-206.

Squire, L.R., Haist, F., & Shimamura, A.P. (1989). The neurology of memory: Quantitative assessment of retrograde amnesia in two groups of amnesic patients. *Journal of Neuroscience, 9,* 828-839.

Wilson, R.S., Kaszniak, A.W., & Fox, J.H. (1981). Remote memory in senile dementia. *Cortex, 17,* 41-48.

16

The Clinical Assessment of Memory Disorders

DEAN C. DELIS[1], J. VINCENT FILOTEO[1],
PAUL J. MASSMAN[2], EDITH KAPLAN[3]
and JOEL H. KRAMER[4]

In the past 25 years, cognitive neuropsychologists have generated a wealth of knowledge on the nature of memory function and dysfunction. At the heart of this quest has been the search for dissociations in dichotomized memory processes. Thus, we have learned that insults to different regions of the brain may selectively disrupt such components of memory as short-term versus long-term memory, anterograde versus retrograde memory, encoding versus retrieval processes, or declarative versus procedural learning. Few researchers have contributed more to our understanding of these fascinating dissociations in different neurologic and psychiatric populations than Nelson Butters. Trained as a clinical psychologist, Nelson was one of the first researchers to embrace a cognitive science approach to the study of amnesia. Throughout his illustrious career as an experimental neuropsychologist, he never strayed from his clinical roots. He has always been a leader in incorporating the latest findings from the experimental laboratory into his clinical evaluations of patients with memory disorders. Those of us who have had the good fortune of working with Nelson, first at the Boston V.A. Medical Center, and later at the San Diego V.A. Medical

[1] DEAN C. DELIS, Ph.D., J. VINCENT FILOTEO, Ph.D. • Department of Veterans Affairs Medical Center, San Diego and Department of Psychiatry, University of California
[2] PAUL J. MASSMAN, Ph.D. • Department of Psychology, University of Houston and Department of Neurology, Baylor College Medicine
[3] EDITH KAPLAN, Ph.D. • Department of Neurology, Boston University School of Medicine
[4] JOEL H. KRAMER, Ph.D. • Department of Psychiatry, University of California, San Francisco, School of Medicine

Neuropsychological Explorations of Memory and Cognition: Essays in Honor of Nelson Butters, edited by Laird S. Cermak, Ph.D. Plenum Press, New York, 1994

Center, have often marveled at his uncanny skill in testing for subtle disruptions in specific memory processes.

In the late 1970s, when the first author was a postdoctoral fellow at the Boston V.A. Medical Center under the supervision of Edith Kaplan, he saw first hand the clinical utility of Nelson's approach to memory assessment. These observations inspired the development of a formal memory test that incorporated multiple principles from cognitive neuroscience into a clinical instrument. In large part, the California Verbal Learning Test (CVLT) is a standardization of many of the principles and procedures that Nelson has used over the years in his research studies and clinical evaluations.

In this chapter, we briefly review several divisions of memory that have been investigated by Nelson and other cognitive neuropsychologists. Next, we describe how this experimental research guided the development of the CVLT. Finally, we review studies that have used the CVLT to characterize the memory deficits of various neurologic and psychiatric patient groups.

DIVISIONS OF MEMORY

In this section, we discuss those dichotomies of memory that have had the most influence in the development of the CVLT. The reader is referred to other chapters in this volume for a more detailed account of these and other memory constructs (e.g., explicit versus implicit memory).

Short-term versus Long-Term Memory

A major distinction within the memory literature is between short- and long-term memory (Atkinson & Shiffrin, 1971; Waugh and Norman, 1965). In general, short-term memory refers to the recall of information immediately after it is presented or during uninterrupted rehearsal of the material. In contrast, long-term memory refers to recall of information after a delay interval in which the examinee's attention is focused away from the target items. The distinction between short-and long-term memory has been demonstrated in various patient populations. Butters and Cermak (1980) found that patients with alcoholic Korsakoff's syndrome performed normally on the first trial of an immediate recall memory test for supra-span material. However, these same patients demonstrated dramatic impairments in their ability to recall material once a delay period was introduced. These findings suggest that short-term memory (if assessed immediately) may be relatively intact in these patients, but that their long-term memory is selectively impaired (Butters, 1984; Butters & Grady, 1977; Butters, Tarlow, Cermak, & Sax, 1976).

Other evidence validating the distinction between short- and long-term memory has come from studies of patients with Alzheimer's disease (AD).

Butters and colleagues have found that AD patients demonstrate rapid rates of forgetting over delay periods (Butters et al., 1988; Hodges, Salmon, & Butters, 1990; Salmon, Granholm, McCullough, Butters, and Grant, 1989; Welsh, Butters, Hughes, Mohs, and Heyman, 1991). Thus, what little information Alzheimer's patients can learn is quickly forgotten. These results suggest that patients with Alzheimer's disease are impaired in encoding and storing new information into long-term memory.

Learning versus Memory
In cognitive neuropsychology, learning refers to the efficiency with which new information is encoded into memory. Learning is typically assessed by asking an individual to recall the same information over repeated trials. An individual's learning efficiency can be evaluated in different ways, including the number of trials to reach a criterion level, the increase in the number of new items recalled over learning trials (i.e., a learning curve), or the consistency with which the same words are recalled across the learning trials. On the other hand, memory refers to the persistence of learned information over time (Squire, 1987).

Learning and memory may place differential demands on cognitive processes (Butters, 1985; Delis, 1989; Squire, 1987). That is, an individual's learning efficiency does not necessarily reflect his or her ability to retain this information over time. Evidence supporting the distinction between learning and memory has come from investigations of several patient populations. For example, although patients with Huntington's disease (HD) tend to demonstrate impaired learning (as reflected by deficient levels of immediate recall), these patients often display normal rates of forgetting. In contrast, alcoholic Korsakoff patients and Alzheimer's patients exhibit abnormally rapid rates of forgetting (Butters et al., 1988; Butters, Wolfe, Martone, Granholm, & Cermak, 1985; Butters, Wolfe, Granholm, & Martone, 1986; Hodges et al., 1990; Troster, Jacobs, Butters, Cullum, & Salmon, 1989; Welsh et al., 1991).

Encoding versus Retrieval
Encoding refers to the process by which physical information is transformed into a stored, mental representation. In contrast, retrieval is the process by which information is brought into conscious awareness. Patients with various forms of brain-damage can demonstrate differential impairment in either of these two components of memory.

For example, Butters and his colleagues have found that Huntington's patients often exhibit normal or close to normal performance on recognition testing but moderately to severely impaired performance on free-recall testing (Butters et al., 1985; Butters et al., 1988; Delis et al., 1991). These findings suggest that Huntington's patients are able to encode information into memory given their good recognition performance, but that they are impaired in retrieving information under free-recall conditions. Other patients with predominantly subcortical involvement also demonstrate better memory performance on recognition testing than free recall (e.g., patients with Parkinson's disease; Fisher, Kennedy, Caine, and Shoulson, 1983). In contrast, Korsakoff patients or Alzheimer's patients demonstrate equivalent levels of impairments on free-recall and recognition testing (Butters et al., 1983, 1985), suggesting that these patients are impaired in encoding and storing new information. This common dissociation, which is found so often in different patient groups, attests to the clinical importance of evaluating whether the locus of a patient's memory disorder is at the encoding and/or retrieval level.

Proactive versus Retroactive Interference
        The ability to learn and recall information may be disrupted by two forms of interference: proactive and retroactive interference. Proactive interference occurs when information learned earlier interferes with the learning of new information. In contrast, retroactive interference occurs when the recall of previously learned information is affected detrimentally by the learning of new material. Although this dichotomy was originally developed based on research with normal subjects (Postman, 1971), neuropsychological studies with different patient groups have provided support for this distinction. For example, although patients with alcoholic Korsakoff's disease may demonstrate normal levels of recall on an initial learning trial, their recall level on subsequent trials may actually decrease (Cermak, Butters, and Moreines, 1974). This pattern of recall suggests that the learning of subsequent information interfered with the learning of new information in these patients, and that alcoholic Korsakoff's patients may be especially susceptible to the effects of proactive interference.
        Another manner in which proactive interference may evidence on memory tests is in the form of intrusion errors. An intrusion error is a response given on a recall trial that is not on the target list, and may reflect problems in discriminating relevant from irrelevant responses (Fuld, Katzman, Davies, & Terry, 1982). Several studies have indicated that intrusion errors are characteristic of the memory deficits exhibited by certain patient groups. For example, both Alzheimer's and alcoholic Korsakoff's patients tend to make a large number of intrusion errors when recalling verbal material (Butters & Cermak, 1980; Fuld et al., 1982).

Semantic versus Serial-Order Clustering
        An important advancement in memory research has been the study of how individuals encode new information. Research with normals has indicated that information will be remembered better if it is learned using some organizing

structure (Craik, 1981; Hunt & Love, 1972). Specifically, subjects will tend to retain more information over time if they recall consecutive words from the same semantic category. This type of learning strategy is called semantic clustering (Bousfield, 1953). If a subject is able to make use of the semantic qualities of verbal information through semantic clustering, they will better be able to recall this information at a later point.

An alternative learning strategy is serial-order clustering. Individuals who utilize this strategy tend to recall words in the same order as they were presented. In general, serial-order clustering is considered to be an ineffective learning strategy because it correlates with poor delayed recall.

Studies from cognitive neuropsychology have indicated that certain patient groups may be differentially impaired in using semantic information when encoding verbal material. Cermak and Butters (1972) and Cermak et al. (1973) found that alcoholic Korsakoff's patients were able to utilize phonemic cues when recalling information, but that they were unable to benefit from semantic cues. These results may suggest that alcoholic Korsakoff's patients are differentially impaired in encoding new verbal information. As Butters and Miliotis (1985) have pointed out, however, alcoholic Korsakoff's patients' deficits in encoding the semantic aspects of verbal material may be due to a general impairment in analyzing complex material per se. Nevertheless, the work by Nelson and Laird Cermak suggests that employing tasks which allow the examinee to utilize efficient (e.g., semantic clustering) or less efficient (e.g., serial clustering) encoding strategies could be beneficial in identifying deficits in various learning strategies.

Primacy versus Recency Recall

Recalled words can be characterized in terms of their positions in the original word list or story to be remembered. It is more difficult to recall items from the beginning of a list or story (primacy regions) than it is to recall information from the end of the list or story (recency region) because primacy words must be held in memory while the remaining stimuli are presented. Words that are recalled from the primacy region of the word list are thought to be encoded into long-term storage (Atkinson & Schiffrin, 1968; Klatzky, 1980). In contrast, recency words can be echoed back as soon as they are presented, and therefore may not be encoded into memory.

Studies of neurological patients have provided construct validation for the distinction between primacy and recency memory effects. For example, patients with Alzheimer's disease tend to demonstrate dramatic impairments in recalling information from the primacy region on both verbal and nonverbal memory tests (Diesfeldt, 1978; Bigler, Rosa, Shultz, Hall, & Harris, 1989). These findings suggest that patients with Alzheimer's disease have impaired long-term storage, with relatively less impaired short-term storage. Previous studies examining primacy and recency effects in patients with Huntington's disease also demonstrated that these patients are relatively impaired in recalling items from the primacy region of the word list (suggesting impaired long-term storage) as compared to items from the recency region. However, it has been demonstrated that this effect in patients with Huntington's disease is dependent on how memory is assessed. Specifically, it has been found that Huntington's patients will not demonstrate a decrease in primacy word recall if they are assessed using recognition memory tests (Massman, Delis, and Butters, 1993).

DEVELOPMENT OF THE CVLT

Historically, clinical tests have tended to assess only an individuals overall level of performance. That is, traditional memory tests have almost exclusively examined the level, or amount, of information recalled or recognized, and they have not incorporated principles and procedures developed in cognitive neuroscience. The traditional approach to the assessment of memory fails to provide sensitive measures of the various component processes of memory that can be differentially impaired following brain damage.

The CVLT (Delis, Kramer, Kaplan, & Ober, 1987) was designed to incorporate numerous memory constructs from cognitive neuropsychology. On the CVLT, a 16-word target list (List A) is read to the examinee over five immediate free-recall trials. The target list is comprised of four words from each of four semantic categories. After the five learning trials, an interference list (List B) is presented for a single, immediate free-recall trial. Free and category-cued recall of target lists are then tested (termed the "short delay" trials). After a 20-minute interval involving nonverbal testing, free recall, cued recall, and recognition of the target list are assessed.

The CVLT scoring system goes well beyond the conventional measure of the total number of correct words recalled or recognized. In addition to tabulating the level or amount of an examinee's recall, the CVLT quantifies and provides normative data for numerous additional indices, including (a) semantic clustering; (b) primacy and recency effects; (c) rate of acquisition across trials; (d) consistency of item recall across trials; (e) measures of vulnerability to proactive and retroactive interference; (f) retention over short and longer delays; (g) intrusion and perseveration rates; and (h) signal detection parameters (discriminability and response bias) of recognition performance.

STUDIES USING THE CVLT

Since its development, the CVLT has been employed in over 100 studies to characterize memory function and dysfunction in a wide range of patient populations. We will review some of the key studies.

Construct Validity of the CVLT

In a study with a large sample of normal and neurological patients (Delis, Kramer, Freeland, Kaplan, 1988), we examined the construct validity of the CVLT using factor analytic techniques. This analysis yielded a six-factor solution. The first factor was a general verbal learning factor, with the highest loadings occurring for the recall and recognition measures. The second factor was comprised of measures of intrusions and false positive errors, and was labeled a response discrimination factor. The third factor reflected learning strategy, because only the semantic and serial clustering indices loaded on it. These two clustering strategies had inverse loadings on the third factor, indicating that when the use of one strategy is increased, use of the other strategy decreases. The fourth and fifth factors represented effects associated with proactive interference and serial position, respectively. Recall from the primacy and recency regions of the list showed inverse loadings on the fifth factor, a finding consistent with the distinction that greater primacy recall reflects more active learning (e.g., rehearsal), whereas greater recency recall indicates more passive recall. The final factor loaded on the learning slope variable, which supports the value of analyzing the rate at which examinee's learn a list independent of their total recall score. The finding that these six orthogonal components emerged from subjects' performances on the CVLT provides further validation for the memory constructs described earlier in this chapter. In a second study which examined the criterion-related validity of the CVLT (Delis, Cullum, Butters, Cairns, & Prifitera, 1988), we administered both the CVLT and the Wechsler Memory Scale- Revised (WMS-R; Wechsler, 1987) to a group of normal individuals and a mixed neurologic patient group. Correlational analyses revealed several strong relationships between the indices derived from the CVLT and the WMS-R, including measures from both tests which assess total level of immediate and delayed recall. Consistent with the previously described memory constructs, semantic clustering indices from the CVLT correlated robustly with the majority of the WMS-R variables, whereas serial clustering scores did not. Similarly, percent recall from the primacy and middle regions of the CVLT word lists correlated with many of the WMS-R, validating the notion that words recalled from the earlier portion of material may be stored in long-term memory. In contrast, percent recall from the recency region of the CVLT word list were not positively associated with the WMS-R indices. Measures from the CVLT reflecting vulnerability to proactive and retroactive interference were also not associated robustly with any measures derived from the WMS-R. Overall, these results provide further construct validation for the measures obtained from the CVLT. Furthermore, this study suggests that the CVLT is more sensitive for the assessment of certain memory constructs (i.e., interference effects), which may be differentially impaired in certain memory disorders (see below).

Other studies providing evidence for the construct validity of the CVLT have indicated that the CVLT is: (1) sensitive to sex differences in verbal memory (Kramer, Delis, & Daniel, 1988), which have previously been reported in the experimental literature (see Maccoby & Jacklin, 1974); and (2) a robust measure of proactive interference in normal subjects (Kramer & Delis, 1991).

Taken together, these studies suggest that the CVLT is a sensitive test of an individual's learning and memory. In addition, these studies provide support for the memory models spoken of earlier in this chapter.

Studies of Dementia and Amnesia

In recent years, the CVLT has been used extensively in studies attempting to differentiate the pattern of memory deficits exhibited by patients with a "cortical" dementia, such as Alzheimer's disease, or a "subcortical" dementia, such as Huntington's disease. As described above, research in cognitive neuropsychology has indicated that patients with Alzheimer's disease typically display a pattern of memory deficits which is qualitatively different than the deficits exhibited by patients with Huntington's disease (e.g., Butters, 1985; Salmon and Butters, 1987). This is thought to be related to an encoding/storage deficit in patients with Alzheimer's disease, and a retrieval deficit in patients with Huntington's disease. The differences in their memory profiles are believed to due to neuropathological changes in different brain regions. Alzheimer's disease is characterized by damage to the hippocampus, association cortices, and the basal forebrain (Arendt, Bigl, Arendt, & Tennstedt, 1983; Cummings & Benson, 1992), whereas Huntington's disease is characterized by damage primarily to the caudate nucleus within the basal ganglia (Cummings and Benson, 1992; Folstein, Brandt, & Folstein, 1990).

In a recent study (Delis, Massman, Butters, Salmon, Cermak, and Kramer, 1991), we contrasted the verbal learning and memory profiles of patients with Alzheimer's disease, Huntington's disease, and alcoholic Korsakoff's syndrome using the CVLT. The results of this study were strikingly similar to past studies which have contrasted the memory patterns of these patient groups (for reviews see Butters, 1985; and Salmon & Butters, 1987). Specifically, both the Alzheimer's and Korsakoff's patients displayed severely impaired immediate recall, flat learning rates across trials, inconsistent recall across trials, ineffective use of semantic clustering, a tendency to recall words passively from the recency region of the word list, poor retention over delay intervals, high intrusion rates, poor recognition discriminability, high false positive rates, a positive response bias on recognition measures, and no improvement on recognition testing relative to free-recall.

In contrast to the performances of the Alzheimer's and alcoholic Korsakoff's patients, the Huntington's disease patients displayed better retention on delayed recall, lower intrusion rates on the free- and cued-recall trials, a trend toward less proactive interference, lower false-positive rates on recognition testing, higher recognition discriminability, and greater improvement on recognition testing relative to free recall. These findings are consistent with past studies that have also demonstrated this pattern of memory impairment in patients with Huntington's disease (Butters et al., 1976, 1985, 1986).

In order to provide a more rigorous test of the CVLT's ability to differentiate the memory profiles exhibited by these patient groups, we next conducted a discriminant function analysis using two key variables from the CVLT on which the three groups most differed. These indices were: (1) percent cued recall intrusions; and (2) recognition discriminability versus the last learning trial. A jackknifed discriminant function analysis was first applied to the data of the Alzheimer's and Huntington's patients. This procedure correctly classified 85% of the Alzheimer's patients and 84% of the Huntington's patients, indicating that the discriminant function equation had good sensitivity in differentiating between the two groups. This same discriminant function was then applied to the data of the alcoholic Korsakoff's patients. The analysis classified 100% of the Korsakoff's patients as Alzheimer's patients and none as Huntington's disease. These findings suggest that the pattern of memory deficits exhibited by Korsakoff's patients is similar to the profile of memory impairments exhibited by Alzheimer's patients, whereas the memory disorder observed in patients with Huntington's disease is qualitatively different.

The CVLT has also been used to examine similarities and differences in the memory profiles of different subcortical dementias. In a recent study (Massman, Delis, Butters, Levin, & Salmon, 1990), the CVLT performances of patients with Huntington's disease or Parkinson's disease were compared. The results of this study were intriguing because they indicated that the memory deficits exhibited by these two patient groups were remarkably similar. Specifically, both groups demonstrated impaired immediate memory spans, inconsistency of recall across trials, deficient use of a semantic clustering learning strategy, normal retention of information over delay periods, normal vulnerability to proactive or retroactive interference, elevated intrusion rates on delayed recall, impaired recognition memory, and normal types of intrusions (i.e., intrusions semantically related to target words). These results suggest that subcortical dysfunction is associated with mildly deficient encoding, intact storage, and marked difficulty initiating systematic retrieval strategies.

The results also indicated that the Huntington's and Parkinson's patients differed on a few of the CVLT measures. Specifically, the Huntington's patients displayed a greater level of impairment on free recall, a more deficient learning slope across trials, reduced primacy and increased recency effects, and an increased perseveration rate. In addition, the Huntington's patients clearly showed a supranormal improvement on recognition testing compared with free-recall, whereas the Parkinson's patients only demonstrated a trend toward disproportionate improvement on the recognition measure. These differences between the two groups appeared to be more quantitative than qualitative in nature. That is, the pattern of their memory deficits were similar, and when the two groups did differ, it was only in terms of the level of their impairment. These findings indicate that the retrieval deficit characteristic of subcortical dementia may be more prominent in patients with Huntington's disease.

In another study (Kramer, Levin, Brandt, & Delis, 1990), patients with Parkinson's, Huntington's, or Alzheimer's disease were administered the CVLT. An initial set of analyses indicated that the Alzheimer's patients recall level across the five learning trials was significantly lower than both the Parkinson's patients and Huntington's patients, whereas the two subcortical groups did not differ. Next, the Parkinson's and Huntington's patients were subgrouped based on their scores from the immediate recall trials. Those Parkinson's patients who recalled greater than thirty items on the five learning trials were classified as the high-functioning Parkinson's, and those who recalled less than thirty were classified as the low-functioning Parkinson's. The same division of subjects was applied to the Huntington's patients. This classification scheme yielded five patient groups: the Alzheimer's group, the high-Parkinson's group, the low-Parkinson's group, the high-Huntington's group, and the low-Huntington's group.

In order to examine the similarities and differences in the pattern of memory profiles, a discriminant function analysis was applied to the data of the five groups. This analyses correctly classified 75% of the patients into their respective groups. The variables that best differentiated these subjects were the ratio of intrusion errors to total responses (highest in Alzheimer's patients), total perseverations (highest in Alzheimer's and Huntington's patients), and rate of forgetting (highest in Alzheimer's and Parkinson's patients). An examination of the subgroup classifications indicated that the memory performances of the Parkinson's and Huntington's were distinguishable in that there was a high degree of accuracy in classifying patients in these two groups. Moreover, when the patients from the subcortical group were misclassified, the patients were equally likely to be misclassified as an Alzheimer's patient as they were to be misclassified into the wrong subcortical group. Taken together, these results suggest that, although the subcortical-cortical distinction may provide a good initial distinction between the memory profiles exhibited by demented patients, a more detailed analysis may be necessary in order to distinguish the memory profiles of different subcortical patient groups.

In recent years, a growing area of research has been the early detection and diagnosis of individuals who are at risk for Alzheimer's disease. Bondi et al. (1993) examined longitudinally the CVLT performances of normal individuals with a positive family history (FH+) for Alzheimer's disease (i.e., the subject had a first degree relative with known Alzheimer's disease), normal individuals with a negative family history (FH-) for Alzheimer's disease, and patients diagnosed with Alzheimer's disease. Discriminant function analysis was applied to subjects' data using the following CVLT indices as discriminating variables: (1) total recall across the five learning trials, (2) degree of semantic clustering, (3) percent long-delay recall saving, (4) and number of cued recall intrusions. For the purposes of the discriminant function analysis, the FH+ and FH-subjects were collapsed into one group. The results from subjects' annual CVLT performances indicated that a subsample of the normal controls displayed similar learning and memory profiles as Alzheimer's patients. In following this subsample of normal subjects over three years, it was found that a large percentage of these individuals subsequently went on to develop Alzheimer's disease. Furthermore, those normal controls who had memory performances similar to Alzheimer's patients and who subsequently went on to develop the disease also had a positive family history for Alzheimer's disease. Taken together, the results of this study suggest that individuals with a positive family history of this disease may be at risk for developing Alzheimer's disease. Furthermore, the results of this study also suggest that the CVLT may be sensitive to the early changes observed in individuals who are exhibiting preclinical cognitive changes associated with dementia.

Studies examining the performances of individuals who test positive for HIV have indicated that the CVLT is sensitive to the memory changes often observed in these patients. Peavey et al. (in press) administered the CVLT to a group of symptomatic HIV positive (HIV+) patients, asymptomatic HIV+ patients, and HIV negative (HIV-) controls. The results indicated that the symptomatic HIV+ patients performed significantly worse than the asymptomatic HIV+ patients and the HIV- controls on the majority of the CVLT indices. Furthermore, the performance of the asymptomatic HIV+ patients fell between the performances of the symptomatic HIV+ patients and the HIV- controls, suggesting that, although these patients were asymptomatic, they nevertheless experienced some alteration in their memory abilities.

Using discriminant function analysis, the CVLT profiles of the HIV patients were compared to the profiles of patients with Alzheimer's or Huntington's disease. The results of this analysis indicated that 32% of the symptomatic HIV+ patients and 16% of the asymptomatic HIV+ patients were classified as Huntington's patients. In contrast, only 3% of the symptomatic HIV+ patients and 1% of the asymptomatic HIV+ patients were classified as Alzheimer's patients. These findings suggest that not all symptomatic and asymptomatic patients with HIV will demonstrate memory deficits, but if they are impaired in memory, the pattern of their deficits will most likely resemble that seen in patients with subcortical pathology (i.e., Huntington's disease). This assertion is consistent with previous reports that have identified subcortical neuropathology in patients with HIV infection (Grant et al., 1987, 1988; Olsen, Longo, Mills, & Normal, 1988).

Studies of Head-Injured Patients

The CVLT has also been used in studies examining the effects of head-injury on memory functioning. Crosson, Novack, Trenerry, and Craig (1988) found that patients with blunt head-injuries were significantly impaired on several of the CVLT indices. Specifically, this study indicated that, compared to a normal control group, head-injured patients recalled less words across the five learning trials, made more intrusions on both free- and cued-recall trials, were less efficient at utilizing a semantic clustering strategy, retained less information across the delay period, and were less able to discriminate target items from nontarget items on recognition testing. In contrast, the head-injured patients displayed disproportionate improvement on the cued recall trials relative to free recall. Overall, the results suggested that blunt head-injury can result in deficits at both the encoding and retrieval levels.

There is some evidence to suggest that head-injuries which affect primarily the left temporal lobe will result in a very specific pattern of memory performance on the CVLT. Crosson and colleagues (Crosson, Sartor, Jenny, Nabors, & Moberg, 1993) administered the CVLT to a small group (n=10) of head-injured patients with various lesion sites (as determined by Magnetic Resonance Imaging). The performances of the head-injured patients were contrasted with cut-off scores derived from a sample of twenty neurologically normal individuals for the following indices: (1) the total number of correct responses on the short- and long-delay free-recall trials; (2) the total number of correct responses on the short- and long-delay cued-recall trials; and (3) the total number of intrusions reported on all delay trials. The results indicated that, although many of the head-injured patients demonstrated impairments on the CVLT, only those patients with left temporal lesions demonstrated an abnormally large number of intrusions on the delayed-recall trials; in contrast, the other patients without left temporal lesions did not demonstrate this deficit. Furthermore, 74% of the intrusions made by patients with left temporal lesions were within category intrusions (i.e., items from the same semantic categories as the target items but not appearing on any of the target word lists). In contrast, patients who had involvement outside of the left temporal lobe (e.g., diencephalic atrophy) tended to intrude more items that were from the distracter list of the CVLT, suggesting more of a source memory deficit in these latter patients. A second experiment reported in this same study examined the pattern of memory performance on the CVLT in temporal lobe patients whose lesions were not due to traumatic brain injuries. The results of this second experiment also suggested that pathology of the temporal lobes may be related to elevated rates of intrusions.

In summary, the studies of head-injured patients using the CVLT suggest (1) that these patients tend to experience both encoding and retrieval deficits; and (2) the tendency to report extra-test intrusion errors may be related to involvement in the left temporal lobe.

Studies of Psychiatric Disorders

It is well known that patients with depression can demonstrate impaired performances on memory tests (Cummings & Benson, 1992). In a recent study (Massman, Delis, Butters, Dupont, and Gillan, 1992), we compared the learning and memory profiles of unipolar depressives and bipolar depressives with those of patients with Huntington's disease, Alzheimer's disease, and normal controls. Based on the results from previous investigations (Butters et al., 1985, 1988; Delis et al., 1991; Kramer et al., 1988, 1989), we selected three indices from the CVLT which would likely prove successful in differentiating the normal controls, Huntington's patients, and Alzheimer's patients. These indices were: (1) the standard score on the measure of total recall over the five learning trials; (2) the standard score on the measure of number of intrusions occurring on the two cued recall trials; and (3) the difference between the standard scores obtained on recognition discriminability and free recall on the fifth learning trial. Using these three indices, we conducted a discriminant function analysis in order to differentiate the pattern of memory performances in the normal controls, Huntington's patients, and Alzheimer's patients. Consistent with previous studies (Delis et al., 1988, 1991), the results of the discriminant function analyses differentiated the memory performance of the three groups in that 90% of the subjects were classified correctly.

Next, this same discriminant function equation was applied to the data of the depressed patients. The results of this analysis classified 70% of the unipolar depressives as normal, 30% as Huntington's patients, and none as Alzheimer's patients. This analysis also classified 44% of the bipolar depressed patients as normal, 56% as Huntington's patients, and none as Alzheimer's patients. These results have several important implications. First, not all patients with depression will demonstrate learning and memory deficits. This was demonstrated by the finding that, on average, 65% of the memory performances of the depressed patients in this study were classified as normal. Second, if depressed patients do demonstrate learning and memory impairments, the pattern of their deficits will likely resemble those of patients with Huntington's disease and not patients with Alzheimer's disease. Third, these results suggest that depression may be related to subcortical dysfunction. The similarities in the memory impairments exhibited by depressed and Huntington's disease patients is consistent with recent neuroimaging studies which have identified subcortical abnormalities in these patients (Baxter et al., 1985; Dupont et al., 1990).

CONCLUSION

We are entering an exciting era of neuropsychological assessment in which clinical instruments are designed to parse the spared and impaired components of cognition. As with the CVLT, the pioneering research of Nelson Butters will always leave a lasting imprint on the design and structure of the clinical memory tests of the future.

REFERENCES

Arendt, T., Bigl, V. Arendt, A., & Tennstedt, A. (1983). Los of neurons in the nucleus basalis of Meynert in Alzheimer's disease, paralysis agitans and Korsakof's syndrome. *Acta Neuropathologica, 61*, 101-108.

Atkinson, R. C., & Schiffrin, R. M. (1968). Human memory: A proposed system and its control processes. In K. W. Spence & J. T. Spence (Eds.), *The psychology of learning and motivation*, (Vol. 2, pp. 89-195). New York: Academic.

Atkinson, R. C., & Schiffrin, R. M. (1971). The control of short-term memory. *Scientific American, 224*, 82-90.

Baxter, L. R., Phelps, M. E., Mazziotta, J. C., Schwartz, J. M., Gerner, R. H., Selin, C. E., & Sumida, R. M. (1985). Cerebral metabolic rates for glucose in modd disorders: Studies with positron emission tomography and fluorodeoxyglucose F18. *Archives of General Psychiatry, 46*, 243-250.

Bigler, E. D., Rosa, L., Schultz, F., Hall, S., & Harris, J. (1989). Rey-Auditory Verbal Learning and Rey-Osterrieth Complex Figure Design performance in Alzheimer's disease and closed head injury. *Journal of Clinical Psychology, 45*, 277-280.

Bondi, M. W., Monsch, A. U., Galasko, D., Butters, N., Salmon, D. P., & Delis, D. C. (1993). Preclinical cognitive markers of dementia of the Alzheimer Type. *Manuscript submitted for publication.*

Bousfield, W. A. (1953). The occurrence of clustering in therecall of randomly arranged associates. *Journal of General Psychology, 49*, 229-240.

Butters, N. (1984). The clinical aspects of memory disorders: Contributions from experimental studies of amnesia and dementia. *Journal of Cliniecal Neuropsychology, 1*, 17-36.

Butters, N. (1985). Alcoholic Korsakoff's syndrome: Some unresolved issues concerning etiology, neuropathology, and cognitive deficits. *Journal of Clinical and Experimental Neuropsychology, 7*, 181-210.

Butters, N., Albert, M. S., Sax, D. S., Miliotis, P., Nagode, J., & Sterste, A. (1983). The effect of verbal mediators on the pictorial memory of brain-damaged patients. *Neuropsychologia* , *21*, 307-323.

Butters, N., & Cermak, L. S. (1980). *Alcoholic Korsakoff Syndrome: An information processing approach.* New York: Academic Press.

Butters, N., & Grady, L. S. (1977). Effect of predistractor delay on the short-term memory performance of patients with Korsakoff's and Huntington's disease. *Neuropsychologia*, *13*, 701-705.

Butters, N., & Miliotis, P. (1984). Amnesic disorders. In K. M. Heilman & E. Valenstein, *Clinical Neuropsychology* (pp. 403-451). New York: Oxford University Press.

Butters, N., Salmon, D. P., Cullum, M. M., Cairns, P., Troster, A. I., Jacobs, D., Moss, M., & Cermak, L. S. (1988). Differentiation of amnesic and demented patients with the Wechsler Memory Scale- Revised. *The Clinical Neuropsychologist, 2*, 133-148.

Butters, N., Tarlow, S., Cermak, L. S., & Sax, D. (1976). A comparison of the information processing deficits of patients with Huntington's Chorea and Korsakoff's syndrome. *Cortex, 12*, 134-144.

Butters, N., Wolfe, J., Granholm, E., & Martone, M. (1986). An assessment of verbal recall, recognition, and fluency abilities in patients with Huntington's disease. *Cortex, 22*, 11-32.

Butters, N., Wolfe, J., Martone, M., Granholm, E., & Cermak, L. S. (1985). Memory disorders associated with Huntington's disease: Verbal recall, verbal recognition, and procedural memory. *Neuropsychologia, 23*, 729-743.

Cermak, L. S., & Butters, N. (1972). The role of interference and encoding in the short-term memory deficits of Korsakoff patients. *Neuropsychologia, 10*, 89-96.

Cermak, L. S., Butters, N., & Gerrein, J. (1973). The extent of the verbal encoding ability of Korsakoff patients. *Neuropsychologia, 11*, 85-94.

Cermak, L. S., Butters, N., & Moreines, J. (1974). Some analyses of the verbal encoding deficit of alcoholic Korsakoff patients. *Brain and Language, 1*, 141-150.

Craik, F. I. M. (1981). Encoding and retrieval effects in human memory: A partial review. In J. Long & A. D. Baddely (Eds.), *Attention and performance, IX..* Hillsdale, N. J.: Erlbaum.

Crosson, T. A., Novack, T. A., Trenerry, M. R., & Craig, P. L. (1988). California Verbal Learning Test (CVLT) performance in severely head-injured and neurologically normal adult males. *Journal of Clinical and Experimental Neuropsychology, 10*, 754-768.

Crosson, B., Sartor, K. J., Jenny, A. B., Nabors, N. A., & Moberg, P. J. (1993). Increased intrusions during verbal recall in traumatic and nontraumatic lesions of the temporal lobe. *Neuropsychology, 7*, 193-208.

Cummings, J. L., & Benson, D. F. (1992). *Dementia: A clinical approach.* Boston: Butterworth-Heinemann.

Delis, D. C. (1989). Neuropsychological assessment of learning and memory. In F. Boller & J. Grafman (Eds.), *Handbook of Neuropsychology*, (Vol 3. pp. 3-33). Amsterdam: Elsevier Science Publishers.

Delis, D. C., Cullom, C. M., Butters, N., & Cairns (1988). Wechsler Memory Scale- Revised and California Verbal Learning Test: Convergence and Divergence. *The Clinical Neuropsychologist, 2*, 188-196.

Delis, D. C., Freeland, J., Kramer, J. H., & Kaplan, E. (1988). Integrating clinical assessment with cognitive neuroscience: Construct validation of the California Verbal Learning Test. *Journal of Consulting and Clinical Psychology, 56*, 123-130.

Delis, D. C., Massman, P. J., Butters, N., Salmon, D. P., Cermak, L. S., and Kramer, J. H. (1991). Profiles of demented and amnesic patients on the California Verbal Learning Test: Implications for the assessment of memory disorders. *Psyhcological Assessment, 3*, 19-26.

Delis, D. C., Kramer, J. H., Kaplan, E., & Ober, B. A. (1987). *The California Verbal Learning Test- Research Edition.* New York: Psychological Corporation.

Diesfeldt, H. F. A. (1978). The distinction between long-term and short-term memory in senile dementia: An analysis of free recall and delayed recognition. *Neuropsychologia, 16*, 115-119.

Dupont, R. M., Jernigan, T. L., Butters, N., Delis, D., Hesselink, J. R., Heindel, W., & Gillin J. C. (1990). Subcortical abnormalities detected in bipolar affective disorder using magnetic resonance imaging: Clinical and neuropsychological significance. *Archives of General Psychiatry, 47*, 55-59.

Fisher, J. M., Kennedy, J. L, Caine, E. D., & Shoulson, I. (1983). Dementia in Huntington disease: A cross-sectional analysis of intellectual decline. In R. Mayeux & W. G. Rosen (Eds.), *The dementias*, (pp. 229-238). New York: Raven Press.

Folstein, S. E., Brandt, J., & Folstein, M. F. (1990). Huntington's disease. In J. L. Cummings (Ed.), *Subcortical dementia*, (pp. 87-107). New York: Oxford University Press.

Grant, I., Atkinson, J. H., Hesselink, J. R., Kennedy, C. J., Richman, D. D., Spector, S. A., & McCutchan, J. A. (1987). Evidence of early central nervous system involvement in the acquired immunodeficiency symdrome (AIDS) and other human immunodeficiency virus (HIV) infections. *Annals of Internal Medicine, 107*, 828-836.

Grant, I., Atkinson, J. H., Hesselink, J. R., Kennedy, C. J., Richman, D. D., Spector, S. A., & McCutchan, J. A. (1988). Human immunodeficiency virus-associated neurobehavioural disorder. *Journal of the Royal College of Physicians of London, 22*, 149-157.

Hodges, J. R., Salmon, D. P., & Butters, N. (1990). Differential impairment of semantic and episodic memory in Alzheimer's and Huntington's disease: A controlled prospective study. *Journal of Neurology, Neurosurgery, and Psychiatry, 53*, 1089-1095.

Hunt, E., & Love, T. (1972). How good can memory be? In A. W. Melton & E. Martin (Eds.), *Coding processes in human memory.* Washington, D. C.: Winston & Sons.

Klatzky, R. L. (1980). *Human memory: Structure and processes.* San Francisco: Freeman.

Kramer, J. H., & Delis, D. C. (1991). Interference effects on the California Verbal Learning Test: A construct validation study. *Psychological Assessment, 3*, 299-302.

Kramer, J. H., Delis, D. C., & Daniel, M. (1988). Sex differences in verbal learning. *Journal of Clinical Psychology, 44*, 907-915.

Kramer, J. H., Levin, B. E., Brandt, J., & Delis, D. C. (1989). Differentiation of Alzheimer's, Huntngton's, and Parkinson's disease patients on the basis of verbal learning characteristics. *Neuropsychology*, *3*, 111-120.

Maccoby, E. E., & Jacklin, C. N. (1974). *The psychology of sex differences.* Stanford, CA: Stanford University Press.

Massman, P. J., Delis, D. C., and Butters, N. (1993). Does impaired primacy recall equal impaired long-term storage?: Serial position effects in Huntington's disease and Alzheimer's disease. *Developmental Neuropsychology*, *9*, 1-15.

Massman, P. J., Delis, D. C., Butters, N., Dupont, R. M., and Gillin, J. C. (1992). The subcortical dysfunction hypothesis of memory deficits in depression: Neuropsychological validation in a subgroup of patients. *Journal of Clinical and Experimental Neuropsychology, 5*, 687-706.

Massman, P. J., Delis, D. C., Butters, N., Levin, B. E., and Salmon, D. P. (1990). Are all subcortical dementias alike?: Verbal learning and memory in Parkinson's and Huntington's disease patients. *Journal of Clinical and Experimental Neuropsychology, 12*, 729-744.

Olsen, W. L., Longo, F. M., Mills, C. M., & Norman, D. (1988). White matter disease in AIDS: Findings at MR imaging. *Radiology, 169*, 445-448.

Peavy, G., Jacobs, D., Salmon, D. P., Butters, N., Taylor, M., Massman, P., Stout, J., Heindel, W. C., Kirson, D., Kirson, D., Atkinson, J. H., Chandler, J. L., Grant, I., and the HNRC Group (in press). Verbal memory performance in patients with Human Immunodeficiency Virus Infection: Evidence for subcortical dysfunction. *Journal of Clinical and Experimental Neuropsychology.*

Postman, L. (1971). Transfer, interference and forgetting. In J. W. Kling & L. A. Riggs (Eds.), *Experimental psychology*, (pp. xx-xx). New York: Holt, Rinehart, and Winston.

Salmon, D. P., & Butters, N. (1987). The etiology and neuropathology of alcoholic Korsakoff's syndrome: Some evidence for the role of the basal forebrain. In M. Galanter *Ed.), *Recent developments in alcoholism*, pp. 27-58). New York: Plenum Press.

Salmon, D. P., Granholm, E., McCullough, D., Butters, N., & Grant, I. (1989). Recognition memory span in mildly and moderately demented patients with Alzheimer's disease. *Journal of Clinical and Experimental Neuropsychology, 11*, 429-443.

Squire, L. R. (1987). *Memory and brain.* New York: Oxford University Press.

Troster, A. I., Jacobs, D., Butters, N., Cullum, C. M., & Salmon, D. P. (1989). Differentiation of Alzheimer's disease from Huntington's disease with the Wechsler Memory Scale-Revised. *Clinics in Geriatric Medicine, 5*, 611-632.

Waugh, N. C., & Norman, D. A. (1965). Primary memory. *Psychological Review, 72*, 89-104.

Welsh, K., Buters, N., Hughes, J., Mohns, R., & Heyman, A. (1991). Detection of abnormal memory decline in mild cases of Alzheimer's disease using CERAD neuropsychological measures. *Archives of Neurology, 48*, 278-281.

17

Differential Neuropsychology

Identifying Risk Factors for Cognitive Dysfunction in Medically Ill Patients

CHRISTOPHER M. RYAN[1]

REMINISCENCE

When I went to Boston as a post-doctoral fellow in 1977, it was to work with Laird Cermak and apply principles from cognitive psychology to understand what aspects of memory were disrupted in alcoholics without Korsakoff's syndrome. Although I was familiar with the name 'Nelson Butters,' it was typically as the second, or third author on papers published by Laird; I assumed Nelson was a post-doctoral fellow or graduate student. On my first day at the VA, Nelson intercepted me, ushered me into his tiny cluttered office with its 1950s metal furniture, talked briefly about some skin condition he was struggling with and lambasted the entire field of dermatology ("Anyone can be a dermatologist: when it's wet, you dry it; when it's dry, you wet it!"), and then told me he would supervise me because Laird was busy, and never supervised post-doctoral fellows. Further, Nelson had a study for me, and as he described it, I found it to be so similar to the one I had proposed in my application that I couldn't refuse his offer. He brought me into the next room which housed most

[1] CHRISTOPHER M. RYAN, Ph.D. • Western Psychiatric Institute and Clinic, Department of Psychiatry, University of Pittsburgh School of Medicine

Neuropsychological Explorations of Memory and Cognition: Essays in Honor of Nelson Butters, edited by Laird S. Cermak, Ph.D. Plenum Press, New York, 1994

of his research assistants, gave me a stool and some file drawer space, and in that way inducted me, so to speak, into the ranks of his students.

Nelson became the most important person in my life. (This may sound melodramatic, but is true nevertheless.) That is not to say that working with him was always easy. He alternated (often from minute to minute) between mentor, parent, and good cop / bad cop. Indeed, an innocent comment could trigger an outburst of rage during which Nelson would carry on for 5 minutes, and then, abruptly, stop. In retrospect, this certainly toughened those of us who experienced these "mad dog" outbursts and prepared us to deal with all kinds of unpleasant situations. At the time, however, it made the fourteenth floor of the VA a very lively place, since everyone on the floor could hear Nelson screaming ("This paper sh*ts -- rewrite it," as he flings the manuscript across the room). Many of his students, I have subsequently come to discover, experienced a similar rite of passage.

Nelson taught me many things. He made me aware of the politics of academic medicine and taught me how to write (and "market") grant applications. He also modeled optimal paper writing skills. He would go to the Countway Library at Harvard Medical School in the morning, armed with a pad and some data, and return, several hours later, with a complete manuscript written out in longhand. "Don't obsess, he would counsel; just do it." And he did. Most important, however, is that he taught me how to serve as a mentor to students and post-docs. Despite the occasional bouts of yelling, Nelson genuinely respected and supported his students, and provided us with a tremendous degree of autonomy. He did not micromanage, but trusted us to work independently, calling on him only when we had problems we couldn't easily resolve. Actually, he encouraged us to call on him for all sorts of problems (professional and personal) and relished the role of paterfamilias. Even now, as he struggles to speak, he has advice to give me about my career and my life.

Nelson also taught me about clinical research, and it is to that topic that I now wish to turn. While others will praise Nelson's skill as a theoretician and the master of the deductive approach to science, I saw a very different side: the inductive opportunist. He taught me to observe behavior and let the data speak. Our strategy, in our studies of alcoholics, was to administer a very extensive battery of cognitive tests to large numbers of subjects and then see what kinds of relationships would appear. In fact, it was this approach that led to our papers on premature aging in alcoholics (Ryan & Butters, 1980a; Ryan, 1982; Ryan & Butters, 1984). Our study had not been designed initially to test the premature aging hypothesis, but the results fell out in that manner when we found that both age and duration of drinking were potent predictors of impairment. Without realizing it at the time, I had begun a line of research that would, over the next 15 years, seek to explain individual differences in cognitive functioning within populations of medically ill patients. In the remainder of this chapter I would like to illustrate the value of "inductive opportunism" by summarizing some of my research that has sought to identify risk factors for neuropsychological impairment in individuals with insulin-dependent diabetes mellitus.

DIABETES-RELATED NEUROPSYCHOLOGICAL IMPAIRMENT

The Disease of Diabetes

At first glance, individuals with insulin dependent (or Type 1) diabetes mellitus seem to be unlikely candidates for neuropsychological impairment. These individuals have a disorder of carbohydrate metabolism that is characterized by an inability to secrete or adequately utilize insulin, a hormone produced by the beta cells of the pancreas. Medical management of this disease is directed at maintaining blood glucose levels as close to the normal range as possible by balancing food intake, exercise, and exogenously supplied insulin. It now appears, however, that both the *treatment* of this disease and the *failure* to treat it can have an adverse impact on the central nervous system. If too much insulin is taken, or if the patient fails to balance insulin dose against food intake and energy expenditure, blood glucose levels may drop too low and directly impair brain function. Glucose is the primary fuel used by the CNS, and because the brain can neither produce nor store enough glucose to supply its needs, even a brief insulin-induced reduction in circulating plasma blood glucose will quickly disrupt neuronal metabolism and produce an acute (but reversible) decrement in mental efficiency. More prolonged episodes of hypoglycemia may lead to neuronal necrosis, or seizures, coma, and (rarely) death. On the other hand, chronic hyperglycemia -- found in those patients who are in consistently poor metabolic control because they have failed to treat their disease adequately -- can lead to an increased risk of biomedical complications which are mediated by damage to small and large blood vessels and to peripheral nerves. Visual problems (retinopathy) and sensory motor disorders (polyneuropathy) are relatively early complications of chronic hyperglycemia; kidney failure and stroke tend to be later complications of this disorder.

Given these facts, it would not be at all surprising to find evidence of brain damage in individuals who had diabetes for a relatively long period of time and had begun to develop clinically significant biomedical complications. Indeed, a series of studies published in the 1960s provided both neuropathological (Reske-Nielsen, Lundbaek, & Rafaelsen, 1965) and (weaker) neuropsychological (Rennick et al., 1968) evidence for a "diabetic encephalopathy" in adults with diabetes of long duration. There was, however, no evidence of diabetic encephalopathy -- or even subtle neuropsychological impairments -- in children or young adults with insulin-dependent diabetes. Most pediatric diabetologists maintained, in fact, that while their young patients might have more psychological distress than children without a chronic medical disease, they were at least as smart, if not smarter than their healthy peers -- a clinical impression that was buttressed by several studies measuring IQ in groups of diabetic and nondiabetic children (e.g., Hiltmann & Låking, 1966; Kubany, Danowski, & Moses, 1956).

Age at Onset and the Development of Cognitive Dysfunction

My own interest in this area was piqued by Alan Drash, a pediatric diabetologist at the University of Pittsburgh who was concerned that despite very high quality medical care, many of his diabetic patients seemed to be less successful as young adults than their nondiabetic siblings. To determine whether his clinical impressions were correct, Arthur Vega and I initiated a study to test the hypothesis that diabetic children were more likely to perform poorly on a battery of neuropsychological tests than their siblings or peers. Our plan was to administer an extensive battery of tests to adolescents 10 to 19 years of age who had been diagnosed with diabetes at least two years earlier, and to compare their performance with a group of demographically similar nondiabetic peers, the majority of whom would be recruited from family members and close friends of the diabetic subjects.

In retrospect, we asked the wrong question and designed the wrong study. I would now argue that any effort to simply compare one patient population with another will almost always yield results that are distorted and are largely irrelevant to the phenomenon of interest because of the biomedical heterogeneity characteristically found within any medically ill patient population. This becomes a real issue for the neuropsychologist if (as is almost always the case) the central nervous system is adversely affected by a relatively limited number of disease-related biomedical variables, and further, if (as is almost always the case) those relevant biomedical disturbances are not necessarily an attribute of all patients with a particular illness. We were not, however, sensitized to this issue when we initiated our study of diabetic youngsters.

Preliminary between-group comparisons, early on in the study, yielded no evidence of any significant neuropsychological impairment in the group of diabetic subjects. As we were about to conclude that there probably was not a significant effect of diabetes on cognitive functioning, we made a very serendipitous finding. Two of our diabetic subjects performed quite poorly on virtually all cognitive tests -- far worse than any of the other diabetic subjects seen to date. Subsequent review of medical records indicated that in both instances, these children had developed diabetes very early in life -- within the first five years of birth. None of our other subjects had such an early onset of diabetes, but this was not surprising since the modal age at onset of diabetes in Pittsburgh occurs between the ages of 9 and 11 years (Drash et al., 1983). As a consequence, we began to oversample children from the Pittsburgh Diabetes

Registry who had been diagnosed with diabetes during the first several years of life. Simple comparisons between 125 diabetic subjects and 83 demographically similar nondiabetic comparison subjects continued to reveal no compelling evidence of significant cognitive impairments for the diabetic sample as a whole. However, when we stratified the diabetic group into two subgroups based on age at onset, we found that those adolescents who developed diabetes during the first five years of life performed more poorly in all cognitive domains as compared to either later onset diabetic subjects or nondiabetic control subjects (Ryan, Vega, & Drash, 1985). To determine the extent to which these statistically significant between-group differences might also be of clinical significance, we operationally defined a "case" of clinically significant impairment as an individual with three or more test scores that were 2 or more standard deviation units below the mean for nondiabetic comparison subjects. Whereas 24% of the subjects in the early onset group met this criterion, only 6% of the later onset diabetic subjects and 6% of the nondiabetic comparison subjects met that criterion.

Age at onset cannot *cause* cognitive impairments in any group of subjects. Rather, it must be a marker or surrogate for some other process that can affect the brain. We hypothesized that age at onset serves as a proxy for the occurrence of multiple episodes of severe hypoglycemia acting on an immature nervous system. We know that children who experience hypoglycemic seizures early in life are likely to manifest significant CNS damage (Hirabayashi, Kitahara, & Hishida, 1980; Ingram, Stark, & Blackburn, 1967), and that those who experience nonhypoglycemic seizures or otherwise sustain brain damage early in life are more likely to show information processing deficits than those who incur such damage later in life (Dikmen, Matthews, & Harley, 1975; Fitzhugh & Fitzhugh, 1965; Teuber & Rudel, 1962). Moreover, children who develop diabetes early in life have a higher frequency of severe hypoglycemia, which has, in turn, been attributed to their heightened sensitivity to the physiological effects of insulin (Ternand et al., 1982). One could further speculate that parents of very young diabetic children might have particular difficulty in discriminating the adrenergic symptoms of hypoglycemia (e.g., sweating, restlessness, generalized discomfort) from other nonspecific disorders of childhood and hence fail to recognize and treat hypoglycemic events until they become quite serious.

If this explanation is correct, one would expect to find an association between the hypoglycemic event rate and the severity of neuropsychological dysfunction. Our failure to find a statistically significant correlation between those variables in our sample of subjects may have been a due to our inability to obtain completely accurate information on the number of hypoglycemic events from our subjects' parents, who were asked to estimate, retrospectively, the number of such episodes during their child's lifetime. However, when parents' responses were classified dichotomously into no episodes versus one or more, we did find that a significantly greater proportion (46%) of the early onset subjects had at least one severe hypoglycemic event than did later onset subjects (25%).

This age at onset effect has subsequently been replicated by other investigators who used a variety of cognitive measures to evaluate very young diabetic children (Golden et al., 1989), school age diabetic children (Rovet et al., 1988), and diabetic children and adolescents (Hagen et al., 1990). All other things being equal, children who developed diabetes during the first 4 or 5 years of life are more likely to manifest cognitive impairments whereas no, or only trivial differences, are typically found between later onset diabetic subjects and nondiabetic controls. Moreover, subjects with early onset diabetes almost invariably have a significantly higher frequency of severe hypoglycemic events than later onset subjects. These findings have important implications for the treatment of the very young diabetic patient. Because intensive insulin therapy is associated with a greatly elevated risk of severe hypoglycemia (DCCT, 1991), and because hypoglycemia increases the risk of cognitive impairment in children under the age of 5, an intensive insulin regimen ought to be avoided in this patient population (Golden et al., 1985).

Our identification of age at onset as an important predictor of neuropsychological dysfunction in diabetic youngsters would have been missed by us had we not stratified subjects on age at diagnosis. We would not have done this had we not made the (chance) clinical observation that the two research subjects who were most impaired were those who developed diabetes during the first years of life. Had we blindly followed our initial experimental design, we would have concluded that diabetic subjects perform as well, or nearly as well, as nondiabetic individuals since our sample of diabetic subjects would have been comprised almost entirely of individuals who developed diabetes somewhat later in life. In contrast, the use of age at onset as a surrogate "risk factor" for impairment led to a striking conclusion: a small subset of diabetic youngsters may manifest *clinically significant* neuropsychological impairments.

Academic Achievement and "Absence" in Later Onset Diabetic Adolescents

One approach to clinical research that was used by Nelson and me in Boston in the late 1970s was to assemble small groups of medically homogeneous patients, match the groups on a variety of demographic variables, and then compare their performance on various neuropsychological measures. Our early study on the so-called "borderline" Korsakoff patient (Ryan & Butters, 1980b) reflects that strategy.

In an effort to understand whether later onset diabetes was associated with any cognitive sequelae, my colleagues in Pittsburgh and I undertook a study using that same approach. That is, we took a relatively homogeneous group of later onset diabetic adolescents and matched each one (on the basis of age, gender, socioeconomic status, and parental education) to a nondiabetic comparison subject (Ryan, Vega, Longstreet, & Drash, 1984). We found that these two groups differed on several measures requiring rapid responding (which we attributed to a more cautious response style on the part of the diabetic subject), but more importantly, differed on measures of verbal intelligence. The verbal intelligence finding was unexpected, and because performance on this measure was not correlated with performance on other neuropsychological tests, we hypothesized that the diabetic subjects' lower scores on Wechsler subtests like Information, Vocabulary, and Arithmetic might be secondary to school absence. These subtests draw on knowledge that is typically acquired in the classroom, and because diabetic adolescents have a chronic disease, they are more likely to miss school than their nondiabetic peers. To examine that possibility, we subsequently interviewed parents about their children's school history and not only found that diabetic youngsters miss almost twice as much school as their nondiabetic friends (and siblings), but that their performance on subtests from the Wide Range Achievement Test can be predicted, in part, by number of school absences (Ryan, Longstreet, & Morrow, 1985). This same pattern of results has been largely replicated in a recent prospective study that followed school-aged diabetic children over a seven year period, beginning with diagnosis. The decline over time in WISC-R Vocabulary seen in those children was paralleled by a decline in school grades, and both of these were related to school absence (Kovacs, Goldston, & Iyengar, 1992). Our detailed analyses of academic achievement indicated that the magnitude of differences between diabetic and nondiabetic subjects on the WRAT is typically on the order of somewhat less than one half standard deviation (e.g., WRAT Reading Standard Score of 121 vs 115). This is certainly not large enough to be clinically significant, but may (for example) be sufficient to adversely affect the child's admission to a particular college.

As used here, school absence has been operationally defined in terms of the child's failure to *attend* school. On the other hand, a child may actually be present in the classroom yet be "absent" if that diabetic child is experiencing an episode of mild to moderately severe hypoglycemia, and if that hypoglycemic event is associated with a transient period of inattentiveness or reduced mental efficiency. Because of the nature of diabetes and its treatment, plasma glucose levels tend to fluctuate widely over the course of the day. Unfortunately, because the majority of diabetic individuals (especially diabetic children and adolescents) fail to monitor their plasma glucose levels systematically, they are often unaware of these fluctuations and hence have a heightened risk of experiencing mild to moderately severe periods of hypoglycemia. Could these periods of even mild hypoglycemia have an adverse effect on mental efficiency and in that way contribute (at least to some extent) to the somewhat lower performance on academic achievement tests that seems to be characteristic of many diabetic teenagers?

Numerous studies have demonstrated that moderately severe hypoglycemia can disrupt performance on a wide range of cognitive measures in both diabetic (Hoffman et al., 1989; Holmes, Koepke, & Thompson, 1986) and nondiabetic (Mitrakou et al., 1991; Steven et al., 1989) *adults*. Furthermore, this reduction in mental efficiency may persist long after restoration of the euglycemic state (Herold et al., 1985). To determine whether a similar relationship would be evident in children, we undertook a series of studies in which we experimentally induced hypoglycemia by means of the hyperinsulinemic clamp technique. Briefly, this procedure entails the intravenous infusion of insulin at a constant rate and the simultaneous intravenous infusion of a 10% dextrose-water solution. Plasma glucose values are sampled every five minutes by drawing blood from an catheter inserted in the nondominant dorsal hand vein. Based on results from the plasma glucose assay, the endocrinologist periodically changes the amount of dextrose infused in an effort to reach (and then maintain or "clamp") a targeted plasma glucose value. In the typical experimental paradigm, a euglycemic state (ca. 100 mg/dl) is clamped for at least 30 minutes, plasma glucose levels are quickly brought down to a hypoglycemic nadir and are clamped at that level for 60 to 90 minutes, and then brought back up to euglycemia.

When we used this technique to induce "mild" hypoglycemia (plasma glucose level of 60-65 mg/dl) in a group of diabetic adolescents, we found a significant deterioration in performance, relative to the euglycemic baseline level of performance, on measures of simple and choice reaction time, on the Stroop Color Word Interference Test, and on the Trail Making Test (Ryan et al., 1990). These decrements in performance were quite dramatic. For example, it took these subjects nearly twice as long to complete Part B of the Trail Making Test during the hypoglycemic state, as compared to the euglycemic state. Moreover, 6 of the 11 children met our criterion for clinically significant impairment on this measure insofar as their hypoglycemic Trail Making scores exceeded the euglycemic mean value by more than 2 standard deviations. Certain performances, like Trail Making, recovered immediately upon restoration of euglycemia. Other performances, like choice reaction time, required more than 30 minutes of euglycemia before they fully recovered. We were particularly struck by the vast individual differences in responsivity to hypoglycemia, with some subjects showing extremely large decrements in performance, whereas for others, no decrement in functioning occurred.

These findings are consistent with our hypothesis that at *least for some diabetic children*, an episode of even mild hypoglycemia may produce a significant decline in mental efficiency, as indexed by measures of attention and mental flexibility. The child may be present in the classroom but not completely attentive and for that reason may be experiencing episodes of *absence* that may be quite similar to the *absence* seen in children with petit mal epilepsy. Why some diabetic children are so sensitive to mild hypoglycemia whereas others are not remains unknown. In our efforts to discover the physiological basis for these individual differences, we have begun to measure changes in regional cerebral blood flow during experimentally induced hypoglycemia (Jarjour, Becker, & Ryan, 1993) and to measure the secretion of hormones like epinephrine, norepinephrine, and pancreatic polypeptide (Gschwend, Ryan, Atchison, & Becker, 1993). Very preliminary results from our hormone studies indicate that there is a robust relationship between decrements on measures like Trail Making and changes in release of the gut hormone, pancreatic polypeptide. Indeed, knowing the children's age, and their relative increase (from baseline) in pancreatic polypeptide secretion, we can account for more than 65% of the variance in Trail Making. Pancreatic polypeptide is considered by some experts to be a marker of autonomic nervous system activity, particularly parasympathetic activity, but the exact mechanism responsible for hypoglycemic-induced cognitive decrements has not yet been identified.

Effects of Chronic Hyperglycemia on Mental Efficiency in Diabetic Young Adults

Work with children and adolescents has emphasized the potentially deleterious effects of hypoglycemic events on cognitive functioning. Although there is no doubt that severe hypoglycemia, at any age, can have a profound effect on the structural and functional integrity of the central nervous system, a series of studies conducted by our research group on a large cohort of diabetic young adults has suggested that chronic severe *hyperglycemia* may also be a very potent risk factor for cognitive dysfunction (Ryan, Williams, Orchard, & Finegold, 1992). To date, we have administered an extensive battery of cognitive tests to more than 140 Type 1 diabetic adults who were drawn from the Children's Hospital of Pittsburgh Diabetes Registry. Each subject was asked to invite a nondiabetic friend or family member to participate in this study as well, and in that way a group of more than 100 demographically similar nondiabetic comparison subjects was assembled. This is a most unusual group of diabetic subjects, not only for its size, but for the fact that all were diagnosed before 17 years of age, and had the disease of diabetes for more than 25 years, on average. Because approximately half the subjects manifested significant biomedical complications of diabetes, we were able to determine the extent to which certain markers of chronic hyperglycemia could have an impact on neuropsychological functioning.

Our results demonstrated that for the most part, diabetic adults show relatively few clinically significant cognitive impairments. Nevertheless, a subset of our subjects were impaired, relative to nondiabetic control subjects, on measures of psychomotor efficiency and spatial information-processing. The most potent predictor of lower scores in these cognitive domains was degree of chronic hyperglycemia, as indicated by the presence of complications like distal symmetrical polyneuropathy. Indeed, the statistical model that we developed indicated that previous episodes of severe hypoglycemia had no direct impact on functioning, but served merely to moderate the effects of the primary predictor, chronic hyperglycemia (Ryan, Williams, Finegold, & Orchard, 1993). In its present form, this risk factor model is able to account for a relatively small (but statistically significant) proportion of the variance in cognitive test scores, but we have not yet examined the effects of other disease states, like hypertension, that are commonly associated with diabetes of long duration and are also known to adversely affect neuropsychological functioning (Waldstein, Manuck, Ryan, & Muldoon, 1991).

    This emphasis on the importance of hyperglycemia in the etiology of neuropsychological dysfunction in young and middle aged diabetic adults is counter to the conventional wisdom that diabetes-related cognitive impairments are solely a consequence of severe hypoglycemia (Langan, Deary, Hepburn, & Frier, 1991; Wredling, Levander, Adamson, & Lins, 1990). There is, however, increasing support for our hypothesis that diabetic peripheral neuropathy -- a common biomedical complication associated with chronic hyperglycemia (Greene, Lattimer, Ulbrecht, & Carroll, 1985) -- may also be a marker for a metabolically-mediated "central neuropathy" that is characterized by the kind of psychomotor slowing seen in our patients (Ryan et al., 1992). Indirect evidence for that hypothesis comes from a series of brainstem auditory evoked potential studies that demonstrate that diabetic adults show longer latencies on these measures than healthy control subjects (Harkins, Gardner, & Anderson, 1985; Khardori et al., 1986). Moreover, diabetic individuals with peripheral neuropathy have a much higher rate of structural lesions within the brain, as indicated by magnetic resonance imaging, than do age matched nondiabetic comparison subjects (Dejgaard et al., 1991).

    The mechanism underlying this "hyperglycemic encephalopathy" remains unknown. One possibility is that the metabolic disturbances which are associated with clinically significant diabetic neuropathy (e.g., changes in peripheral nerve Na+-K+-ATPase activity and the resulting reduction in *myo*-inositol and sorbitol metabolism; Greene et al., 1985) may disrupt the cell transport of metabolites and substrates within both the peripheral and central nervous systems. Alternately, chronic hyperglycemia may adversely affect brain function by inducing a loss of neocortical neurons and/or by leading to a shortening the neocortical capillary network (Jakobsen et al., 1987). It is also possible that chronic hyperglycemia may lead to cerebral *hypo*glycemia by reducing the transport of glucose across the blood-brain barrier (Gjedde & Crone, 1981). Although the exact mechanism underlying this central neuropathy remains obscure, the identification of this type of deficit has important (and immediate) implications for patient care. Preventing chronic hyperglycemia by implementing an intensive insulin therapy regimen (DCCT, 1993) may serve not only to retard the development of clinically significant peripheral neuropathy in the diabetic adult, but it may serve to prevent or reduce the severity of the psychomotor slowing which is the hallmark of central neuropathy.

EXPLAINING COGNITIVE VARIABILITY IN MEDICALLY ILL PATIENTS: TOWARDS A DIFFERENTIAL NEUROPSYCHOLOGY

Two conclusions can be drawn from this research on the relationship between cognitive functioning and diabetes. First, not all individuals with the disease manifest significant (or even subtle) neuropsychological deficits. Second, the risk factors responsible for impairment may change across the lifespan (Ryan, in press). In fact, it appears that not only do the risk factors vary, but the phenomenology of impairment -- the nature and extent of the neurobehavioral dysfunction -- differ, depending on the individual's age at assessment. Very young children with an early onset of diabetes tend to have deficits that are primarily visuospatial in nature whereas adolescents with the same type of medical history tend to show impairments in all cognitive domains. These deficits have been attributed to repeated episodes of hypoglycemia that presumably affect the structural and functional integrity of the CNS. On the other hand, children and adolescents with a later onset of diabetes show the greatest cognitive deficits on measures of academic achievement and verbal intelligence, and this, in turn, seems to be associated with "absences" -- defined in terms of school attendance, and in terms of transient episodes of inattention secondary to mild neuroglycopenia. As we move into the young adult diabetic population, the relative salience or biomedical risk factors, as well as the behavioral manifestations of dysfunction change again. Cognitive deficits are largely, but not entirely, psychomotor in nature, and these are best predicted not by hypoglycemia but by severe hyperglycemia, as indexed by the presence of certain medical complications, like distal symmetric polyneuropathy. It is interesting to note that in the elderly adult with *Type 2* (i.e., non-insulin dependent) diabetes, the best predictor of cognitive dysfunction is also degree of chronic *hyper*glycemia (Ryan & Williams, 1993).

As I think about other medical (and neurological) disorders, I see a need to take a similar approach and incorporate in experimental designs those biomedical (and psychosocial) variables that may help explain why certain patients manifest a particular pattern of cognitive impairment, whereas others are completely intact. I have previously used the term "neurobehavioral epidemiology" to characterize a strategy where investigators would administer comprehensive biomedical, psychosocial and neuropsychological assessment batteries to large numbers of subjects drawn from a particular population of interest. By exploring the inter-relationships between test scores and various medical, demographic, and psychosocial variables, one would be able to identify salient risk factors for cognitive impairment (Ryan, Morrow, Bromet, & Parkinson, 1987). It is critical to take a truly epidemiologic approach and conduct such an assessment on a large sample drawn randomly (to the extent that is possible) from the population of interest. In this way, we will be closer in reaching the goal of being able to explain the individual variability found within any patient population, and that, in turn, will provide us with important insights into the etiology of neuropsychological dysfunction in the medically ill individual.

As my mentor, Nelson emphasized both the value of collecting enormous amounts of data on each subject, and more importantly, the need to search for meaningful relationships within a diverse data set. Allowing data to speak is a critical feature of "inductive opportunism." Another critical feature is this: be prepared for the unexpected, and exploit it. While I have certainly learned many things from Nelson, I consider this maxim to be his legacy to me.

REFERENCES

DCCT Research Group. (1993). Effect of intensive treatment of diabetes on the development and progression of long-term complications in insulin-dependent diabetes mellitus. *New England Journal of Medicine, 329*, 977-986.

DCCT Research Group. (1991). Epidemiology of severe hypoglycemia in the Diabetes Control and Complications Trial. *American Journal of Medicine, 90*, 450-459.

Dejgaard, A., Gade, A., Larsson, H., Balle, V., Parving, A., & Parving, H. (1991). Evidence for diabetic encephalopathy. *Diabetic Medicine, 8*, 162-167.

Dikmen, S., Matthews, C., & Harley, J.P. (1975). The effect of early versus late onset of major motor epilepsy on cognitive-intellectual performance. *Epilepsia, 16*, 73-81.

Drash, A.L., LaPorte, R.E., Becker, D.J., Orchard, T.J., Wagener, D.K., Rabin, B., & Kuller, L.H. (1983). Epidemiological studies in children with diabetes mellitus and their families: The Allegheny County Registry Experience. In: G. Chiumello & M. Sperling, Eds. *Recent Progress in Pediatric Endocrinology.* New York: Raven Press, pp 125-136

Fitzhugh, K.B. & Fitzhugh, L.C. (1965). Effects of early and later onset of cerebral dysfunction upon psychological test performance. *Perceptual and Motor Skills, 20*, 1099-1100.

Gjedde, A., & Crone, C. (1981). Blood-brain glucose transfer: repression in chronic hyperglycemia. *Science, 214*, 456-457.

Golden, M., Ingersoll, G., Brack, C., Russell, B., Wright, J., & Huberty, T. (1989). Longitudinal relationship of asymptomatic hypoglycemia to cognitive function in IDDM. *Diabetes Care, 12*, 89-93.

Golden, M., Russell, B., Ingersoll, G., Gray, D., & Hummer, K. (1985). Management of diabetes mellitus in children younger than 5 years of age. *American Journal of Diseases in Children, 139*, 448-452.

Greene, D., Lattimer, S., Ulbrecht, J., & Carroll, P. (1985). Glucose- induced alterations in nerve metabolism: Current perspective on the pathogenesis of diabetic neuropathy and future directions for research and therapy. *Diabetes Care*, *8*, 290-299.

Gschwend, S., Ryan, C., Atchison, J., & Becker, J. (1993). Changes in cognitive function during glycemic variations are associated with ANS stimulation in adolescents with IDDM. *Diabetes*, *42* (Suppl. 1), 198A.

Hagen, J.W., Barclay, C.R., Anderson, B.J., Feeman, D.J., Segal, S.S., Bacon, G., & Goldstein, G.W. (1990). Intellective functioning and strategy use in children with insulin-dependent diabetes mellitus. *Child Development*, *61*, 1714-1727.

Harkins, S., Gardner, D., & Anderson, R. (1985). Auditory and somatosensory far-field evoked potentials in diabetes mellitus. *International Journal of Neuroscience*, *28*, 41-47.

Herold, K.C., Polonsky, K.S., Cohen, R.M., Levy, J., & Douglas, F. (1985). Variable deterioration in cortical function during insulin-induced hypoglycemia. Diabetes, 34, 677-685.

Hiltmann, H. & Låking, J. (1966). Die intelligenz bei diabetischen kindern im schulalter. *Acta Paedopsychiatrica*, *33*, 11-24.

Hirabayashi, S., Kitahara, T., & Hishida, T. (1980). Computed tomography in perinatal hypoxic and hypoglycemic encephalopathy with emphasis on follow-up studies, *4*, 451-456. *Journal of Computer Assisted Tomography*

Hoffman, R.G., Speelman, D.J., Hinnen, D.A., Conley, K.L., Guthrie, R.A., & Knapp, R.K. (1989). Changes in cortical functioning with acute hypoglycemia and hyperglycemia in type I diabetes. *Diabetes Care*, *3*, 193-197.

Holmes, C., Koepke, K., & Thompson, R. (1986). Simple versus complex performance impairments at three different glucose levels. *Psychoneuroendocrinology*, *11*, 353-357.

Ingram, T.T.S., Stark, G.D., & Blackburn, I. (1967). Ataxia and other neurological disorders as sequels of severe hypoglycemia in childhood. *Brain*, *90*, 851-862.

Jakobsen, J., Sidenius, P., Gundersen, H., & Osterby, R. (1987). Quantitative changes of cerebral neocortical structure in insulin-treated long-term streptozocin-induced diabetes in rats. *Diabetes*, *36*, 597-601.

Jarjour, I.T., Becker, D.J., & Ryan, C.M. (1993). Asymmetrical increases in regional cerebral blood flow during hypoglycemia in children with insulin-dependent diabetes mellitus. *Annals of Neurology*, *34*, 466-467.

Khardori, R., Soler, N., Good, D., DevlescHoward, A., Broughton, D., & Walbert, J. (1986). Brainstem auditory and visual evoked potentials in Type I (insulin-dependent) diabetic patients. *Diabetologia*, *29*, 362-365.

Kovacs, M., Goldston, D., & Iyengar, S. (1992). Intellectual development and academic performance of children with insulin-dependent diabetes mellitus: a longitudinal study. *Developmental Psychology*, *28*, 676-684.

Kubany, A., Danowski, T., & Moses, C. (1956). The personality and intelligence of diabetics. *Diabetes*, *5*, 462-467.

Langan, S., Deary, I., Hepburn, D., & Frier, B. (1991). Cumulative cognitive impairment following recurrent severe hypoglycaemia in adult patients with insulin-treated diabetes mellitus. *Diabetologia*, *34*, 337-344.

Mitrakou, A., Ryan, C., Veneman, T., Mokan, M., Jenssen, T., Kiss, I., Durrant, J., Cryer, P., & Gerich, J. (1991). Hierarchy of glycemic thresholds for counterregulatory hormone secretion, symptoms, and cerebral dysfunction. *American Journal of Physiology, 260*, E67-E74.

Rennick, P., Wilder, R., Sargent, J., & Ashley, B. (1968). Retinopathy as an indicator of cognitive-perceptual-motor impairment in diabetic adults [Summary]. Proceedings of the 76th Annual Convention of the American Psychological Association, p 473-474.

Reske-Nielson, E., Lundbaek, K., & Rafaelsen, O. (1965). Pathological changes in the central and peripheral nervous system of young long-term diabetics. *Diabetologia, 1*, 232-241.

Rovet, J., Ehrlich, R., & Hoppe, M. (1988). Specific intellectual deficits associated with the early onset of insulin-dependent diabetes mellitus in children. *Child Development, 59*, 226-234.

Ryan, C. (1982). Alcoholism and premature aging: A neuropsychological perspective. *Alcoholism: Clinical and Experimental Research, 6*, 22-30.

Ryan, C. (in press). Effects of diabetes on neuropsychological functioning: A lifespan approach. In Adams, K.M. & Grant, I., (Eds): *Neuropsychological Assessment of Neuromedical Disorders*. New York: Oxford University Press.

Ryan, C., Atchinson, J., Puczynski, S., Puczynski, M., Arslanian, S., & Becker, D. (1990). Mild hypoglycemia associated with deterioration of mental efficiency in children with insulin-dependent diabetes mellitus. *Journal of Pediatrics, 117*, 32-38.

Ryan, C., & Butters, N. (1980a). Learning and memory impairments in young and old alcoholics: Evidence for the premature-aging hypothesis. *Alcoholism: Clinical and Experimental Research, 4*, 288-293.

Ryan, C., & Butters, N. (1980b). Further evidence for a continuum-of-impairment encompassing male alcoholic Korsakoff patients and chronic alcoholic men. *Alcoholism: Clinical and Experimental Research, 4*, 190-198.

Ryan, C., & Butters, N. (1984). Alcohol consumption and premature aging: A critical review. In: M. Galanter, Ed. *Recent Developments in Alcoholism, 2*. Plenum Publishing Corporation, pp 223-250.

Ryan, C., Longstreet, C., & Morrow, L. (1985). The effects of diabetes mellitus on the school attendance and school achievement of adolescents. *Child: Care, Health and Development, 11*, 229-240.

Ryan, C., Morrow, L., Bromet, E., & Parkinson, D. (1987). Assessment of neuropsychological dysfunction in the workplace: Normative data from the Pittsburgh Occupational Exposures Test Battery. *Journal of Clinical and Experimental Neuropsychology, 9*, 665-679.

Ryan, C., Vega, A., & Drash, A. (1985). Cognitive deficits in adolescents who developed diabetes early in life. *Pediatrics, 75*, 921-927.

Ryan, C., Vega, A., Longstreet, C., & Drash, A. (1984). Neuropsychological changes in adolescents with insulin-dependent diabetes. *Journal of Consulting and Clinical Psychology, 52*, 335-342.

Ryan, C., & Williams, T.M. (1993). Effects of insulin-dependent diabetes on learning and memory efficiency in adults. *Journal of Clinical and Experimental Neuropsychology,* *15,* 685-700.

Ryan, C., Williams, T.M., Finegold, D.N., & Orchard, T.J. (1993). Cognitive dysfunction in adults with Type 1 (insulin-dependent) diabetes mellitus of long duration: effects of recurrent hypoglycaemia and other chronic complications. *Diabetologia, 36,* 329-334.

Ryan, C., Williams, T., Orchard, T., & Finegold, D. (1992). Psychomotor slowing is associated with distal symmetrical polyneuropathy in adults with diabetes mellitus. *Diabetes, 41,* 107-113.

Stevens, A.B., McKane, W.R., Bell, P.M., Bell, P., King, D.J., & Hayes, J.R. (1989). Psychomotor performance and counterregulatory responses during mild hypoglycemia in healthy volunteers. *Diabetes Care, 12,* 12-17.

Ternand, C., Go, V., Gerich, J., & Haymond, M. (1982). Endocrine pancreatic response of children with onset of insulin-requiring diabetes before age 3 and after age 5. *Journal of Pediatrics, 101,* 36-39.

Teuber, H.-L. & Rudel, R. (1962). Behavior after cerebral lesions in children and adults. *Developmental Medicine and Child Neurology, 4,* 3-20.

Waldstein, S.R., Manuck, S.B., Ryan, C.M., & Muldoon, M.F. (1991). Neuropsychological correlates of hypertension: Review and methodologic considerations. *Psychological Bulletin, 110,* 451-468.

Wredling, R., Levander, S., Adamson, U., & Lins, P. (1990). Permanent neuropsychological impairment after recurrent episodes of severe hypoglycaemia in man. *Diabetologia, 33,* 152-157.

18

Procedural Memory and Rehabilitation

GERALD GOLDSTEIN[1]

In his 1984 APA Division 40 Presidential Address, Nelson Butters presented evidence of a double dissociation in the memory function of patients with Huntington's disease and alcoholic Korsakoff's syndrome (Butters, 1984). The Huntington's disease patients were found to have relatively normal verbal recognition memory but poor skill learning, while the reverse was true for the alcoholic Korsakoff patients. Of particular interest for our present purposes was that the skill learning of the alcoholic Korsakoff patients, using a mirror-reading task, was accomplished at a rate comparable to that of the normal controls. Despite their failure to recognize features of the task following training, their performance nevertheless improved over three days of training.

This report confirmed the earlier findings of Cohen and Squire (1980) indicating that severely amnesic patients can learn new information. Since that time an extensive literature has emerged documenting and delineating the existence of a preserved memory system in Korsakoff type amnesia, now generally characterized as implicit memory (Schacter, 1990). A series of studies using priming paradigms, skill learning, repetitive instruction with vanishing cues (Glisky, Schacter, & Tulving, 1986) and related methodologies have continued to demonstrate relatively normal performance by severely amnesic patients on tasks of these types in the presence of severe memory failure on free recall or other declarative memory tasks.

Clinicians responsible for the care of amnesic patients have traditionally been perhaps understandably pessimistic about the outcome for patients with

[1] GERALD GOLDSTEIN, Ph.D. • Department of Veterans Affairs Medical Center, Pittsburgh and Unversity of Pittsburgh

Neuropsychological Explorations of Memory and Cognition: Essays in Honor of Nelson Butters, edited by Laird S. Cermak, Ph.D. Plenum Press, New York, 1994

these disorders. Typically, these amnesias are dense, persistent, and substantially disabling. They do not remit spontaneously, nor does any form of treatment or rehabilitation appear to be effective in restoring memory. As a neuropsychologist interested in rehabilitation, the description and experimental verification of a preserved memory system was very exciting to me, and I am pleased to acknowledge the major impact of Nelson Butters and his colleagues on the work my collaborators and I have been doing in memory rehabilitation for patients with severe amnesia. The idea we had was a very simple one. If amnesic patients can learn new skills on experimental tasks, perhaps they can also learn information significant for their everyday lives. While such new learning would not be expected to "cure" or reverse their amnesias, it might provide skills that are of some adaptive significance. In what follows, I would like to review our progress in pursuing that idea.

INITIAL CASE STUDIES WITH BEHAVIOR THERAPY

The first approach taken to rehabilitation involved not so much memory training itself, but a form of behavior modification with amnesic patients designed to reduce the incidence of disruptive behaviors. Some years ago, we published two case studies utilizing operant conditioning methodology for reduction of disruptive behaviors in severely amnesic patients (Goldstein & Ruthven, 1987). Initially, we were skeptical about the potential efficacy of these procedures, thinking that the patients would not have the capacities to encode and retrieve their reinforcement histories. However, both of these patients showed reasonably typical operant conditioning learning curves. One of them was taught to refrain from continually making inappropriate verbal requests (for candy and chewing gum), and the other showed a marked reduction in frequent, daily episodes of fecal incontinence. In both cases, single-subject designs were employed with adequate baseline measurement and systematic application of reinforcers under well controlled conditions. The learning curves were no different from what one would expect from a normal subject.

MEMORY TRAINING STUDIES

Subsequently, we applied conditioning strategies to two more patients, this time within the context of more formal memory training. The first case was a man with alcoholic Korsakoff's syndrome who we attempted to teach functionally useful items of information, such as the name of his ward, through an application of the Premack recency principle (Premack, 1965). In this application, we paired items in the patient's intact long term memory, such as his wife's name, with the items to be learned. The patient was administered a series of daily repetition trials over a period of three days. The training was conducted in the morning, and probes were made by ward staff members in the morning and afternoon. For example, a pair might be Jane (wife's name retained by the patient) with 2-3 West (the ward name). The probe would be an inquiry concerning the ward name. If the patient responded incorrectly, he would be given the stimulus word (Jane). We found that the patient did learn and retain the new material, and made mostly correct responses to the probes, both in the morning and the afternoon. However, when he failed to remember, the stimulus word was rarely effective in producing a correct response. It now seems clear that we were doing a form of skill learning with this patient, and thereby tapping into his preserved procedural knowledge system.

As an experimental demonstration of this kind of skill acquisition learning, we trained a patient whose amnesia was produced by an episode of cardiac arrest to improve his performance on the Luria-Nebraska Neuropsychological Battery (Golden, Hammeke, & Purisch, 1980) Memory Processes Scale. As anticipated, the patient performed extremely poorly on this scale initially, only passing immediate repetition type items. However, with daily administration of the scale over twenty sessions, performance gradually improved to the point of an almost perfect performance. An alternate form of the scale was improvised, and he was trained on it as well. Learning occurred at the same rate as was the case for the original scale, without savings.

We serendipitously received support for the idea that procedural knowledge was what was being learned in these patients when we attempted to train an amnesic patient with a method that would appear to involve declarative memory. The patient, a 52 year old severely amnesic man, received training utilizing a paired-associate learning method stressing imagery and verbal mediation. Thus, for example, if the word pair was "tree-grocery" the patient was taught to make up a sentence like, "The bright green tree stood in front of the Italian grocery store." While the patient did an excellent job of producing sentences with high imagery, there was no improvement in his associative memory ability. It now seems apparent that this failure may well have been related to reliance on the ability to form new associations; i.e. a declarative memory ability not in the patient's repertoire. Interestingly, in a study involving head-injured patients with relatively mild amnesia, imagery methods were found to be effective (Goldstein, McCue, Turner, Spanier, & Malec, 1988). This difference in outcome is supportive of Nelson Butters' concept of different types of amnesia described in his 1984 address and in Butters, Miliotis, Albert, & Sax (1984). Thus, it now appears that the heterogeneity of amnesia has implications for differential treatment planning dependent on the type and severity of memory loss.

We then went on to a more direct attempt to teach new information in the manner of skill acquisition. The first patient we worked with was a 52 year old man with the diagnosis of alcoholic amnestic disorder. Because of the profound nature of his amnesia, we determined that we would attempt to teach this patient basic orientation items such as the name of his ward and his room number. We used the same method described above involving pairing an old memory with a to-be-learned item over a number of daily sessions. However, this time we used a multiple baseline design in which one item was trained at a time. A total of five items was selected, and so the patient was trained on one item and probed on all five in order to demonstrate the specific effects of the training. One probe was made every day following training, and one was made every afternoon. Baseline data were collected to establish that the patient did not already have the to-be-taught information in his repertoire. We were able to effectively teach this patient three of the five items trained. He learned, and consistently recalled upon request the name of his ward, the location of the canteen, and the name of the trainer. He did not learn his room number or the hospital visiting hours, both of which were sequences of numbers.

Since the introduction of the old memory stimulus word did not produce recall when spontaneous recall did not occur, we abandoned the paired associate method and, in subsequent studies, simply used daily repetition of the material to be learned. We completed a study utilizing this repetition method in a multiple baseline design with five patients, all of whom met the Butters and Cermak (1980) psychometric criteria for Kosakoff's syndrome (Goldstein & Malec, 1989). Patients were asked to do 20 repetitions of the item trained every day, with two probes a day, as described above. With few exceptions, each of these patients learned all of the items trained. All of the patients learned some of the items. The multiple baseline design effectively demonstrated that recall was restricted to the trained items. There were no spontaneous recalls of untrained items.

As might be anticipated, the patients who participated in the studies described above, while generally successful at learning specific material by repetition, remained as amnesic as ever in other respects. The rehabilitation problem therefore became one of finding some means of obtaining generalization to new materials. Otherwise, one would only have recourse to teaching patients every individual new item one wanted them to learn. A case study mentioned above indicated that severely amnesic patients do not appear to benefit from use of mnemonic aids such as imagery or verbal elaboration. Thus, the application of so-called "strategy learning" techniques appeared to be inappropriate. The implicit or procedural learning we were employing appeared to be learning without generalization or transfer. The issue of transfer in memory impaired patients has recently been considered by M. Butters, Glisky, & Schacter (1993) who report that the evidence for transfer is conflicting, and may vary depending upon the severity of the amnesia. In their own study, their severely impaired patients showed less transfer than their mildly and moderately impaired patients. It was suggested that failure of transfer may result from too few learning trials.

If that were the case, however, it would still be necessary to expend extensive efforts on teaching of specific material.

A MEMORY PROTHESIS

Our proposed solution to the problem involved taking a prosthetic approach. Several considerations contributed to our reasoning. First, most amnesic patients retain the ability to read, and have sufficient motor skill to operate simple devices. Second, we were aware of the common practice used in rehabilitation hospitals involving having anomic or amnesic patients maintain lists of words or things to do that they cannot remember. Third, while the list method can be quite effective in some cases, densely amnesic patients would be likely to forget about the existence of the list itself, and would probably have to be continually reminded to use it. Thus, the idea of designing a simple device emerged in which information could be stored. The device would have the appearance of a pocket computer which patients could carry with them. The device could also be programmable, such that the information could be changed when necessary.

In and of itself, providing patients with a device would not be sufficient because, like lists, the device would readily be forgotten. The problem therefore became one of teaching patients to remember to use the device. Actual operation of it could be reasonably assured by making it quite simple, containing only a window display for the items and two push-buttons for moving the item list forward or backward. We did not feel that the commonly available "personal reminders" incorporated into pocket computers or wrist watches would work, because of their complexity. The possible solution to the problem was once again inspired by the work of Nelson Butters, who showed that very amnesic patients can acquire skills or learn procedures.

We are now in the process of teaching patients with Korsakoff's syndrome to use such a device. The device contains information customized for each patient, and may contain such materials as the patient's address, names of medication, and names of significant people. The teaching procedure utilizes a conditioning paradigm in which a question requesting information is the unconditioned stimulus, a tone is the conditioned stimulus, and the movements required to access and operate the device is the conditioned response. Preliminary data indicate that, as anticipated, patients can operate the device. Initial results with field trials are promising, and indicate that patients can learn to reach for and use the device when asked a question. Planned future research will also look at generalization across questioners and settings in which the device is used.

SUMMARY AND CONCLUDING COMMENTS

In summary, we have tried to show how studies done and theories developed within the framework of experimental neuropsychology can not only provide new knowledge concerning human memory, but can also quickly become relevant to patient care considerations. Nelson Butters is particularly adept at formulating scientific insights in a way that has direct relevance to human problems. To him, the disciplines of "experimental" and "clinical" neuropsychology are not separate entities, divided on each side by sometimes elitist boundaries, but rather represent a process in which observation of patients leads to scientific investigation and discoveries, with these discoveries subsequently aiding in the understanding and treatment of patients. It has been my personal observation over the years that Nelson Butters is not interested in amnesic patients solely because they are particularly good subjects for studying memory. He became genuinely interested in his Korsakoff patients, and could tell you a great deal about their lives and about how they were as people. In his recent work, he has also become quite concerned with the development of scientifically sound clinical assessment instruments (e.g., Jacobs, Tröster, Butters, Salmon, & Cermak, 1990).

Nelson Butters and I never collaborated on a study, and we never had a student-teacher or co-worker relationship. Nevertheless, he has had a remarkable impact on my career, the material presented above being only one example of many that could have been given. We served on many boards and committees together, and worked hard to get clinical neuropsychology established in the Veterans Administration and with the psychological establishment. Nelson Butters' career spanned the founding of the International Neuropsychological Society (INS) and the National Academy of Neuropsychology (NAN), the establishment of the Division of Clinical Neuropsychology in the American Psychological Association, and the establishment of diplomate status for clinical neuropsychology through the American Board of Professional Psychology. I'm sure that others contributing
to this volume will also comment on this aspect of Nelson Butters' career, but I would like to do so as well since it is important to recognize that his contributions to our discipline were not only those of a scientist and clinician, but also that of an effective, articulate, and dedicated leader.

REFERENCES

Butters, M. A., Glisky, E. L. & Schacter, D. L. (1993). Transfer of new learning in memory-impaired patients. *Journal of Clinical and Experimental Psychology, 15,* 219-230.

Butters, N. (1984). The clinical aspects of memory disorders: Contributions from experimental studies of amnesia and dementia. *Journal of Clinical Neuropsychology, 6*, 17-36.

Butters, N., & Cermak, L. S. (1980). Alcoholic Korsakoff's syndrome: An information-processing approach to amnesia. New York: Academic Press.

Butters, N., Miliotis, P., Albert, M. S., & Sax, D. (1984). Memory assessment: Evidence of the heterogeneity of amnesic symptoms. In G. Goldstein (Ed.), *Advances in clinical neuropsychology, Vol. 1.* New York: Plenum Press.

Cohen, N., & Squire, L. R. (1980). Preserved learning and retention of pattern analyzing skills in amnesia: Dissociation of knowing how and knowing that. *Science, 210*, 207-210.

Glisky, E. L., Schacter, D. L., & Tulving, E. (1986). Learning and retention of computer-related vocabulary in memory-impaired patients: Method of vanishing cues. *Journal of Clinical and Experimental Neuropsychology, 8*, 292-312.

Golden, C. J., Hammeke, T. A., & Purisch, A. D. (1980). The Luria-Nebraska Neuropsychological Battery: Manual. Los Angeles: Western Psychological Services.

Goldstein, G. & Malec, E. A. (1989). Memory training for severely amnesic patients. *Neuropsychology, 3*, 9-16.

Goldstein, G., McCue, M., Turner, S., Spanier, C. & Malec, E. (1988). An efficacy study of memory training for patients with closed head injury. *The Clinical Neuropsychologist, 2*, 251-259.

Goldstein, G., & Ruthven, L. (1987). Rehabilitation of the brain-damaged adult. New York: Plenum Press.

Jacobs, D., Tröster, A. I., Butters, N., Salmon, D. P. & Cermak, L. (1990). Intrusion errors on the visual reproduction test of the Wechsler Memory Scale and the Wechsler Memory Scale-Revised. *The Clinical Neuropsychologist, 4*, 177-191.

Premack, D. (1965). Reinforcement theory. In D. Levin (Ed.). Nebraska symposium on motivation. Lincoln, Nebraska: University of Nebraska Press.

Schacter, D. L. (1990). Toward a cognitive neuropsychology of awareness: Implicit knowledge and anosognosia. *Journal of Clinical and Experimental Neuropsychology, 12*, 155-178.

19

Psychodynamic Phenomena, Cognitive Science, and Neuroscience

BARBARA PENDLETON JONES[1]

I met Nelson Butters waiting for the elevator on the 14th floor of the Boston VA Hospital. At the time, I was a research assistant for a couple of neurologists, taking psychology courses at night and applying to graduate programs in clinical psychology. I had taken but a single psychology course as an undergraduate, not being very interested in the reigning behaviorism, but had caught fire studying abnormal psychology. Subsequently, a year as a research assistant at Oxford's Department of Experimental Psychology (while my husband, a classmate of Bill Clinton's, finished a scholarship) had had the unexpected result of sparking my interest in the brain. So by the time I met Nelson, I already had my unorthodox dual interest in psychopathology and cognitive processes. Nelson encouraged me to apply to the Boston University clinical program and offered to supervise my master's and doctoral research if I wanted to specialize in neuropsychology. I did, and he did, and we published several papers on my work on olfactory deficits in Korsakoff syndrome patients and chronic alcoholics. This work evoked mostly skepticism and bemusement at the time but was replicated and helped to open up a whole new area of research within neuropsychology. Then and always Nelson was a superb teacher and supported and encouraged me even when I did not undertake a traditional career in academic neuropsychology. He was amused and pleased to see some of my interests--e.g., repression and dissociation--

---

[1] BARBARA PENDLETON JONES, Ph.D. • Laboratory of Psychology and Psychopathology, National Institute of Mental Health

Neuropsychological Explorations of Memory and Cognition: Essays in Honor of Nelson Butters, edited by Laird S. Cermak, Ph.D. Plenum Press, New York, 1994

become respectable again as researchers discovered the parallels between these phenomena and the phenomena of implicit memory.

Now I am back to the subject that started my career in psychology--psychodynamic phenomena involving alterations of consciousness--but in the meantime have become a board-certified neuropsychologist and a fully trained psychoanalyst. This paper will address several psychodynamic phenomena involving alterations of consciousness and summarize current attempts to model these phenomena in terms of brain functioning.

As this audience hardly needs to be reminded, there has been a paradigm shift over the past few decades in the way psychologists view thinking (e.g., Baars, 1986; Gardner, 1985 (1987); Sperry, 1993). In the development often termed the cognitive revolution, psychologists abandoned the position of the behaviorists and began to study the organization of thought in new and fruitful ways. Among important contributions to the cognitive revolution are those from the disciplines of artificial intelligence, neuroscience, philosophy, and social psychology.

For the most part, cognitive psychologists have not had very much to say about psychodynamic phenomena, perhaps because most cognitive psychologists are not clinicians. Lacking the clinician's intensive and rich experience with such psychodynamic phenomena as repression, many cognitive and experimental psychologists are not very knowledgeable about these phenomena and are often not convinced of their reality (e.g., Holmes, 1990). However, some individuals have begun to employ the insights of cognitive psychology and neuroscience to psychodynamic phenomena (see, for example, Horowitz, 1987, 1988, 1991; Jones, 1993; Jones, in press; Kihlstrom, 1990; Kihlstrom, Tataryn, & Hoyt, 1993). It will be the goal of this brief paper to summarize some current models of psychodynamic phenomena; this paper will draw in part from my recent papers (Jones, 1993; Jones, in press).

Since many neuropsychologists will have a limited familiarity with psychodynamic phenomena involving alterations of consciousness, it is useful to begin with some terms and definitions.

Repression refers to the exclusion from consciousness of an idea. Although experimental psychologists have tended to study repression in paradigms involving the exclusion of memories from consciousness, Freud saw repression as operating most importantly to exclude from consciousness psychic representations of libidinal or aggressive drives. Thus, repression is defined as:

> A defensive process by which an idea is excluded from consciousness. The ideational content repressed carries potentially troublesome instinctual drive derivatives and their impulses. These threaten overexcitation, anxiety, or conflict, which bring painful affects (Moore & Fine, 1990, p. 166).

Dissociative phenomena include depersonalization and derealization, psychogenic amnesia, psychogenic fugue, and multiple personality disorder.

Depersonalization is a symptom involving a feeling of unreality and strangeness involving the self. It is typically accompanied by emotional numbing, is experienced as uncomfortable, and does not involve impaired insight or delusional elaboration (Ackner, 1954). Depersonalization may be the main feature of a transient or chronic psychiatric syndrome (transient depersonalization syndrome or depersonalization disorder) or may appear as part of another psychiatric disorder. Derealization, a symptom in which the individual feels that the world is strange and unfamiliar, may accompany depersonalization. It has been found that depersonalization often appears in the wake of extreme trauma (e.g., life-threatening events, physical or sexual abuse, political imprisonment) (Jacobson, 1959; Noyes & Kletti, 1977; Noyes, Hoenk, & Kuperman, 1977; Spiegel, 1984).

Psychogenic amnesia involves an acute inability to remember important information about the self which is too extensive to be ascribed to ordinary forgetfulness and which is not due to an organic mental disorder. Psychogenic fugue is characterized by sudden, unexpected travel from one's customary environment, with an inability to recall one's past and assumption of a new identity (American Psychiatric Association, 1987), although Kihlstrom and his colleagues maintain that the essential feature is an extensive functional retrograde amnesia with a loss of personal identity (Kihlstrom et al., 1993). Most studies of psychogenic amnesia and psychogenic fugue have supported the view that these conditions appear in situations of overwhelming stress and intolerable emotions (Loewenstein, 1991).

The essential feature of multiple personality disorder (MPD) is the presence within an individual of two or more discrete personalities or personality states, each with its own consistent pattern of perceiving, relating to, and thinking about the self and the world (American Psychiatric Association, 1987). At least two personalities alternate in taking full control of the individual's behavior. It is quite likely that the recent burgeoning in the number of reported cases of MPD represents not a true increase in the incidence of the disorder, but rather the effect of popular presentations of this disorder, suggestibility on the part of some patients with hysteroid and dissociative features, and unintentional cuing by overzealous therapists. A majority of patients diagnosed with MPD have a history of severe emotional trauma in childhood, often physical or sexual abuse (Putnam, Guroff, Silberman, Barban, & Post, 1986).

Hypnosis is also for the most part viewed as a dissociative experience. Hypnosis is an experience in which an individual enters into an altered state which is characterized by intense absorption, dissociation, and extreme suggestibility (Spiegel, 1990). According to Tellegen and Atkinson (1974), the essence of the hypnotic experience is "a disposition for having episodes of single 'total' attention that fully engage one's representational [i.e., perceptual, enactive, imaginative, and ideational] resources."

NEUROBIOLOGICAL MODELS OF REPRESSION

Rosenblatt and Thickstun

Rosenblatt and Thickstun (1970) sketched a neurobiological model of repression which appears to have been inspired by Hebb's (1949) postulates concerning the nervous system. Hebb proposed that the brain operated as a complex neural network in which complex cognitive operations were executed via the formation of cell assemblies--organized groups of linked neurons. According to Rosenblatt and Thickstun (1970),

> ...such neural nets or circuits as constitute a memory or fantasy may stimulate firing of other cortical networks, resulting in the subjective consciousness of such memories or ideation, this irradiation being influenced by the reticular activating system. This irradiation may also be subject to inhibition through other neural circuits or through some other biochemical alteration in conductivity effected when the previous irradiation to conscious cortical "centres" was accompanied by stimulation of certain affect systems (p. 275).

Although this very brief sketch foreshadowed a number of features of current neurobiological models of repression, it appears not to have attracted much attention.

Galin

Much more attention was paid to the so-called right-hemisphere hypothesis of the unconscious articulated by Galin (1976). This hypothesis grew out of the famous series of callosectomies carried out by P. Vogel and J. E. Bogen in the 1960s for the treatment of intractable epilepsy. As every neuropsychologist knows, the study of this series of patients resulted in an accumulation of welcome knowledge about the functions of the two hemispheres in isolation from each other, but also in a less fortunate overelaboration of views about functional hemispheric specialization. Galin (1976) noted that the right hemisphere mode of functioning shares important attributes of what psychoanalysts call primary process: nonverbal image representation, nonsyllogistic logic, and an emphasis on simultaneity rather than on temporal sequencing. As he goes on to theorize:

> These similarities suggest the hypothesis that in normal intact people mental events in the right hemisphere can become disconnected functionally from the left hemisphere (by inhibition of neural transmission across the corpus callosum) and can continue a life of their own. This hypothesis offers a neurophysiological mechanism for at least some instances of repression, and an anatomical locus for the unconscious mental contents (p. 42).

This kind of "functional commissurotomy" repression might occur in the case of conflicting messages, e.g., when a child receives a positive verbal message from his mother and a negative nonverbal message from her facial expression. Galin felt that the engrams in the right hemisphere could be functionally disconnected from the left and continue a life of their own, influencing subsequent perceptions, expectations, evaluation, and responses. Ledoux, Wilson, and Gazzaniga (1977) found some evidence for this hypothesis in the study of a callosectomy patient who had sufficient linguistic abilities in his right hemisphere to carry out a series of rating tasks; the left and right hemispheres in this patient differed considerable in their evaluations of certain people and concepts.

Schwartz
Schwartz (1987, 1988, 1992) has articulated a model of repression in which affect-based associative learning is paramount. In his model representational processes which are linked with dysphoric affects (anxiety/fear, sadness/depression, disgust, embarrassment/shame, anger/contempt) may, through classical conditioning, become inhibited and no longer available to conscious awareness. Schwartz also finds in the paradigm of state-dependent learning a powerful explanation for the phenomena of repression. Neuropsychologists are familiar with the findings of experiments demonstrating that information presented to an individual in a particular state (e.g., ethanol intoxication, anxiety, sadness) is best recalled, and in some cases, may only be recalled, when the person is in the same state as that prevailing during presentation of the information (for a review, see Weingartner, 1978).

Luborsky and His Colleagues
Luborsky and his colleagues (Luborsky, 1967, 1988; Luborsky, Sackeim, & Cristoph, 1979) have addressed one type of repression, namely, momentary forgetting in a psychotherapy session. Luborsky has found that the content of the momentary forgetting is consistently related to what he terms the patient's core conflictual relationship theme (CCRT). The CCRT is deduced from the analysis of either psychotherapy transcripts or a special interview designed to elicit relationship anecdotes. Raters identify three components of the CCRT:

> (a) the patient's main wishes, needs, or intentions toward the other person in the narratives; (b) the responses of the other person; and (c) the responses of the self. (Luborsky, Crits-Cristoph, Friedman, Mark, & Schaffler, 1991, p. 169)

In the phenomenon of momentary forgetting during a psychotherapy session, the forgotten content is consistently similar to one of the three components of the CCRT; moreover, the patient is experiencing at that moment in the relationship with the therapist some aspect of the danger involved in the CCRT.

EXPERIMENTAL AND COGNITIVE PSYCHOLOGISTS

Among experimental and cognitive psychologists who have addressed the phenomenon of repression, Holmes (1990) represents one extreme, holding that after 60 years of research, "...there is no controlled laboratory evidence supporting the concept of repression" (p. 96). The problem of most of the studies reviewed by Holmes is that they utilize normal control subjects, for many of whom repression might not be an important defense mechanism. Further, the nature of the materials may simply not be such as to mobilize signal anxiety and significant defensive operations in the subjects. Clinicians know that the same stimulus may have an entirely different meaning or valence for different subjects. Bower (1990) argues that there is no necessity for the concept of motivated forgetting of aversive emotional material. He emphasizes that there are well-documented mechanisms to explain forgetting, including motivated nonlearning (via inattention, nonrehearsal, or automatized avoidance of unpleasant thoughts) learning different associations to the same cues, or failures in retrieval due, e.g., to an ineffective cue. However, it is unclear why the possibility of motivated forgetting is any less plausible than motivated nonlearning.

Kihlstrom (1987; Kihlstrom & Hoyt, 1990) proposes that repression results from the automatization of the process of suppressing conscious thoughts. Since automatic procedures are by definition invariably activated by certain inputs and expend little in the way of cognitive resources, they are themselves unconscious. Thus both the process of repression and the target of its operation would be unavailable to consciousness, as Freud required in order for repression to serve as a useful defense.

Erdelyi (1974, 1985) has outlined three models of repression, pointing out how any scientific model is in effect an analogy. In his sociopolitical model of repression, he models repression on censorship. Repression, like censorship, may be achieved through the deletion of material; through its toning down through hints, modifications, and allusions; through displacement of emphasis; through destruction of the offending agency; or through withdrawal of resources from the offending agency. In his neobehavioristic model, he postulates that like laboratory animals attempting to escape from aversive stimuli, consciousness will tend to avoid memories previously associated with trauma or even thoughts associated with trauma. In his information processing model, he renders Freud's repression/censorship model as an information processing model in which the censors or screens that control access to the preconscious or conscious are rendered as decision nodes. Freud's ego is replaced by executive processes; consciousness by working memory; and psychic structure by routines, programs, and software.

Greenwald (1992) reviews the evidence for unconscious cognition and concludes that the evidence leaves little doubt for perception without conscious awareness. Greenwald departs from the psychoanalytic definition of repression as operating most importantly on ideas which are derivatives of libidinal or aggressive drives; rather, he conceives of repression as operating only on memories. In Greenwald's view, repression may be understood as a phenomenon of implicit memory:

> A simpler account of repression uses empirically established phenomena of implicit memory as the basis for understanding apparent instances of recovery of repressed memories (see also Kihlstrom, Barnhardt, & Tataryn, 1992). Explanations of implicit memory assume that memory traces of an attended event are often preserved despite inability to recall the event. Because these unconscious traces influence conscious experience (as manifestations of implicit memory), they can provide a basis for recovering the otherwise unretrievable event. (p. 773)

Implicit memory phenomena are of course familiar to neuropsychologists. Schachter (1987) has traced the development of the concept of implicit memory from early roots in psychical research, psychiatry, philosophy, and experimental psychology and has described relevant findings from studies of savings during relearning, subliminal perception, learning without awareness, repetition, priming, and amnesia. It has been demonstrated that different forms of implicit memory are intact in patient populations that have impaired explicit memory; different forms of implicit memory are probably subserved by distinct neuroanatomical systems. A psychodynamic approach would not deny that some instances of repression might represent implicit memory phenomena; it would simply add emotional considerations to the list of conditions that can result in implicit memory phenomena (e.g., the threat of intolerable anxiety or depressive affect).

Parallel Distributed Processing

Within the domain of cognitive science proper, the model of human information processing known as parallel distributed processing (PDP), connectionism, or neural network modeling (McClelland, Rumelhart, & the PDP Research Group, 1986; Rumelhart, McClelland, & the PDP Research Group, 1986) lends itself well to an understanding of repression. PDP posits a very large number of processing units within the brain, each devoted to a specific task, and each connected to many other units. With activation of a particular unit, other units with which it is linked will be excited or inhibited. A perception, thought, or impulse results from the alteration of the strength of the connections among processing units. Learning can occur in one network and can influence subsequent thought or action without conscious awareness or global action. In the PDP model if a set of units concerned with a sexual impulse has become associatively linked with a set of units having to do with anxiety or guilt, then the excitation of the latter units when the first is activated might effectively shut down the former, or at least inhibit their activations of units having to do with attention or conscious awareness.

NEUROBIOLOGICAL MODELS OF DISSOCIATIVE PHENOMENA AND HYPNOSIS

Hilgard (1977, 1986) has proposed a neodissociation model to account for hypnotic and dissociative phenomena. He posits multiple subsystems, or cognitive control systems, the activation of which corresponds to specialized skills, attitudes, interests, habits, etc. Once activated, these subsystems can operate relatively autonomously and automatically. In addition, he posits an "executive ego or central control structure" with executive and monitoring functions. Parallel processing is an inherent feature of this model. In hypnosis, Hilgard feels, the hypnotic procedure fosters a dissociative experience by restricting attentional focus, promoting extreme absorption, distorting reality orientation, and stimulating the imagination. The executive function is shared with the hypnotist, and the monitoring function is divided. Hilgard regards most of the other dissociative phenomena as reflecting the operation of one or more subsystems, operating relatively autonomously and without the full engagement of the executive and monitoring functions.

Horowitz's Role Relationship Models Configurational Analysis

Like most researchers in the interface between psychodynamics and cognitive science, Horowitz and his colleagues assume the operation of organized knowledge structures, including schemata. A representative definition of schemata is as follows:

> The basic idea is that schemata are data structures for representing the genetic concepts stored in memory. There are schemata for generalized concepts underlying objects, situations, events, sequences of events, actions, and sequences of actions. Roughly, schemata are like models of the outside world. To process information with the use of a schema is to determine which model best fits the incoming information. Ultimately, consistent configurations of schemata are discovered which, in concert, offer the best account for the input. This configuration of schemata together constitutes the interpretation of the input. (Rumelhart, Smolensky, McClelland, & Hinton, 1986, p. 18)

Horowitz and others use the concept of person schemas or self schemas in modeling a number of different psychodynamic phenomena. A person schema is a schema or meaning structure which contains knowledge about the self and others; person schemas are assumed to operate both consciously and unconsciously to organize moods, thoughts, self-evaluations, and actions. Role-relationship models are structures of meaning that combine a self schema, a schema for another person or persons, and a "script" of interactions. In their method known as role-relationship models configurational analysis, Horowitz and his colleagues (Horowitz, 1987, 1988, 1991) have developed a means of analyzing psychodynamic phenomena and psychic change. Trained raters analyze material (usually tapes, transcripts, or process notes of psychotherapy sessions) to formulate a pattern of role-relationship models. Configurational analysis assumes that any situation or event may be unconsciously processed and interpreted simultaneously in parallel channels in terms of quite different role relationship models. Whereas conscious experience is usually dominated by one schematic representation of the self and the interaction, other role relationship models may be unconsciously activated. A particular role relationship model may be wished for, dreaded, or may be a compromise of wished and feared self schemas. Unconscious control processes act to inhibit dreaded role-relationship models and facilitate other role-relationship models.

Horowitz (1991) postulates that in normal development, self schemas become progressively differentiated and integrated, leading ultimately to supraordinate self schemas which provide a secure sense of identity and stability of the self. In his view, the failure to develop a supraordinate self schema can lead to depersonalization or MPD; he also notes that childhood trauma can lead to dissociation or identity diffusion.

PDP

PDP seems to lend itself quite well to modeling dissociative phenomena. Spiegel (1990) highlights the features of PDP models which are particularly well suited to this purpose. These include the property of "local learning via changes in connection weights without overarching global knowledge" (p. 122; cp. the notion of information processing in separate subsystems without automatic access to consciousness). Further, PDP nets function independently and result in outputs that may compete with the outputs of other nets. In the PDP model a unified sense of the self would not be a given, but would have to be achieved through the progressive assimilation of a variety of schemas existing in the interconnections among a number of different nets. Spiegel (1990) sketches the application of the PDP model to MPD:

> An analogy can be drawn between these dissociated mental
> states in multiple personality disorder and separate nets in a
> PDP model. This theoretical approach presupposes a pattern
> of storage of information organized into coherent subunits.
> The coherence of these subunits may include networks of
> meaning or connections between affect and content. The
> activation of one network tends to inhibit the activation of

another competing network. Dissociation fits this model neatly in that it postulates the organization of stored information into coherent subunits that have their own rules of organization and interaction with other subunits. Thus an analogy between PDP nets and the extreme dissociation seen in multiple personality disorder, for example, in which each personality has a fairly exclusive store of memories, experiences, and identities that become manifest as a given personality obtains access to consciousness. (p. 128)

Baars's Global Workspace Theory

Baars's (1988) global workspace theory adds the concept of a global workspace or a kind of central information exchange to the PDP model. In addition to a large number of specialized processing units operating relatively autonomously, in parallel, and out of consciousness, he posits a global workspace which provides access to consciousness, processes serially, and allows for information from one processing unit to be broadly disseminated. Baars relates hypnosis to the ideomotor theory in his model; this theory, originated by William James, holds that "a single conscious goal-image, if it does not meet with competition, may suffice to set off a complex, highly coordinated, largely unconscious action (Baars, 1988, p. 259). Absorption, widely held to be one of the central characteristics of hypnosis (Spiegel, 1990), would mean the elimination of all but one goal-image with greatly reduced competition for the workspace. Baars's theory also includes a self (system), which he defines as the "overarching context of experience" (p. 387); a context for Baars is a set of specialized processors that serve to "evoke and shape global messages without themselves broadcasting any message" (p. 372). Baars relates psychogenic fugue, multiple personality, and depersonalization disorder to a disruption of the self system due to shocking events which violate dominant contexts.

Dennett's Multiple Drafts Model

Dennett (1991), a philosopher with an extensive knowledge of both neuroscience and cognitive science, has developed what he calls the Multiple Drafts theory of consciousness. The essential points of his model are as follows:

1) There is no one, definitive "stream of consciousness" because there is no "Cartesian Theater" (place/time in the brain where "it all comes together" to be presented in consciousness).

2) There are instead multiple channels of "specialist circuits" creating multiple drafts of experience as they go.

3) Some of these drafts "get promoted to further functional roles...by the activity of a virtual machine in the brain" (Dennett, 1991, p. 254). A virtual machine is a "temporary set of highly structured regularities imposed on the

underlying hardware [in this case, the brain] by a program: a structured recipe of hundreds of thousands of instructions that give the hardware a huge, interlocking set of habits or dispositions to react" (Dennett, 1991, p. 216; material in brackets added).

4) The serial character of this virtual machine is not hard-wired but has resulted from a progression of linkages of these specialist circuits.

Dennett believes that consciousness evolved with the development of language and in effect involved "talking to oneself," through which information available to one or more specialist circuits became available to other circuits. In Dennett's theory a self is a representation of a person (to himself and to others) and is a kind of narrative or fiction about a set of experiences and tendencies. Each individual has a number of unconsciously created selves. Ordinarily one of these selves "represents" the person and controls the language system. However, in MPD childhood trauma reinforces the inherent tendency in human beings toward a multiplicity of selves and prevents the dominance of a single self.

Hemispheric Approaches

For most right-handers the left hemisphere appears to play a predominant role in language expression, analysis, and comprehension; gestural communication; temporal sequencing; verbal abstraction ability; mathematical ability; and control of purposeful motor output. The mode of information processing by the left hemispheric appears to be one of sequential analysis, selection of relevant details, and categorization by means of linguistic labels. The right hemisphere appears to play a predominant role in spatial processing, apprehension of the gestalt of visual stimuli, the perception of tactile and proprioceptive information, maintenance of the body image, emotional processing (discerning facial emotions and mediating emotional arousal and expression), and the production and perception of tonal patterns, intonational contours, and melody. Thus the right hemisphere appears to be dominant for the processing of non-linguistic, non-sequential sensory information arising from the external or internal environment.

More surprising is some evidence for complementary hemispheric specialization for the processing of emotionally charged stimuli, depending on whether the emotional valence is positive or negative (Davidson, Schwartz, Saron, Bennett, & Goleman, 1979; Dimond & Farrington, 1977; Dimond, Farrington, & Johnson, 1976; Fox & Davidson, 1986; Natale, Gur, & Gur, 1983; Reuter-Lorenz & Davidson, 1981; Reuter-Lorenz, Givis, & Moscovitch, 1983). Studies on the spontaneous experience or expression of emotion are less equivocal in demonstrating a right-hemisphere specialization for negative affect (Ahern & Schwartz, 1985; Davidson & Tomarkin, 1989; Gainotti, 1979; Tucker, Stenslie, Roth, & Shearer, 1981).

Joseph (1982) has speculated on the ramifications of several facts--the relative right-hemisphere specialization for emotional encoding and expression, the greater abundance of right-hemisphere reciprocal connections with the limbic system, and the fact that interhemispheric communication seems to be nonexistent before age three (Salamy, 1978), very limited before age 5 (Galin, Johnstone,Nakell, & Herron, 1979), and incomplete until at least age ten (Yakovlev & Lecours, 1967).

> In that the emerging human organism is asymmetrically arranged, with apparently little interaction and informational exchange between the cerebral hemispheres, the effects of early "socializing" experiences could have potentially profound effects indeed. As a good deal of this early experience is likely to have its unpleasant if not traumatic moments, it is fascinating to consider the later ramifications of the early emotional learning occurring in the right hemisphere unbeknownst to the left; learning and associated emotional responding which may later be completely unaccessible to the language centers of the brain even when extensive interhemispheric transfer is possible...(p. 24)

If there is, for most right-handers, relative right-hemisphere specialization for the encoding of negative emotion, then experiences of overwhelming trauma, shame, or guilt would have a potential not only for differential activation of and encoding by the right hemisphere, but might even be refractory to left hemisphere or linguistic encoding and thus awareness.

Physiological Approaches

Shevrin and his colleagues have studied electroencephalographic correlates--specifically, event-related potential (ERP) correlates--of unconscious activity. Having demonstrated ERP correlates of subliminal stimulation (Shevrin & Rennick, 1967; Shevrin, Smith, & Fritzler, 1969, 1970), and the relationship between these ERP correlates and repression (Shevrin, Smith, & Fritzler, 1969, 1970), this group has gone on to study ERP correlates of words which are consciously or unconsciously related to a subject's neurotic conflicts, presented either subliminally or supraliminally (Shevrin, 1988). Shevrin feels that their findings indicate that the dynamic unconscious is capable of "highly complex, highly spontaneous, affective, motivational, and cognitive processing" (p. 155). In a recent review of the issue of a "smart or dumb" unconscious, Loftus and Klinger (1992) found the current consensus to be that there can no longer be any doubt of the reality of unconscious cognitive processes, but that "...there seems to be a general consensus that the unconscious may not be as smart as previously believed" (p. 764). It should be noted that proponents of a dumb unconscious are not clinicians; one also wonders what they make of Kekule's discovery of the structure of the benzene ring via an image in a hypnagogic state (Gruber, 1989).

Another physiological approach to psychodynamic phenomena involving alterations of consciousness is the study of physiological indices of the dissociated states in MPD (for reviews, see Braun, 1983b; Coons, 1988; Putnam, 1984). These studies have documented consistent differences in physiological indices across different personalities and support the view that different personalities in MPD patients are discrete, complex, and differentiated states of consciousness.

A Synthesis

I would like to offer a synthesis of what I feel are the most compelling features of the various approaches and close by applying the synthesis to each of the major psychodynamic phenomena of interest here. Most current researchers in the field accept that information processing in the brain is massive and parallel, so we begin with a very large number of specialized processing units, functioning automatically and largely autonomously except for interconnected circuits. Some circuits contain in their connections a representation of the person (to himself and to others), a kind of narrative of the self and its experiences, or self schema. Some processing units (in the left hemisphere for most right-handed persons) specialize in linguistic functions and/or analytic, sequential, detail-oriented modes of information processing. Other processing units (in the right hemisphere for most right-handed people) specialize in visuospatial analysis and representation; maintenance of the body image; decoding of nonverbal sounds, prosody, and some aspects of music; emotional processing, expression, and experience; and somesthetic and proprioceptive information. Right-hemisphere circuits may be predominant in non-analytic, holistic, and Gestalt-oriented modes of processing. There are almost undoubtedly self-schemas encoded in left-hemisphere units and circuits (containing linguistically coded, conscious narratives about the self) and other, separate self schemas encoded in right hemisphere units and circuits (containing non-linguistically coded, unconscious representations of the self, the body, and various emotional states).

Following Dennett (1991), I see the origin of consciousness as a kind of silent "talking to oneself" which occurs automatically and confers the advantage of keeping other specialist circuits informed of how the "self" feels. Consciousness would thus correspond to the activity of certain left-hemisphere circuits containing linguistically coded narratives about the self.

Normally, a self schema develops which is dominant, consists of a narrative about the individual's experience and dispositions, and "does most of the talking" for the individual (Dennett, 1991). Even in the context of normal development, however, one sees psychodynamic phenomena involving alterations of consciousness, with unexpected omissions or intrusions into the stream of consciousness.

Repression occurs when the life experiences of the individual have led to the production of (or expectation of) a danger signal (anxiety or depressive affect [Brenner, 1975]) when derivatives of certain impulses (sexual, aggressive) are experienced. The memory or idea or feeling which becomes the target of repression is something that is incompatible with the dominant self schema. Some of these incompatible thoughts, feelings, or memories probably involve the activation of certain right-hemisphere units or nets (in part because of the differential activation of the right hemisphere during negative emotional states). In our PDP-like system, repression can take place automatically, as a result of the reciprocal connections among sets of specialized circuits. I would also agree with Freud (1932) in that another way in which the earliest kind of repression comes about is in situations in which the individual is exposed to excessively strong impulses; repression, like dissociation, serves to protect the self from feeling overwhelmed.

Depersonalization, which is a frequent finding in persons who have suffered physical or sexual abuse, political imprisonment, etc. (Jacobson, 1959; Spiegel, 1984), seems to result from a mismatch between the representation of the self (and its familiar store of memories, expectations, and dispositions) and the knowledge of the terrifying events to which one has in fact been exposed (cp. Horowitz et al., 1991). Depersonalization disorder, which is characterized by a chronic feeling of unreality and of detachment from the self or body, seems to correspond to a failure in the consolidation of a self schema. This might result from a child's being reared in such a way that experiences which validated his sense of being a unique, complex-but-coherent human being were lacking. E.g., the child is responded to in a highly inconsistent way which has little to do with his behavior and therefore fails to reinforce a sense of consistency about the self; or the child is not really responded to as a human being with real feelings, and develops a self schema with feelings of unreality.

I would follow Kihlstrom in positing that psychogenic amnesia comes about when the memories for a whole set of events or an entire period to the individual's life become disconnected from the self schema (Kihlstrom et al., 1993). This may be the result of trauma or of actions which violate the individual's own moral or ethical codes. Psychogenic fugue, which involves an extensive psychogenic amnesia, often sudden travel from one's usual environment, and the assumption of a new identity, seems to involve a walling off of the old self schema with its collection of autobiographical memories and the formation of a new self schema (Kihlstrom et al., 1993). Schachter, Wang, Tulving, and Friedman (1982) studied a patient with psychogenic fugue and found a dissociation between episodic memory and semantic memory. During the fugue state, autobiographical memories stemmed almost exclusively from the period covered by the fugue. After the resolution of the amnesia, autobiographical memories stemmed almost exclusively from the pre-fugue period.   These findings support the concept of separate self schemas with their own associated stores of autobiographical memories.

MPD comes about when early trauma potentiates the inherent capacity for dissociation in our PDP-like system.   In addition, some or even most recent cases of MPD may have developed from dissociative tendencies to a full-blown picture of separate personalities because of unintentional cuing by overzealous therapists.   I believe that some cases develop without the influence of the therapist and are due to the failure of the normal tendency for one self schema to become dominant.   The alternate self or selves arise when a significant body of experience--e.g., trauma or abuse--cannot be assimilated within the dominant self schema.

Hypnosis is a less striking form of dissociative phenomenon which can be induced in those with an unusual capacity for absorption and suggestion.   The experiences hidden behind the amnesic barrier at the hypnotist's suggestion may be subsequently recalled at the hypnotist's suggestion because the original dissociation was voluntary and was not dictated by the necessity of avoiding overwhelming anxiety or depressive affect.

CONCLUSION

Psychodynamic phenomena involving alterations of consciousness have attracted scientific attention for more than a century.   Recent advances in the domains of cognitive science and neuroscience have provided new ways of modeling these phenomena.   Under the reign of behaviorism, psychology, like a patient with psychogenic amnesia, segregated these phenomena from its awareness.   In the last several decades, the cognitive revolution has made it possible for psychology to reclaim these phenomena as appropriate objects of its contemplation and understanding.

ACKNOWLEDGEMENT.   I would like to thank Petra Moosleitner for assistance in researching the literature on this topic.

REFERENCES

Ackner, B. (1954). Depersonalization, I. Aetiology and phenomenology. *Journal of Mental Science, 100*, 838-853.

Ahern, G. L., & Schwartz, G. E. (1985). Differential lateralization for positive and negative emotion in the human brain: EEG spectral analysis. *Neuropsychologia, 23*, 745-756.

American Psychiatric Association. (1987). *Diagnostic and statistical manual of mental disorders* (3rd ed.). Washington, DC: Author.

Baars, B. J. (1986). *The cognitive revolution in psychology.* New York: Guilford.

Baars, B. J. (1988). *A cognitive theory of consciousness*. Cambridge: Cambridge University Press.

Bower, G. H. (1990). Awareness, the unconscious, and repression: An experimental psychologist's perspective. In J. L. Singer (Ed.), *Repression and dissociation: Implications for personality theory, psychopathology, and health* (pp. 209-232). Chicago: University of Chicago Press.

Braun, B. G. (1983). Psychophysiological phenomena in multiple personality and hypnosis. *American Journal of Clinical Hypnosis, 26*, 124-137.

Brenner, C. (1975). Affects and psychic conflict. *Psychoanalytic Quarterly, 44*, 528.

Coons, P. M. (1988). Psychophysiologic aspects of multiple personality disorder: A review. *Dissociation, 1*, 47-53.

Davidson, R. J., Schwartz, G. E., Saron, C., Bennett, J., & Goleman, D. (1979). Frontal versus parietal EEG asymmetry during positive and negative affect. *Psychophysiology, 16*, 202-203.

Davidson, R. J., & Tomarkin, A. J. (1991). Laterality and emotion: Anelectrophysiological approach. In F. Boller & J. Grafman (Eds.), *Handbook of neuropsychology* (Vol. 3, pp. 419-441). Amsterdam: Elsevier.

Dennett, D. C. (1991). *Consciousness explained*. Boston: Little Brown.

Dimond, S. J., & Farrington, L. (1977). Emotional response to films shown to the right or left hemisphere of the brain measured by heart rate. *Acta Psychologia, 41*, 255-260.

Dimond, S. J., Farrington, L., & Johnson, P. (1976). Differing emotional response from right and left hemispheres. *Nature, 261*, 690-692.

Erdelyi, M. H. (1974). A new look at the New Look: Perceptual defense and vigilance. *Psychological Review, 81*, 1-25.

Erdelyi, M. H. (1985). *Psychoanalysis: Freud's cognitive psychology*. New York: W. H. Freeman & Co.

Fox, N. A. & Davidson, R. J. (1986). Taste-elicited changes in facial signs of emotion and the asymmetry of brain electrical activity in human newborns. *Neuropsychologia, 24*, 417-422.

Freud, S. (1932). New introductory lectures on Psychoanalysis. *The standard edition of the complete psychological works of Sigmund Freud* (Vol. XXII). London: Hogarth.

Gainotti, G. (1972). Emotional behavior and hemispheric side of lesion. *Cortex, 8*, 41-55.

Galin, D. (1976). The two modes of consciousness and the two halves of the brain. In P. R. Lee, R. E. Ornstein, D. Galin, A. Deikman, & C. T. Tart (Eds.), *Symposium on consciousness* (pp. 26-52). New York: Viking.

Galin, D., Johnstone, J., Nakell, L., & Herron, J. (1979). Development of the capacity for tactile information transfer between hemispheres in normal children. *Science, 204*, 1330-1332.

Gardner, H. (1985 [Epilogue, 1987]). *The mind's new science: A history of the cognitive revolution*. New York: Basic Books.

Greenwald, A. G. (1992). New Look 3: Unconscious cognition reclaimed. *American Psychologist, 47*, 766-779.

Gruber, H. E. (1989). The evolving systems approach to creative work. In D. B. Wallace & H. E. Gruber (Eds.), *Creative people at work* (pp. 3-24). New York: Oxford University Press.

Hebb, D. O. (1949). *The organization of behavior*. New York: Wiley.

Hilgard, E. R. (1977). *Divided consciousness: Multiple controls in human thought and action*. New York: John Wiley & Sons.

Hilgard, E. R. (1986). *Divided consciousness: Multiple controls in human thought and action* (Rev. ed.). New York: Wiley-Interscience.

Holmes, D. (1990). The evidence for repression: an examination of sixty years of research. In J. L. Singer (Ed.), *Repression and dissociation: Implications for personality theory, psychopathology, and health* (pp. 85-102). Chicago: University of Chicago Press.

Horowitz, M. J. (1987). *States of mind: Configurational analysis of individual psychology* (2nd ed.). New York: Plenum Press.

Horowitz, M. J. (1988). Psychodynamic phenomena and their explanation. In M. J. Horowitz (Ed.), *Psychodynamics and cognition*, (pp. 3-20). Chicago: University of Chicago Press.

Horowitz, M. J. (Ed.). (1991). *Person schemas and maladaptive interpersonal patterns*. Chicago: University of Chicago Press.

Jacobson, E. (1959). Depersonalization. *Journal of the American Psychoanalytic Association, 7*, 581-610.

Jones, B. P. (1993). Repression: The evolution of a psychoanalytic concept from the 1890's to the 1990's. *Journal of the American Psychoanalytic Association, 41*, 63-93.

Jones, B. P. (in press). Psychodynamic phenomena involving alterations of consciousness. In F. Boller & J. Grafman (Eds.), *Handbook of Neuropsychology* (Vol. 10). New York: Elsevier.

Joseph, R. (1982). The neuropsychology of development: Hemispheric laterality, limbic language, and the origin of thought. *Journal of Clinical Psychology, 38*, 4-33.

Kihlstrom, J. F. (1987). The cognitive unconscious. *Science, 237*, 1445-1452.

Kihlstrom, J. F. (1990). The psychological unconscious. In L. Pervin (Ed.), *Handbook of personality: Theory and research* (pp. 445-464). New York: Guilford.

Kihlstrom, J. F., Barnhardt, T. M., & Tataryn, D. J. (1992). The psychological unconscious: Found, lost, and regained. *American Psychologist, 47*, 788-791.

Kihlstrom, J. F., & Hoyt, I. P. (1990). Repression, dissociation, and hypnosis. In J. L. Singer (Ed.), *Repression and dissociation: Implications for personality theory, psychopathology, and health* (pp. 181-208). Chicago: University of Chicago Press.

Kihlstrom, J. F. , Tataryn, D. J., & Hoyt, I. P. (1993). Dissociative disorders. In P. B. Sutker & H. E. Adams (Eds.), *Comprehensive handbook of psychopathology* (pp. 203-234). New York: Plenum Press.

Ledoux, J. E., Wilson, D. H., & Gazzaniga, M. S. (1977). A divided mind: Observations on the conscious properties of the separated hemispheres. *Annals of Neurology, 2*, 417-421.

Loewenstein, R. J. (1991). Psychogenic amnesia and psychogenic fugue: A comprehensive review. In A. Tasman & M. Goldfinger (Eds.), *Review of Psychiatry* (Vol. X) (pp. 189-221).

Loftus, E. F., & Klinger, M. R. (1992). Is the unconscious smart or dumb? *American Psychologist, 47*, 761-765.

Luborsky, L. (1967). Momentary forgetting during psychotherapy and psychoanalysis: A theory and research method. *Psychological Issues, 5* (2, 3), monograph 18/19, 177-217.

Luborsky, L. (1988). Recurrent momentary forgetting: Its content and its context.InM. J. Horowitz (Ed.), *Psychodynamics and cognition* (pp. 223-251). Chicago: University of Chicago Press.

Luborsky, L., Sackeim, H., & Cristoph, P. (1979). The state conducive to momentary forgetting. In J. Kihlstrom & F. Evans (Eds.), *Functional disorders of memory* (pp. 325-353). Hillsdale, NJ: Erlbaum.

Luborsky, L., Crits-Cristoph, P., Friedman, S. H., Mark, D., & Shaffler, P. (1991). Freud's transference template compared with the core conflictual relationship theme (CCRT): Illustrations by the two specimen cases. In M. J. Horowitz (Ed.), *Person schemas and maladaptive interpersonal patterns* (pp. 167-195). Chicago: University of Chicago Press.

McClelland, J. L., Rumelhart, D. E., & the PDP Research Group (Eds.). (1986). *Parallel distributed processing: Explorations in the microstructure of cognition. Vol. 2: Psychological and biological models.* Cambridge, MA: MIT Press.

Moore, B. E., & Fine, B. D. (1990). *Psychoanalytic terms and concepts.* New Haven: The American Psychoanalytic Association and Yale University Press.

Natale, M., Gur, R. E., & Gur, R. C. (1983). Hemispheric asymmetries in processing emotional expressions. *Neuropsychologia, 21*, 555-565.

Noyes, R., Jr., & Kletti, R. (1977). Depersonalization in response to life threatening danger. *Comprehensive Psychiatry, 18*, 375-384.

Noyes, R., Jr., Hoenk, P., & Kuperman, S. (1977). Depersonalization in accident victims and psychiatric patients. *Journal of Nervous and Mental Disease, 164*, 401-407.

Putnam, F. H. (1984). The psychophysiologic investigation of multiple personality disorder: A review. *Psychiatric Clinics of North America, 7*, 31-39.

Putnam, F. W., Guroff, J. J., Silberman, E. K., Barban, L., & Post, R. M. (1986). The clinical phenomenology of multiple personality disorder: Review of 100 recent cases. *Journal of Clinical Psychiatry, 47*, 285-293.

Reuter-Lorenz, P., & Davidson, R. J. (1981). Differential contributions of the two cerebral hemispheres to the perception of happy and sad faces. *Neuropsychologia, 19*, 609-613.

Reuter-Lorenz, P., Givis, R. P., & Moscovitch, M. (1983). Hemispheric specialization and the perception of emotion: Evidence from right-handers and from inverted and non-inverted left-handers. *Neuropsychologia, 21*, 687-692.

Rosenblatt, A. D., & Thickstun, J. T. (1970). A study of the concept of psychic energy. *International Journal of Psychoanalysis, 51*, 265-278.

Rumelhart, D. E., McClelland, J. L., & the PDP Research Group. (1986). *Parallel distributed processing: Explorations in the microstructure of cognition. Vol. 1: Foundations.* Cambridge, MA: MIT Press.

Rumelhart, D. E., Smolensky, P., McClelland, J. L., & Hinton, G. (1986). Schemata and sequential thought processes in PDP models. In J. L. McClelland, D. E. Rumelhart, and the PDP Research Group (Editors), *Parallel distributed processing. Explorations in the microstructure of cognition. Vol. 2. Psychological and biological models* (pp. 7-57). Cambridge, MA: MIT Press.

Salamy, A. (1978). Commissural transmission: Maturational changes in humans. *Science, 200*, 1409-1411.

Schachter, D. L. (1987). Implicit memory: History and current status. *Journal of Experimental Psychology, 13*, 501-518.

Schachter, D. L., Wang, P. L., Tulving, E., & Friedman, M. (1982). Functional retrograde amnesia: A quantitative case study. *Neuropsychologia, 20*, 523-532.

Schwartz, A. (1987). Drives, affects, behavior--and learning: Approaches to a psychobiology of emotion and to an integration of psychoanalytic and neurobiologic thought. *Journal of the American Psychoanalytic Association, 35*, 467-506.

Schwartz, A. (1988). Reification revisited: Some neurobiologically-filtered views of "psychic structure" and "conflict." *Journal of the American Psychoanalytic Association, 36* (Suppl.): 359-385.

Schwartz, A. (1992). Not art but science: Applications of neurobiology, experimental psychology and ethology to psychoanalytic technique. I: Neuroscientifically guided approaches to interpretive "what's" and "when's." *Psychoanalytic Inquiry, 12*, 445-474.

Shevrin, H. (1988). Unconscious conflict: A convergent psychodynamic and electrophysiological approach. In M. J. Horowitz (Ed.), *Psychodynamics and cognition* (pp. 117-167).. Chicago: University of Chicago Press.

Shevrin, H., & Rennick, P. (1967). Cortical response to a tactile stimulus during attention, mental arithmetic, and free association. *Psychophysiology, 3*, 381-388.

Shevrin, H., Smith, W. H., & Fritzler, D. (1969). Repressiveness as a factor in the subliminal activation of brain and verbal responses. *Journal of Nervous and Mental Disease, 149*, 261-269.

Shevrin, H., Smith, W. H., & Fritzler, D. (1970). Subliminally stimulated brain and verbal responses of twins differing in repressiveness. *Journal of Abnormal Psychology, 76*, 39-46.

Sperry, R. (1993). The impact and promise of the cognitive revolution. *American Psychologist, 48*, 878-885.

Spiegel, D. (1984). Multiple personality as a post-traumatic stress disorder. *Psychiatric Clinics of North America, 7*, 101-110.

Spiegel, D. (1990). Hypnosis, dissociation, and trauma. In J. L. Singer (Ed.), *Repression and dissociation: Implications for personality theory, psychopathology, and health* (pp. 121-142). Chicago: University of Chicago Press.

Tellegen, A., & Atkinson, G. (1974). Openness to absorbing and self-altering experiences ("absorption"), a trait related to hypnotic susceptibility. *Journal of Abnormal Psychology, 83*, 268-277,.

Tucker, D. M., Stenslie, C. E., Roth, R. s., & Shearer, S. L. (1981). Right frontal lobe activation and right hemisphere performance decrement during a depressed mood. *Archives of General Psychiatry, 38*, 169-174.

Weingartner, H. (1978). Human state-dependent learning. In B. T. Ho, D. W. Richards, & D. C. Chute (Eds.), *Drug discrimination and state-dependent learning* (pp. 361-382). New York: Academic Press.

Yakovlev, P. I., & Lecours, A. (1967). The myelinogenetic cycles of regional maturation of the brain. In A. Minkowski (Ed.), *Regional development of the brain in early life* (pp. 404-491). London: Blackwell.

20

Applying the Neuropsychology of Memory Disorders to Post-Traumatic Stress Disorder

JESSICA WOLFE[1]

Working with Nelson Butters changed my career. In 1981, I had just completed an unparalleled two years of postdoctoral training in clinical neuropsychology with Edith Kaplan. Eager to learn more about neuropsychological research, I asked Edith for a training recommendation and, always correct in her judgment, she unequivocally recommended Nelson Butters. Nelson took me on as a clinical research trainee with considerable clinical neuropsychological background but limited research experience. Over the next two years, through trials and tribulations, admonitions and exhortations, I managed to generate actual scientific research in areas of mutual interest, and Nelson and I came to be lasting colleagues and very close friends.

Although I had approached Nelson with an interest in evaluating the memory changes associated with major depression, Nelson recognized the importance of a solid grounding in basic memory paradigms if one were to study memory disturbance. Consequently, our first paper together focused on examining the retrieval and procedural learning deficits purportedly associated with the memory problems of Huntington's Disease (HD) patients. This set of studies (Butters, Wolfe, Martone, Granholm, & Cermak, 1985) represented an

[1] JESSICA WOLFE, Ph.D. • Department of Veterans Affairs, Boston and Tufts University School of Medicine

Neuropsychological Explorations of Memory and Cognition: Essays in Honor of Nelson Butters, edited by Laird S. Cermak, Ph.D. Plenum Press, New York, 1994

extension of Nelson's work in the performance-based memory dissociations of certain neurologic groups. In our first experiment, we administered a series of verbal recall and recognition tests to HD patients, amnesics, and normal control (NC) subjects. As predicted, although the performance of NCs surpassed both patient groups, the performance of HD patients was superior to that of the amnesics on the recognition task. This finding supported earlier results showing the relatively preserved memory capacities of HD patients, especially in cases where their performance did not require extensive use of retrieval processes.

The second experiment in this study entailed an investigation of procedural learning skills using the famed "Tower of Hanoi" test (Corkin, 1984). It yielded less definitive results: On the skill acquisition component of this task, early HD patients and NC subjects solved the difficult puzzle at approximately the same rate, but more advanced HD patients and amnesics showed little improvement over repeated trials. On a subsequent recognition task tapping factual information about the Tower, both EHD and AHD patients demonstrated learning that was superior to the amnesics. Overall, these findings added support to an existing retrieval deficit hypothesis for HD patients; however, the data also suggested that the use of motor-based procedural tasks with advanced HD patients was likely to confound behavioral performance and impede research efforts to demonstrate the sought after "double dissociation" between the memory abilities of HD patients and other amnesic individuals.

A second study of ours (Granholm, Wolfe, & Butters, 1985) examined the role of affective-arousal factors in alcoholic Korsakoff amnesics (AKs) and HD patients' abilities to learn and retain prose passages. Earlier research had shown that AK patients suffered from arousal and motivational defects which secondarily influenced their anterograde memory (Butters, Lewis, Cermak, & Goodglass, 1973). However, there was little research on affective-arousal factors to indicate what impact the latter had on the performance of other memory-disordered patients (e.g., HD patients). To evaluate differences in memory disorders further, we administered a series of passages to HD, AK, and NC subjects to assess their verbal retention skills. As anticipated, HD patients evidenced pronounced learning deficits when retrieval processes were tapped but, like normal control subjects, these individuals demonstrated minimal forgetting between immediate and delayed recall. As predicted, the memory performance of AK subjects was selectively enhanced when the semantic content of the material reflected sexual themes, suggesting that activation played some role in the memory capacities of these amnesics..

In a third study (Butters, Wolfe, Granholm, & Martone, 1986), we found that early and late-stage HD patients were capable of superior recognition memory compared to AK subjects when list learning paradigms or passages were employed. As expected, both groups showed substantial impairment on recall tasks, though for differing reasons: Retrieval deficits in HD patients were found in HD patients' significantly worse performance on a letter fluency task whereas

AK patients had marked perseverative errors, consistent with their pronounced susceptibility to proactive interference.

To study these distinctions among memory disorders further, we (Butters, Wolfe, Granholm, & Martone, 1986) then contrasted the memory impairments of AK and HD patients with the performance of early Alzheimer (AD) patients. Because of obvious cognitive limitations, all patients in this study were matched for dementia severity. Using passage recall to evaluate episodic memory, all three patient groups demonstrated substantial memory impairment although the performance of AD and AK patients was distinctively characterized by intrusion errors. On two semantic memory tasks (letter and category fluency), HD and AK patients again exhibited deficits although AD patients were impaired only on category fluency. Overall, these findings suggested that the memory deficits in AD and HD represented processing that was selectively disturbed by differences in neuropathology: In AD, an emerging language deficit and the sensitivity to proactive interference affected their memory performance whereas HD patients were particularly vulnerable on tasks requiring extensive search of active memory.

In our last study together (Wolfe, Granholm, Butters, Saunders, & Janowsky, 1987), we extended the use of the above recall and recognition paradigms to psychiatric patients suffering from either unipolar (UP) or bipolar (BP) depression. Based on prior psychiatric studies, we expected that the verbal learning and fluency of depressed patients would be impaired relative to normal control subjects, primarily due to motivational and behavioral factors. However, we also anticipated that the memory performance of more severely depressed patients might qualitatively resemble patterns found in HD, based on a presumed similarity in subcortical dysfunction. Analysis of our data in fact confirmed that both UP and BP depressed patients did substantially worse than normal control subjects on verbal recall and recognition tasks, with BP patients showing the greatest impairment. Bipolar patients also exhibited more deficits on the verbal fluency task. Qualitative analysis of some of these data suggested certain similarities between the memory disturbances found in bipolar illness and those of HD patients, providing some of the first documentation of memory deficits spanning psychiatric and neurologic groups. Since that time, further work (Massman, Delis, Butters, Dupont, & Gillin, 1992) has offered strong empirical support for a subcortical dysfunction hypothesis in depression; however, this extends only to a subgroup of depressed patients. Additional research is needed to examine the neuropathological and behavioral correlates of these complex syndromes.

More recently, my work has expanded into the fields of behavioral psychology and post-traumatic stress disorder (PTSD). PTSD, which is uniquely characterized by exposure to a recognizable stressor of extreme proportion that is beyond usual human experience and is markedly distressing to almost anyone, also is defined by a set of hallmark symptoms that include cognitive or perceptual reexperiencing (e.g., intrusive thoughts, recollections or nightmares of the traumatic event), behavioral avoidance and affective numbing (on exposure to cues that resemble the event), and physiological hyperreactivity and hyperarousal (present at baseline and enhanced on cue re-exposure).

Although PTSD was first regarded as an affective disturbance, both the DSM-III and DSM-III-R subsequently classified PTSD as an anxiety disorder. Ongoing debate about PTSD's exact diagnostic nomenclature and the disorder's validity led many researchers in the 1980's to spend considerable time attempting to delineate the parameters of the disorder. With my colleagues in Boston, my early work in this area focused on efforts to define PTSD that would differentiate it from closely associated illnesses, for example, major depression (Keane, Wolfe, & Taylor, 1987; Wolfe, Keane, Lyons, & Gerardi, 1987). We also focused on defining the requisite components of a multimodal assessment battery that would provide more objective evaluation of stress symptomatology through the use of behavioral, emotional, cognitive, and laboratory-based psychophysiological measures (Lyons, Gerardi, Wolfe, & Keane, 1988; Wolfe & Keane, 1990). These efforts contributed to the development of a valid, comprehensive functional assessment protocol for PTSD that is now in widespread use in this field. This battery, which helps distinguish behavioral, emotional, and cognitive components of PTSD, aids clinicians with their diagnostic evaluation of patients and also has helped promote more widespread support for PTSD as a distinct clinical entity that, despite high rates of comorbidity, is separate and unique from other anxiety and affective disorders (Wolfe & Keane, 1990).

Although the explosion in behavioral, psychophysiological, genetic, and biological PTSD research has been considerable (see Wolfe & Charney, 1991; Wolfe & Keane, 1993, for a review), the pathophysiology and exact pathogenesis of this disorder still are poorly understood. This is of particular concern given the disorder's frequently debilitating and chronic course as well as its high rate of association with depression, panic disorder, and substance abuse. More recent research has been directed at examining aspects of PTSD that are especially problematic, for example, the genesis and exacerbation of painful, intrusive trauma recollections and the frequent fluctuations in PTSD patients' abilities to access and retrieve trauma memories. This interest is best reflected in a growing fascination with memory functions and information processing networks in PTSD (Wolfe & Charney, 1991).

Recently, some authors have suggested that PTSD symptoms involving both intrusive thoughts and intermittent psychogenic amnesia reflect the existence of an altered, affectively valence semantic network that is established following severe stressor exposure and subsequent traumatization (Chemtob, Roitblat, Hamada & Carlson, 1988). These changes presumably arise as a result of interlinked, trauma-induced, conditioned associations that are supported by accompanying changes in autonomic arousal. Much of this interest stems from work that has been conducted in affective disorders where paradigms from cognitive psychology and neuropsychology have been used to demonstrate mood consonant attentional, learning, and memory deficits in clinically depressed individuals. To date, results from depression studies have primarily shown deficits on some encoding and retrieval tasks. These deficits appear to reflect problems in activation and motivation (or "resource allocation"; Ellis, Thomas & Rodriguez, 1984; Weingartner & Silberman, 1982; Wolfe, Granholm, et al., 1987) as well as strong effects of mood congruency (Bower, 1981). That is, depressed patients typically display a robust preference for the recall and retention of negatively valence material, consistent with general effects of mood congruence and state dependence on information processing.

Very recently, related research in the anxiety disorders has revealed preferential processing and selective attention to relevant "threat" stimuli (for a review, see Dalgleish & Watts, 1990; Mogg, Mathews & Eysenck, 1992; Rusted & Dighton, 1991), especially in patients with pronounced fear or acquired phobias. In conjunction with empirical findings on the memory problems of depressed patients, these newer data strongly suggested that the application of established neuropsychological and memory paradigms from work by Nelson and others might prove very valuable in defining some aspects of PTSD. In our first empirical study of cognition in PTSD we (Wolfe, Keane, Gerardi, Mora, Butters & Weathers, 1993) administered a modified version of the Rey Auditory Verbal Learning Test (RAVLT) to three groups: male combat veterans with well-diagnosed war-related PTSD, male veterans hospitalized with major depression (but not PTSD), and well-adjusted male combat veterans, all from the Vietnam era. The RAVLT was modified to allow close examination of the effects of word content as well as valence on learning and recall. To accomplish this, we constructed matched lists of four category types: neutral combat, unpleasant combat, neutral noncombat, and unpleasant noncombat words. Using standard RAVLT administration, we found that PTSD and depressed patients both had poorer total recall than war veterans who were stress exposed but well-adjusted, with depressed patients having the largest impairment.

In terms of word type effects, both PTSD and well-adjusted combat veterans showed a distinct preference for learning combat words above all others; moreover, PTSD patients displayed enhanced learning of unpleasant combat words in a way that distinguished them from the two other groups. Examination of the effect of trials indicated that PTSD patients learned at a slightly slower rate than their well-adjusted counterparts. This finding may reflect an individualized interference effect due to the presence of threat cues; alternatively, it may point to a more generalized attentional deficiency as PTSD patients' functioning on a generic continuous performance task in this study showed substantially increased response latencies and more false positive errors than other groups.

The preceding study helped to confirm that the memory and recall abilities of PTSD patients were quantitatively and qualitatively different from that of both well-adjusted individuals and patients with an equally serious but differing Axis 1 disorder. In this case, neuropsychological paradigms helped to delineate important functional differences associated with diagnostic status, raising the possibility that these differences someday may be found to be associated with variations in pathophysiology as well as psychopathology. To extend this work, a more recent study of ours (Wolfe, Weisstein, Clum, Chrestman, & Kaloupek, 1993) explored explicit and implicit memory in female veterans with and without war-related PTSD. Basing our design on research by a number of investigators including, for example, Squire (1992) and Schacter, Chiu, and Ochsner (1993), we constructed a word stem completion task, along with cued recall and recognition conditions, to examine the impact of PTSD status on overall memory and memory for affectively valence material. As before, word lists were derived using the four word categories described above to examine memory processes under conditions involving conscious and unconscious awareness.

Preliminary results from this experiment suggest that the overall recall ability of PTSD "positive" women is not markedly dissimilar from that of PTSD "negative" control subjects. However, our data indicate that women with PTSD allocate less attention to unpleasant military words under explicit (vs. implicit) recall conditions than do their matched counterparts without the disorder (Wolfe & Clum, 1993). Although these results are preliminary and require further verification, it is of note that similar studies with male veterans to date have obtained the opposite finding on explicit memory tasks; that is, males with PTSD have shown enhanced recall of unpleasant combat stimuli compared to non-PTSD men (Zeitlin & McNally, 1991). Further interpretation of this finding requires more detailed investigation; for example, what cognitive, psychological, and behavioral characteristics are associated with these patterns in women? Do women with PTSD have higher rates of avoidant than intrusive symptomatology, a finding that might help to explain their seemingly "biased" performance on the explicit recall task?

In another phase of this study, we examined women's performance on the accompanying recognition task and found roughly comparable abilities in women with and without PTSD. However, women with PTSD committed significantly more false positive errors, preferentially endorsing unpleasant military words as targets. Interestingly, preliminary analysis of implicit memory data in our study showed that PTSD positive women had enhanced priming for unpleasant military words compared to both the well-adjusted women and to their own implicit memory performance on other word categories (Wolfe, 1993). This finding seems to suggest that unpleasant military associations may be more salient (and accessible) in PTSD when conscious recall is not a factor, a conclusion that could support empirical research proposing a uniquely interconnected, readily activated, semantic network in PTSD (Foa, Steketee & Rothbaum, 1989). Detailed analysis of our subjects' response latency and psychophysiological reactivity data will help clarify further the range of domains and factors potentially associated with these processing alterations.

Clearly, the roles of memory bias, conscious awareness, activation and arousal, and efficiency of encoding and retrieval strategies are all critical in assessing some of the unique symptom patterns associated with severe PTSD. Models from neuropsychology studies of amnesic and depressed patients offer a significant opportunity to employ well-established paradigms to advance these investigations. In addition, the breadth of findings obtained from administering these paradigms to various well-defined neurologic patient groups, for example, evidence of performance dissociations and selective sparing of memory systems, encoding and retrieval distinctions, activation phenomena, and fluency and organizational strategies, clearly have enhanced our ability to evaluate the cognitive alterations reported by PTSD patients. Nelson's rare insight into characterizing normal and abnormal memory functions, and his creativity in designing empirical tests related to performance variables, are guiding yet another field in new and critical directions.

REFERENCES

Butters, N., Wolfe, J., Martone, M., Granholm, E., & Cermak, L. S. (1985). Memory disorders associated with Huntington's Disease: Verbal recall, verbal recognition and procedural memory. *Neuropsychologia, 23*, 729-743.

Butters, N., Wolfe, J., Granholm, E., & Martone, M. (1986). An assessment of verbal recall, recognition and fluency abilities in patients with Huntington's Disease. *Cortex, 22*, 11-32.

Butters, N., Lewis, R., Cermak, L. S., & Goodglass, H. (1973). Material-specific memory deficits in alcoholic Korsakoff patients. *Neuropsychologia, 11*, 291-299.

Bower, G. H. (1981). Mood and Memory. *American Psychologist, 36*, 129-148.

Corkin, S. (1984). Lasting consequences of bilateral medial temporal lobectomy: clinical course and experimental findings of H. M. *Seminars in Neurology, 4*, 249-259.

Chemtob, C. M., Roitblat, H. L., Hamada, R. S., Carlson, J. G., et al. (1988) A cognitive action theory of post-traumatic stress disorder. *Journal of Anxiety Disorders, 2*, 253-275.

Dalgleish, T. & Watts, F. N. (1990) Biases of attention and memory in disorders of anxiety and depression. *Clinical Psychology Review, 10*, 589-604.

Ellis, H. C., Thomas, R. L., & Rodriguez, I. A. (1984). Emotional mood states and memory: Elaborative encoding, semantics processing, and cognitive effort. *Journal of Experimental Psychology-Learning, Memory and Cognition, 10*, 470-482.

Foa, E. B., Steketee, G. & Rothbaum, B. O. (1989). Behavioral/cognitive conceptualizations of post-traumatic stress disorder. *Behavior Therapy, 20*, 155-176.

Granholm, E., Wolfe, J., & Butters, N. (1985). Affective-arousal factors in the recall of thematic stories by amnesic and demented patients. *Developmental Neuropsychology, 4*, 317-333.

Keane, T., Wolfe., & Taylor, K. (1987). Post-traumatic stress disorder: evidence for diagnostic validity and methods of psychological assessment. *Journal of Clinical Psychology, 43*, 32-43.

Lyons, J. A., Gerardi. R. J., Wolfe, J. & Keane, T. M. (1990). Multidimensional assessment of combat related PTSD: Phenomenological, psychometric and psychophysiological considerations. *Journal of Traumatic Stress, 1*, 373-394.

Mogg, K., Mathews, A. & Eysenck, M. (1992). Attentional bias to threat in clinical anxiety states. *Cognition & Emotion, 6*, 149-159.

Rusted, J. M. & Dighton, K. (1991). Selective processing of threat-related material by spider phobics in a prose recall task. *Cognition and Emotion, 5*, 123-132.

Schacter, D. L., Chiu, C. -Y. P., & Ochsner, K. N. (1993). Implicit memory: A selective Review. *Annual Review of Neuroscience, 16*, 159-182.

Squire, L. R. (1992). Declarative and nondeclarative memory: Multiple brain systems supporting learning and memory. *Journal of Cognitive Neuroscience, 4*, 232-243.

Weingartner, H. & Silberman, E. (1982). Models of cognitive impairment: cognitive changes in depression, *Psychopharmacology Bulletin, 18*, 27-42.

Wolfe, J. (1993, October). *Significance of cognitive changes in PTSD: Implications for survival.* In R. Yehuda (Chair), Memory deficits in war veterans with chronic PTSD. Symposium conducted at the meeting of the International Society for Traumatic Stress Studies, San Antonio.

Wolfe, J. & Charney, D. S. (1991). Use of Neuropsychological Assessment in posttraumatic stress disorder. *Psychological Assessment, 3*, 573-580.

Wolfe, J. & Clum, G. (1993, October). *Memory with and without conscious awareness in female trauma survivors: A functional model.* In D. Bremner (Chair), Stress and memory. Symposium conducted at the meeting of the International Society for Traumatic Stress Studies, San Antonio.

Wolfe, J., Granholm, E., Butters, N., Saunders, E., & Janowsky, D. (1987). Verbal memory deficits associated with major affective disorders: A comparison of unipolar and bipolar patients. *Journal of Affective Disorders, 13*, 83-92.

Wolfe, J. & Keane, T. M. (1990). The diagnostic validity of post-traumatic stress disorder. In M. Wolf, & A. Mosnaim (Eds.), *Post-traumatic stress disorder: Etiology phenomenology, and treatment.* Washington, D. C.: American Psychiatric Press.

Wolfe, J. & Keane, T. M. (1993). New perspectives in the assessment of combat-related post-traumatic stress disorder. In J. Wilson & B. Raphael (Eds.), *The international handbook of traumatic stress syndromes.* New York: Plenum.

Wolfe, J. , Keane, T. M., Gerardi, R. J., Mora, C. A., Butters, M., & Weathers, F. (1993). *Information processing and memory changes associated with combat-related post-traumatic stress disorder.* Manuscript submitted for publication.

Wolfe, J., Keane, T. M., Lyons, J. A., & Gerardi, R. J. (1987). Current trends and issues in the assessment of combat-related posttraumatic stress disorder. *The Behavior Therapist, 10*, 27-32.

Wolfe, J., Weisstein, C., Clum, G. A., Chrestman, K. R. & Kaloupek, D. (1993).Memory and arousal and posttraumatic stress disorder in women veterans. Work in progress.

Zeitlin, S. B. & McNally, R. J. (1991). Implicit and explicit memory bias for threat in post-traumatic stress disorder. *Behavior Research and Therapy, 29*, 451-457.

21

Organismic-Developmental Theory and Neuropsychological Research

GUILA GLOSSER[1] and MORTON WIENER[2]

Nelson Butter's view of neuropsychological problems and his methods of investigation can be seen as his assimilation and transformation of Organismic-Developmental theory (Werner, 1937, 1948), the orientation that was dominant at Clark University during his graduate training in the 1960's. Although his research interests have always been focused on main stream issues and questions, his approach to them has been guided conceptually and methodologically by a less traditional viewpoint, articulated by Heinz Werner. We will try to trace some of the influences of this conceptual framework on Butters' prolific research endeavors, beginning at Clark University, then at the National Institutes of Health, through his tenure at the Boston V.A. Medical Center, and in his current work at the University of California at San Diego.

Werner (1948) claimed that developmental psychology was more than the study of ontogenesis, and it has two basic aims: "One is to grasp the characteristic pattern of each genetic level, the structure peculiar to it. The other, and no less important one, is to establish the genetic relationship between these levels, the direction of development, and the formulation of any general tendency revealed in developmental relationship and direction" (p. 5). Be it describing the developmental unfolding of the individual from childhood to maturity,

[1] GUILA GLOSSER, Ph.D. • Department of Neurology, The Graduate Hospital, Philadelphia
[2] MORTON WIENER, Ph.D. • Department of Psychology, Clark University

Neuropsychological Explorations of Memory and Cognition: Essays in Honor of Nelson Butters, edited by Laird S. Cermak, Ph.D. Plenum Press, New York, 1994

phylogenetic evolution of the nervous system, development of human cultures, or the sequence of behavior change (or the process) during performance of a task, ordering the relationships between different levels is the essence of a "genetic" analysis.

For Werner each developmental level and the relationships between levels are conceived as organic systems that must be explored in their totality, or as a "gestalt." Every event is also considered as an organic process directed to some end-point. Werner (1937) stressed the importance of distinguishing between the means or process (e.g., the different patterns and sequences by which a goal is attained) and the ends or achievement (e.g., whether a response is correct or incorrect) in a "genetic" analysis. This type of analysis combines detailed assessment of component parts or means within a system with an evaluation of the ways in which the different parts are integrated in the achievement of an organized end-product or goal.

The organizing principles of differentiation and hierarchic integration in the development of neurological and behavioral functions constitute another important premise of Werner's Organismic-Developmental approach. He emphasized that developmental change is characterized by movement from a state of homogeneity and uniformity towards increasing heterogeneity. He exemplified this notion of differentiation by contrasting the nervous system of corals, in which a diffuse uncentralized series of nerve cells and branching fibrils run "indiscriminately" throughout the body, to that of a more developed organism, such as the worm, in which peripheral structures become differentiated form a central pole in the nervous system. Along with the increasing specialization within different parts of the nervous system, developmental change is also characterized by increasing hierarchic organization. There is increasingly greater subordination of distinct parts to a coordinated organization of the whole system and to emerging centralized integrative units.

Influences of Organismic-Developmental theory first appear in Butters' Master's thesis (Butters and Wiener, 1962), in which he explored the controversy between the continuity-discontinuity views of verbal learning. In contrast to previous investigators, Butters used response time, rather than measuring only the accuracy of response, in a paired-associate learning paradigm. His examination of the sequences of changes in response times over successive learning trials, enabled him to conclude that these data were consistent with the view that learning can best be characterized as a continuously evolving event. The influence of Werner's theory is also apparent in Butter's dissertation (Butters, 1966), where he again utilized measures other than response accuracy (i.e., response latencies and patterns of response errors) to study the breakdown of discrimination learning in the white rat. In both of these studies conducted at Clark University, Butters employed less common types of dependent measures to evaluate response tendencies and types of errors manifested by subjects en route to learning. These detailed analyses of response patterns were taken as the basis for inferences about the different means by which an organism can either succeed or fail to achieve a goal, inferences that could not have been made using only conventional indexes.

A unifying notion in Werner's Organismic-Developmental theory is the idea that the same developmental stages that are appropriate to distinguish ontogenetic and phylogenetic patterns of behavior change can also be invoked to explore the microgenetic evolution of behavior change during learning. This framework can further be used to analyze the patterns of behavioral "regression" that result from dysfunctions in the nervous system. This account of developmental progression (and regression), which is germane for all categories of behavior and species, enabled Butters to target neurobehavioral research questions that encompassed both humans and animals in normal as well as impaired conditions.

Principles derived from Organismic-Developmental theory, such as Werner's distinctions between different levels of development of cognitive operations, guided Butters' animal studies and his first investigations of brain-damaged patients in the late 1960's and early 1970's. In contrast to the tradition dominant in American neuropsychology at that time, which was concerned principally with identifying relationships between loci of neurological dysfunction and clinical symptomatology, Butters drew on the theoretical model learned at Clark University to examine the different kinds and patterns of cognitive impairments that underlie various behavioral disorders. He was especially interested in impairments of higher order integrative functions such as the capacity to adopt and shift a mental set in learning tasks (e.g., Butters and Rosvold, 1968) and the ability to represent and to manipulate spatial relationships in imagery or abstract thought (e.g., Butters and Barton, 1970).

At the same time that he was exploring problems in the development and dissolution of cognition and behavior in humans, Butters also participated in an active program of animal research. Of particular note is his collaboration with Donald Stein, a physiological psychologist at Clark University, who also assimilated the framework of Organismic-Developmental theory within his experimental work (Stein, 1988). In a series of ground-breaking studies Stein challenged the predominant notion of static relationships between structure and function in the nervous system (Butters, Rosen & Stein, 1974). Following the dynamic-organismic view of neurological and behavioral organization, Stein, in collaboration with Nelson Butters and Jeffrey Rosen, investigated the effects of different factors that moderate relationships between structure and function in the nervous system. For example, they assessed the effects of serial versus single stage ablations of prefrontal cortex on behavioral deficits; they compared sparing of function for different loci of neurological damage; and they explored interactive effects of intact and damaged neural tissue on behavioral symptomatology following brain damage. Consistent with the importance Werner placed on hierarchic integration of functions to explain behavioral and neural organization, Butters' other animal studies were almost all concerned with defining multi-modal integrative association areas in the brain (Rosen, Stein & Butters, 1971; Van Hoesen, Pandya & Butters, 1972).

In the mid 1970's Butters formed a productive collaboration with Laird Cermak. They focused initially on characterizing the exact pattern of deficits underlying the memory disorders of patients with alcoholic Korsakoff's syndrome (Butters & Cermak, 1980). Rigorous experimental methods borrowed from cognitive psychology were applied to analyze the anterograde and retrograde memory problems of Korsakoff's patients. In these studies Butters returned to his earlier interest in mechanisms of new learning in humans.

Concurrent with his investigations of Korsakoff's syndrome, Butters began to examine differences in the memory disorders among other groups of amnesic patients (e.g., those with Huntington's Disease and Herpes encephalitis). These qualitative analyses of symptoms in different patient groups reflected the belief that the same end-product (amnesia) can result from a multiplicity of means or component processes. Butters (1990) summarized this endeavor by stating that in his laboratory "the process-achievement approach has been used to differentiate the global memory impairments manifested by patients with various forms of amnesia and dementia. Although actuarial approaches to neuropsychology have suggested that the severe memory deficits of such patient populations are highly similar when assessed with standardized tests of memory, investigations applying these concepts and models of cognitive neuropsychology have often noted important differences among these superficially (i.e., quantitatively) comparable retention deficiencies" (pp. 99).

Butters' work in the mid-1980's reflected increasing recognition that amnestic deficits in patients with neurological illnesses occur in the context of other cognitive impairments, ones that interact with the memory problems to modify the pattern of the observed amnesia. This thinking seemed to evolve from earlier studies exploring concomitant symptoms of alcoholic Korsakoff's syndrome, such as visuoperceptual disturbance, problem solving difficulties, and impairments in motivational-affective arousal, and their contribution to the memory disorders of these patients (Becker, 1986; Butters & Miliotis, 1985; Granholm, Wolfe & Butters, 1985; Glosser, Butters & Kaplan, 1977). The idea that behavior can be seen as a function of dynamic interactions between different systems is a derivative of the premise in Organismic-Developmental theory that every instance of an action is always a function of the whole integrated system in which it is embedded. Again in the 1980's, Butter's approach contrasted with the predominant view held by cognitive neuroscientists at the time who explained brain-behavior relationships in a much more reductionistic and mechanistic manner. Concern with interactions between deficits in different cognitive domains led to Butters' efforts to characterize the underlying cognitive disturbances in various forms of dementia in the late 1980's and in the 1990's. Although the primary focus of inquiry has remained on different aspects of memory dysfunction, the scope of investigations has broadened to consider the linguistic (Butters, et al., 1987) and conceptual disorders (Chan, et al., 1993a) of patients with dementias such as Alzheimer's Disease.

In recent years Butters' research appears to be moving once again in a direction charted by Organismic-Developmental theory. Werner had particular interest in the structural organization of representations of conceptual knowledge. He was also concerned with the ways in which conceptual and symbolic representations change ontogenetically and as a consequence of brain-damage (Werner & Kaplan, 1963). Similar trends are becoming apparent in Butters' evolving thoughts about the manner in which the structure of semantic knowledge breaks down in patients with Alzheimer's Disease (Chan, et al., 1993b). His investigations of semantic memory disorders in dementia reflect the application of many of the same developmental principles of behavioral evolution and dissolution as those articulated by Werner.

In his statement of goals and directions for *Neuropsychology*, the journal that he edits, Butters (1993) indicates the importance that he, like Werner, places on the interdependence of clinical and cognitive approaches to neuropsychology. Butters' own career is an excellent illustration of this type of integration of theory and practice. Throughout his work, Butters has interwoven threads from clinical neurology and neuropsychology together with methods from physiological psychology and principles from Organismic-Developmental theory to form a rich and elaborate tapestry of knowledge for clinicians and researches alike.

ACKNOWLEDGEMENT. We are grateful to Ina Samuels for sharing her insights about Nelson Butter's work and to Seymour Wapner for sharpening our understanding of Heinz Werner's theory.

REFERENCES

Butters, N. (1966) The effect of LSD-25 on spatial and stimulus perseverative tendencies in rats. *Psychopharmacologia, 8,* 454-460.

Butters, N. (1985) Alcoholic Korsakoff's syndrome: Some unresolved issues concerning etiology, neuropathology, and cognitive deficits. *Journal of Clinical and Experimental Neuropsychology, 7,* 181-210.

Butters, N. (1993) Some comments on the goals and direction of Neuropsychology. *Neuropsychology, 1,* 3-4.

Butters, N. & Barton, M. (1970) Role of the right parietal lobe in the mediation of crossmodal associations and reversible operations in space. *Cortex, 6,* 174-190.

Butters, N. & Cermak, L.S. (1980) *Alcoholic Korsakoff's Syndrome: An Information Processing Approach to Amnesia.* New York: Academic Press.

Butters, N., Granholm, E., Salmon, D.P., Grant, I. & Wolfe, J. (1987) Episodic and semantic memory: A comparison of amnesic and demented patients. *Journal of Clinical and Experimental Neuropsychology, 9*, 479-497.

Butters, N. & Miliotis, P. (1985) Amnesic disorders. In K.M. Heilman & E. Valenstein (Eds.) *Clinical Neuropsychology*, Second Edition (pp 403-452). New York: Oxford University Press.

Butters, N., Rosen J.J. & Stein, D.G. (1974) Recovery of behavioral functions after sequential ablation of the frontal lobes of monkeys. In D.G. Stein, J.J. Rosen & N. Butters (Eds.) *Plasticity and Recovery of Function in the Central Nervous System* (pp 429-466). New York: Academic Press.

Butters, N. & Rosvold, H.E. Effect of caudate and septal nuclei lesions on resistance to extinction and retention of delayed alternation. *Journal of Comparative and Physiological Psychology, 65*, 397-403.

Butters, N., Salmon, D.P. & Heindel, W.C. (1990) Processes underlying the memory impairments of demented patients. In E. Goldberg (Ed.) *Contemporary Neuropsychology and the Legacy of Luria*. Hillsdale, NJ: Lawrence Erlbaum Associates.

Butters, N. & Wiener, M. (1962) The continuity-discontinuity controversy in paired associate learning. *The Journal of Psychology, 54*, 473-483.

Chan, A.S., Butters, N., Paulson, J.S., Salmon, D.P., Swenson, M.R. & Maloney, L.T. (1993a) An assessment of the semantic network in patients with Alzheimer's Disease. *Journal of Cognitive Neuroscience, 5*, 254-261.

Chan, A.S., Butters, N., Salmon, D.P., & McGuire, K.A. (1993b) Dimensionality and clustering in the semantic network of patients with Alzheimer's Disease. *Psychology and Aging, 8*, 411-419.

Granholm, E., Wolfe, J. & Butters, N. (1985) Affective-arousal factors in the recall of thematic stories by amnesic and demented patients. *Developmental Neuropsychology, 1*, 317-333.

Rosen J.J., Stein, D.G. & Butters, N. (1971) Recovery of function after serial ablation of the prefrontal cortex in the rhesus monkey. *Science, 173*, 353-356.

Stein, D.G. (1988) Development and plasticity in the CNS: Organismic and environmental influences. *Heinz Werner Lecture Series*, volume *17*. Worcester, MA: Clark University Press.

Van Hoesen, G.W., Pandya, D.N. & Butters, N. (1972) Cortical afferents to the entorhinal cortex of the rhesus monkey. *Science, 175*, 1471-1473.

Werner, H. (1937) Process and achievement: A basic problem of education and developmental psychology. *Harvard Educational Review, 7*, 353-368.

Werner, H. (1948) *Comparative Psychology of Mental Development*. New York: International Universities Press, Inc.

Werner, H. & Kaplan, B. (1963) *Symbol Formation*. New York: John Wiley & Sons.

22

Growing up in Neuropsychology

MERYL A. BUTTERS[1]

While my endeavors as a neuropsychologist do not yet constitute a true "body of work", I have been active in the field for a number of years. I have been influenced by many mentors and colleagues, (many of whom have contributed to this volume), but no one more so than my father. I have a lifetime of experiences to share, and only a few pages on which to convey them.

Anyone who knows me even slightly, knows that genetic factors notwithstanding, I was probably not destined to become a neuropsychologist. But the seeds were obviously sown at an early age. Growing up with my father was in many ways a unique experience. Some of his personal idiosyncracies have given me a different set of memories than most. For example: Most kids first experience animals on a family outing to the zoo. One of my earliest memories is of the rat lab at Clark University, where as a graduate student, my father was conducting experiments on the effects of LSD on rats. Many children have fathers with conventional professions such as doctors, accountants, and bankers. When their fathers take them to work for the day they visit offices. When my father took me to work we visited the primate lab where I watched monkeys learning which food well to search for reinforcement.

By the time I reached adolescence (which to my father's chagrin turned out to be a rather prolonged period in my life), my interest in things cerebral and academic had diminished severely. I concentrated on my social life, and so it was with great embarrassment that I learned that my father had accepted the invitation of my 10th grade biology teacher and would be lecturing my class. The most

---

[1] MERYL A. BUTTERS, Ph.D. • Department of Psychiatry, Western Psychiatric Institute and Clinic, University of Pittsburgh Medical Center

Psychological Explorations of Memory and Cognition: Essays in Honor of Nelson Butters, edited by Laird S. Cermak, Ph.D. Plenum Press, New York, 1994.

memorable moment: my father passing around a jar that contained a brain preserved in formaldehyde.

Upon college graduation, I moved home, put off searching for a job and announced my plan to spend the summer "lounging" on Cape Cod. My father, horrified by my lack of focus and motivation, conceived a plan that ultimately would have a lasting impact on my life. On Father's Day 1980, he announced that I would not be spending the summer at the beach, because I had a job. I replied that was impossible, because I was not looking for a job. He then explained that he had procured me a position just for the summer, in his lab (though he assured me that I would not be working directly for him), and that if I planned to live at home or in any way sponge off my family, I had to work. Seeing no alternative (I did not even have a resume), I begrudgingly went to work in his lab the following week. An amazing thing happened. At that time he was conducting studies on the memory disorders associated alcoholism and various forms of dementia. For the first time I began to actually learn about what my father did in his professional life, and I found it at worst interesting, and at best fascinating.

I went on to work for other people, and while it took 5 years, I slowly incorporated my father's scientific values and eventually came to want to put forth effort and hard work in order to accomplish my newly formed goals. And so it was that I eventually attended graduate school, majoring in psychology.

Once ensconced in graduate school I began to attend conferences with my father (I claimed that it was largely for the free room and board). For the first several years, much to his dismay, I refused to wear my name tag. While he thought I was embarrassed by him, the truth was that I did not want to become known only as his daughter, but wanted to be known for myself. As that has gradually come to pass, I have proudly revealed my lineage to my colleagues.

Throughout my father's career he has attempted to demonstrate that there are distinct dissociations among cognitive functions within and between patients with various forms of cerebral dysfunction. In my own work, I attempt to exploit the cognitive abilities that remain intact in brain damaged patients, to find ways to maximize their level of functioning, and ultimately their quality of life.

The early work my father conducted with Jeffrey Rosen and Donald Stein on plasticity and recovery of function following injury to the central nervous system in many ways laid the groundwork for my future interest in brain injury. His eventual focus on memory disorders spawned my interest in the most common complaint of individuals who have suffered closed head injuries--memory difficulties. Another influence has been his careful studies with Laird Cermak, in which they manipulated encoding conditions and demonstrated that the amnesic syndrome exhibited by individuals with Alcoholic Korsakoff's Syndrome is fundamentally due to an encoding deficit. They demonstrated that if encoding was ensured, the memory performance of Korsakoff's Syndrome patients improved. I now employ both their general approach and some of their specific techniques in both my clinical work and research. For appropriate brain injured individuals (those with moderate and/or unimodal memory impairment and intact or no more than mildly impaired executive functioning), interventions that increase the amount of material processed and the depth of encoding greatly improves recall in everyday life.

The work my father has done with David Salmon, Bill Heindel and others on the status of procedural memory in various forms of dementia has helped lead to the conclusion that motor skill learning is mediated by the basal ganglia. This attempt at localizing a form of implicit memory greatly enriched the interpretation of results in my doctoral thesis. In that study, I was able to demonstrate that patients with frontal lobe damage could overcome their deficit in memory for temporal order by employing their intact motor memory, which relies on their functioning basal ganglia.

My father's recent work on the breakdown of the structure of semantic memory in Alzheimer's Disease dovetails with my current focus and future pursuits. In a series of particularly creative studies with numerous colleagues, he has shown that compared to individuals with other forms of memory disorder, many of the deficits exhibited by Alzheimer's Disease patients are accounted for by a fundamental breakdown in the structure of semantic memory. Some of my current work centers on exploiting the intact semantic knowledge systems possessed by many amnesic patients. The results have important implications for knowledge acquisition strategies and the generalization of training.

My father has emphasized the process approach to neuropsychological assessment that has been assiduously developed and promoted by Edith Kaplan and Harold Goodglass. In recent years he has contributed to the process approach by demonstrating that with careful observation and inspection of test results, various patient groups may perform quantitatively similarly but qualitatively very different on tasks. This approach not only has contributed to improving diagnostic accuracy, but has induced me to attempt to demonstrate similar dissociations among individuals with Alzheimer's Disease and frontal lobe dementia.

As a neuropsychologist my father has distinguished himself as a concerned mentor and colleague, and his work has helped to set a high standard for the field. He has been unusually successful at integrating neuroanatomy, and cognitive and neuropsychological theory with applied work. His unique combination of intellectual creativity, drive, ambition, irreverence, and the ability to not take himself too seriously, has certainly allowed him to make his mark on the field of neuropsychology, and in particular, on me. His influence is clear, and he continues to advise, cajole, and direct me on my way through the professional maze. Perhaps the best way to mark this occasion, however, is to acknowledge where *he* feels he has made the greatest impact--as a son, husband, father, father-in-law, and grandfather. His example of hard work, loyalty, tolerance, generosity and love has touched us all.

Bibliography of Nelson Butters, Ph.D.

1. N. Butters and M. Wiener: "The Continuity-Discontinuity Controversy in Paired-Associate Learning," *Journal of Psychology*, 54:473-483, 1962.

2. H. Kellner, N. Butters, and M. Wiener: "Mechanisms of Defense: An Alternative Response," *Journal of Personality*, 32:601-621, 1964.

3. N. Butters, M. Wiener, and H. Kellner: "Schedules of Reinforcement and Individual Differences in Learning in Recall," *Psychological Reports*, 17:3-9, 1965.

4. N. Butters: "The Effect of LSD-25 on Spatial and Stimulus Perseverative Tendencies in Rats," *Psychopharmacologia*, 8:454-460, 1966.

5. N. Butters and H.E. Rosvold: "The Effect of Selective Septal Lesions on Resistance to Extinction and Spatial Delayed-Alternation Performance in Monkeys," *Journal of Comparative and Physiological Psychology*, 66:389-395, 1968.

6. N. Butters and B. Brody: "The Role of the Left Parietal Lobe in the Mediation of Intra- and Cross-Modal Associations," *Cortex*, 4:328-343, 1968.

7. N. Butters and H.E. Rosvold: "Effect of Caudate and Septal Nuclei Lesions on Resistance to Extinction and Delayed Afterman," *Journal of Comparative and Physiological Psychology*, 65:397-403, 1968.

8. N. Butters, E. Jones, J. Hoyle, and C. Zsambok: "Effect of Dynamic Verbal and Tonal Stimuli on the Perception of Time," *Perceptual and Motor Skills*, 27:431-437, 1968.

9. N. Butters and B. Brody: "Familiarity as a Factor in the Cross-Modal Associations of Brain-Damaged Patients," *Perceptual and Motor Skills*, 28:68, 1969.

10. N. Butters: "Changes in Equivalence Judgments Following Verbal, Perceptual, or Functional Practice Conditions," *Child Development*, 40:1179-1191, 1969.

11. N. Butters and D. Pandya: "Retention of Delayed-Alternation Effect of Selective Lesions of Sulcus Principalis," *Science*, 165:1271-1273, 1969.

12. N. Butters, M. Barton, and B. Brody: "Role of the Right Parietal Lobe in the Mediation of Cross-Modal Associations and Reversible Operations in Space," *Cortex*, 6:174-190, 1970.

13. N. Butters, I. Samuels, H. Goodglass, and B. Brody: "Short-Term Visual and Auditory Memory Disorders After Parietal and Frontal Lobe Damage," *Cortex*, 6:440-459, 1970.

14. N. Butters and M. Barton: "Effect of Parietal Lobe Damage on the Performance of Reversible Operations in Space," *Neuropsychologia*, 8:205-214, 1970.

15. I. Samuels, N. Butters, and H. Goodglass: "Visual Memory Deficits Following Cortical and Limbic Lesions: Effect of Field of Presentation," *Physiology and Behavior*, 6:447-452, 1971.

16. D. Pandya, P. Dye, and N. Butters: "Efferent Cortico-Cortical Projections of the Prefrontal Cortex in the Rhesus Monkey," *Brain Research*, 31:35-46, 1971.

17. J. Rosen, D. Stein, and N. Butters: "Recovery of Function After Serial Ablation of Prefrontal Cortex in The Rhesus Monkey," *Science*, 173:353-356, 1971.

18. L.S. Cermak, N. Butters, and H. Goodglass: "The Extent of Memory Loss in Korsakoff Patients," *Neuropsychologia*, 9:307-315, 1971.

19. N. Butters, D. Pandya, K. Sanders, and P. Dye: "Behavioral Deficits in Monkeys After Selective Lesions Within the Middle Third of Sulcus Principalis," *Journal of Comparative and Physioloical Psychology*, 76:8-14, 1971.

20. I. Samuels, N. Butters, H. Goodglass, and B. Brody: "A Comparison of Subcortical and Cortical Damage on Short-Term Visual and Auditory Memory," *Neuropsychologia*, 9:293-306, 1971.

21. N. Butters, C. Soeldner, and P. Fedio: "Comparison of Parietal and Frontal Lobe Spatial Deficits in Man: Extrapersonal vs. Personal (Egocentric) Space," *Perceptual Motor Skills*, 34:27-34, 1972.

22. N. Butters, D. Pandya, D. Stein, and J. Rosen: "A Search for the Spatial Engram Within the Frontal Lobes of Monkeys," *Acta Neurobiologiae Experimentalis*, 32:305-330, 1972.

23. W. Pohl, N. Butters, and H. Goodglass: "Spatial Discrimination Systems and Cerebral Lateralization", *Cortex*, 8:304-314, 1972.

24. G. Van Hoeson, D. Pandya, and N. Butters: "Cortical Afferents to the Entorhinal Cortex of the Rhesus Monkey," *Science*, 175:1471-1473, 1972.

25. I. Samuels, N. Butters, and P. Fedio: "Short-Term Memory Disorders Following Temporal Lobe Removals in Humans," *Cortex*, 8:283-298, 1972.

26. L.S. Cermak and N. Butters: "The Role of Interference and Encoding in the Short-Term Memory Deficits of Korsakoff Patients," *Neuropsychologia*, 10:89-95, 1972.

27. N. Butters, D. Sax, B. Tomlinson, and R. Feldman: "Effects of Serial Caudate Lesions and L-Dopa Administration Upon the Cognitive and Motor Behavior of Monkeys," *Advances in Neurology, Volume 1: Huntington's Chorea, 1872-1972*, edited by A. Barbeau, T.N. Chase, and G.W. Paulson, New York: Raven Press, 1973.

28. N. Butters, R. Lewis, L.S. Cermak, and H. Goodglass: "Material-Specific Memory Deficits in Alcoholic Korsakoff Patients", *Neuropsychologia*, 11:291-299, 1973.

29. N. Butters, H. Gardner, F. Boller, and J. Moreines: "Retrieving Information from Korsakoff Patients: Effects of Categorical Cues and Reference to the Task," *Cortex*, 9:165-175, 1973.

30. L.S. Cermak, N. Butters, and J. Gerrein: "The Extent of the Verbal Encoding Ability of Korsakoff Patients," *Neuropsychologia*, 11:85-94, 1973.

31. L.S. Cermak and N. Butters: "Information Processing Deficits of Alcoholic Korsakoff Patients," *Quarterly Journal of Studies on Alcohol*, 34:1110-1132, 1973.

32. L.S. Cermak, R. Lewis, N. Butters, and H. Goodglass: "Role of Verbal Mediation in Performance of Motor Tasks by Korsakoff Patients," *Perceptual and Motor Skills*, 37:259-262, 1973.

33. N. Butters, C. Butter, J. Rosen, and D. Stein: "Behavioral Effects of Sequential and One-Stage Ablations of Orbital Prefrontal Cortex in the Monkey," *Experimental Neurology*, 39:204-214. 1973.

34. I. Samuels, N. Butters, and L. Cermak: "Short-Term Visual Memory: Effects of Visual Field, Serial Position and Exposure Duration," *Perceptual and Motor Skills*, 36:115-121, 1973.

35. D. Stein, J. Rosen, and N. Butters, editors: *Plasticity and Recovery of Function in the CNS*, New York: Academic Press, 1974.

36. L.S. Cermak, N. Butters, and J. Moreines: "Some Analyses of the Verbal Encoding Deficit of Alcoholic Korsakoff Patients," *Brain and Language*, 1:141-150, 1974.

37. N. Butters, J. Rosen, and D. Stein: "Recovery of Behavioral Function After Sequential Ablation of the Frontal Lobes of Monkeys," *Plasticity and Recovery of Function in the Central Nervous System*, edited by D. Stein, J. Rosen, and N. Butters, pp. 429-466. New York: Academic Press, 1974.

38. N. Butters and L.S. Cermak: "The Role of Cognitive Factors in the Memory Disorders of Alcoholic Patients with the Korsakoff Syndrome," *Annals of New York Academy of Sciences*, 233:61-75, 1974.

39. N. Butters and L.S. Cermak: "Some Comments on Warrington and Baddeley's Report of Normal Short-Term Memory in Amnesic Patients," *Neuropsychologia*, 12:283-285, 1974.

40. N. Butters: "Recovery of Function After Sequential Ablation of the Frontal Lobe of Monkeys," *Neurosciences Research Program Bulletin*, 12:269-272, 1974.

41. N. Butters, L.S. Cermak, B. Jones, and G. Glosser: "Some Analyses of the Information Processing and Sensory Capacities of Alcoholic Korsakoff Patients," *Alcohol Intoxication and Withdrawl*, edited by M. Gross, pp. 595-604. New York: Plenum Press, 1975.

42. B. Jones, H. Moskowitz, and N. Butters: "Olfactory Discrimination in Alcoholic Korsakoff Patients," *Neuropsychologia*, 13:173-179, 1975.

43. B. Jones, H. Moskowitz, N. Butters, and G. Glosser: "Psychophysical Scaling of Olfactory, Visual, and Auditory Stimuli by Alcoholic Korsakoff Patients," *Neuropsychologia*, 13:387-393, 1975.

44. D. DeLuca, L.S. Cermak, and N. Butters: "An Analysis of Korsakoff Patients' Recall Following Varying Types of Distractor Activity," *Neuropsychologia*, 13:271-279, 1975.

45. G. Van Hoesen, D. Pandya, and N. Butters: "Some Connections of the Entorhinal (Area 28) and Perirhinal (Area 35) Cortices of the Rhesus Monkey. II. Frontal Lobe Afferents," *Brain Research*, 95:25-38, 1975.

46. N. Butters and L.S. Cermak: "Some Analyses of Amnesic Syndromes in Brain-Damaged Patients," *The Hippocampus*, edited by K. Priham and R. Isaacson, pp. 377-409. New York: Plenum Press, 1975.

47. J. Rosen, N. Butters, C. Soeldner, and D. Stein: "Effects of One-Stage and Serial Ablations of the Middle Third of Sulcus Principalis on Delayed Alternation Performance in Monkeys," *Journal of Comparative and Physiological Psychology*, 89:1077-1082, 1975.

48. M. Oscar-Berman and N. Butters: "Sequential and Single-Stage Lesions of Posterior Association Cortex in Rhesus Monkeys," *Physiology and Behavior*, 17:287-295, 1976.

49. L.S. Cermak and N. Butters: "The Role of Language in the Memory Disorders of Brain-Damaged Patients," *Annals of the New York Academy of Sciences*, 280:857-867, 1976.

50. N. Butters and L.S. Cermak: "Neuropsychological Studies of Alcoholic Korsakoff Patients," *Empirical Studies of Alcoholism*, edited by G. Goldstein and C. Neuringer, pp. 153-193. Cambridge, MA: Ballinger Press, 1976.

51. D. DeLuca, L.S. Cermak and N. Butters: "The Differential Effects of Semantic, Acoustic, and Non-Verbal Distraction on Korsakoff Patients' Verbal Retention Performance," *International Journal of Neuroscience*, 6:279-284, 1976.

52. G. Glosser, N. Butters, and I. Samuels: "Failures in Information Processing in Patients with Korsakoff's Syndrome," *Neuropsychologia*, 14:327-334, 1976.

53. N. Butters, S. Tarlow, L.S. Cermak, and D. Sax: "A Comparison of the Information Processing Deficits of Patients with Huntington's Chorea and Korsakoff's Syndrome," *Cortex*, 12:134-144, 1976.

54. N. Butters: "Visuoperceptive Deficits After Brain Damage in Man," *The International Encyclopedia of Neurology, Psychiatry Psychoanalysis and Psychology, Volume II*, Edited by B. Wolman, pp. 398-401. New York: Human Sciences Press, 1977.

55. N. Butters, L.S. Cermak, K. Montgomery, and A. Adinolfi: "Some Comparisons of the Memory and Visuoperceptive Deficits of Chronic Alcoholics and Patients with Korsakoff's Disease," *Alcoholism: Clinical and Experimental Research*, 1:73-80, 1977

56. M. Mesulam, G. Van Hoesen, and N. Butters: "Clinical Manifestations of Chronic Thiamine Deficiency in the Rhesus Monkey," *Neurology*, 27:239-245, 1977.

57. G. Glosser, N. Butters, and E. Kaplan: "Visuoperceptual Processes in Brain Damaged Patients on the Digit-Symbol Substitution Test," *International Journal of Neuroscience*, 7:59-6, 1977.

58. N. Butters and M. Grady: "Effect of Predistractor Delays on the Short-Term Memory Performance of Patients with Korsakoff's and Huntington's Disease," *Neuropsychologia*, 15:701-706, 1977.

59. N. Kapur and N. Butters: "Visuoperceptive Deficits in Long-Term Alcoholics and Alcoholics with Korsakoff's Psychosis," *Journal of Studies on Alcohol*, 38:2025-2035, 1977.

60. D. Stein, N. Butters, and J. Rosen: "A Comparison of Two-and- Four-Stage Ablations of Sulcus Principalis on Recovery of Spatial Performance in the Rhesus Monkey," *Neuropsychologia*, 15:179-182, 1977.

61. P. Meudell, N. Butters, and K. Montgomery: "The Role of Rehearsal in the Short-Term Memory Performance of Patients with Korsakoff's and Huntington's Disease," *Neuropsychologia*, 16:507-510, 1978.

62. N. Butters, D. Sax, K. Montgomery, and S. Tarlow: Comparison of the Neuropsychological Deficits Associated with Early and Advanced Huntington's Disease," *Archives of Neurology*, 35:585-589, 1978.

63. S. Jacobson, N. Butters, and N. Tovsky: "Afferent and Efferent Subcortical Projections of Behaviorally Defined Sectors of Prefrontal Granular Cortex," *Brain Research*, 159:279-296, 1978.

64. J. Dricker, N. Butters, G. Berman, I. Samuels, and S. Carey: "The Recognition and Encoding of Faces by Alcoholic Korsakoff and Right Hemisphere Patients," *Neuropsychologia*, 16:683-695, 1978.

65. B. Jones, N. Butters, H.R. Moskowitz, and K. Montgomery: "Olfactory and Gustatory Capacities of Alcoholic Korsakoff Patients," *Neuropsychologia*, 16:323-337, 1978.

66. N. Butters: "Amnesic Disorders," *Clinical Neuropsychology*, edited by K. Heilman and E. Valentine, pp. 439-473. Oxford University Press, 1979.

67. M.S. Albert, N. Butters, and J. Levin: "Temporal Gradients in the Retrograde Amnesia of Patients with Alcoholic Korsakoff's Disease," *Archives of Neurology*, 36:211-216, 1979.

68. N. Butters, M.S. Albert, and D. Sax: "Investigations of the Memory Disorders of Patients with Huntington's Disease," *Advances in Neurology*, edited by T. Chase, N. Wexler, and A. Barbeau, pp. 203-213. New York: Raven Press, 1979.

69. I. Samuels, N. Butters, P. Fedio, and C. Cox: "Deficits in Short-Term Auditory Memory for Verbal Material Following Right Temporal Removals in Humans," *International Journal of Neuroscience*, 11:101-108, 1980.

70. M.S. Albert, N. Butters, and J. Levin: "Memory for Remote Events in Chronic Alcoholics and Alcoholic Korsakoff Patients," *Biological Effects of Alcohol*, edited by Henri Begleiter, pp. 719-730. New York: Plenum Publishing Corporation, 1980.

71. C. Ryan, N. Butters, and K. Montgomery: "Memory Deficits in Chronic Alcoholics: Continuities Between the 'Intact' Alcoholic and the Alcoholic Korsakoff Patient," *Biological Effects of Alcohol*, edited by Henri Begleiter, pp. 701-730. New York: Plenum Publishing Corporation, 1980.

72. N. Butters and L.S. Cermak: *Alcoholic Korsakoff's Syndrome: An Information Processing Approach to Amnesia*. New York: Academic Press, 1980.

73. C. Ryan and N. Butters: "Learning and Memory Impairments in Young and Old Alcoholics: Evidence for the Premature-Aging Hypothesis," *Alcoholism: Clinical and Experimental Research*, 4:288-293, 1980.

74. C. Ryan and N. Butters: "Further Evidence for a Continuum-of-Impairment Encompassing Male Alcoholic Korsakoff Patients and Chronic Alcoholic Men," *Alcoholism: Clinical and Experimental Research*, 4:190-198, 1980.

75. H. Potter and N. Butters: "Continuities in the Olfactory Deficits of Chronic Alcoholics and Alcoholics with the Korsakoff Syndrome," *Currents in Alcoholism Vol. 7*, edited by Marc Galanter, pp. 261-271. Grune and Stratton, Inc, 1980.

76. H. Potter and N. Butters: "An Assessment of Olfactory Deficits in Patients with Damage to Prefrontal Cortex," *Neuropsychologia*, 18:621-628, 1980.

77. N. Butters: "Neuropsychology: A Textbook of Systems and Psychological Functions of the Human Brain." *New England Journal of Medicine*, pp. 1128-1129, 1980.

78. C. Ryan, B. DiDario, N. Butters, and A. Adinolfi: "The Relationship Between Abstinence and Recovery of Function in Male Alcoholics," *Journal of Clinical Neuropsychology*, 2:125-134, 1980.

79. M.S. Albert, N. Butters, and J. Brandt: "Memory for Remote Events in Alcoholics," *Journal of Studies on Alcohol*, 41:1071-1081, 1980.

80. N. Butters: "Potential Contributions of Neuropsychology to Our Understanding of the Memory Capacities of the Elderly," *New Directions in Memory and Aging: Proceedings of the George Talland Memorial Conference*, edited by L.W. Poon and J.L. Fozard, pp. 451-459. New Jersey: L. Erlbaum Associates, 1980.

81. D. Rubin and N. Butters: "Clustering by Alcoholic Korsakoff Patients," *Neuropsychologia*, 19:137-140, 1981.

82. D. Rubin, E.H. Olson, M. Richter, and N. Butters: "Memory for Prose in Korsakoff and Schizophrenic Populations," *International Journal of Neuroscience*, 13:81-85, 1981.

83. M.S. Albert, N. Butters, and J. Brandt: "Patterns of Remote Memory in Amnesic and Demented Patients," *Archives of Neurology*, 38:495-500, 1981.

84. M.S. Albert, N. Butters, and J. Brandt: "Development of Remote Memory Loss in Patients with Huntington's Disease," *Journal of Clinical Neuropsychology*, 3:1-12, 1981.

85. N. Butters: "The Wernicke-Korsakoff Syndrome: A Review of Psychological, Neuropathological and Etiological Factors," *Currents in Alcoholism*, edited by M. Galanter, pp. 205-232. New York: Grune and Stratton, 1981.

86. C. Biber, N. Butters, J. Rosen, and L. Gerstman, and S. Mattis: "Encoding Strategies and Recognition of Faces by Alcoholic Korsakoff and Other Brain-Damaged Patients," *Journal of Clinical Neuropsychology*, 3:315-330, 1981.

87. N. Butters and M.S. Albert: "Processes Underlying Failures to Recall Remote Events," *Human Memory and Amnesia*, edited by L.S. Cermak, pp. 257-274, NJ: L. Erlbaum Associates, 1982.

88. J. MacVane, N. Butters, K. Montgomery, and J. Farber: "Cognitive Functioning in Men Social Drinkers," *Journal Studies on Alcohol*, 43:81-95, 1982.

89. M.S. Albert, N. Butters, S. Rogers, J. Pressman, and A. Geller: "A Preliminary Report: Nutritional Levels and Cognitive Performance in Chronic Alcohol Abusers," *Drug and Alcohol Dependence*, 9:131-142, 1982.

90. M. Laine and N. Butters: "A Preliminary Study of the Problem-Solving Strategies of Detoxified Long-Term Alcoholics," *Drug and Alcohol Dependence*, 10:235-242, 1982.

91. B.P. Jones and N. Butters: "Neuropsychological Assessment," *The Clinical Psychology Handbook*, edited by M. Hersen, A. Kazdin and A. Bellack, pp. 377-396. Pergamon Press, 1983.

92. C. Ryan and N. Butters: "Cognitive Deficits in Alcoholics," *The Pathogenesis of Alcoholism*, edited by B. Kissin and H. Begleiter, pp. 485-538. New York: Plenum Press, 1983.

93. D. Sax, B. O'Donnel, N. Butters, L. Menzer, K. Montgomery, H. Kayne: "Computed Tomographic, Neurologic, and Neuropsychological Correlates of Huntington's Disease," *International Journal of Neuroscience*, 18:21-356, 1983.

94. E. Holmes, N. Butters, S. Jacobson, and B.M. Stein: "An Examination of the Effects of Mammillary-body Lesions on Reversal Learning Sets in Monkeys," *Physiological Psychology*, 3:159-165, 1983.

95. F.R. Sparadeo, W. Zwick, and N. Butters: "Cognitive Functioning of Alcoholic Females: An Exploratory Study," *Drug and Alcohol Dependence*, 12:143-150, 1983.

96. J. Brandt, N. Butters, C. Ryan, and R. Bayog: "Cognitive Loss and Recovery in Long-Term Alcohol Abusers," *Archives of General Psychiatry*, 40:435-442, 1983.

97. E.J. Holmes, S. Jacobson, B.M. Stein, N. Butters: "Ablations of the Mamillary Nuclei in Monkeys: Effects on Postoperative Memory," *Experimental Neurology*, 81:97-113, 1983.

98. N. Butters, M.S. Albert, D. Sax, P. Miliotis, J. Nagode, and A. Sterste: "The Effect of Verbal Mediators on the Pictorial Memory of Brain-Damaged Patients" *Neuropsychologia*, 21:307-323, 1983.

99. J. Becker, N. Butters, A. Hermann, and N. D'Angelo: "A Comparison of the Effects of Long-Term Alcohol Abuse and Aging on the Performance of Verbal and Nonverbal Divided Attention Tasks," *Alcoholism: Clinical and Experimental Research*, 7:213-219, 1983.

100. J. Becker, N. Butters, A. Hermann, and N. D'Angelo: "Learning to Associate Names and Faces: Impaired Acquisition on an Ecologically Relevant Memory Task by Male Alcoholics," *Journal of Nervous and Mental Disease*, 171:617-623, 1983.

101. M. Freedman, P. Riviora, N. Butters, D. Sax, and R. Feldman: "Retrograde Amnesia in Parkinson's Disease," *Canadian Journal of Neurological Sciences*, 11:297-301, 1984.

102. N. Butters and C. Ryan: "Alcohol Consumption and Premature Aging: A Critical Review," *Recent Developments in Alcoholism, Volume 2*, edited by G. Galanter, pp. 223-250. New York: Plenum Press, 1984.

103. R. Kenyon, J. Becker, and N. Butters: "Oculomotor Function in Wernicke-Korsakoff's Syndrome: II: Smooth Pursuit Eye Movements," *International Journal of Neuroscience*, 25:67-79, 1984.

104. N. Butters: "The Clinical Aspects of Memory Disorders: Contributions from Experimental Studies of Amnesia and Dementia," *Journal of Clinical Neuropsychology*, 6:17-36, 1984.

105. R. Kenyon, J. Becker, N. Butters, and H. Herman: "Oculomotor Function in Wernicke-Korsakoff's Syndrome: I: Saccadic Eye Movements," *International Journal of Neuroscience*, 25:53-65, 1984.

106. D. Davidoff, N. Butters, L. Gerstman, E. Zurif, I. Paul, and S. Mattis: "Affective/Motivational Factors in the Recall of Prose Passages by Alcoholic Korsakoff Patients," *Alcohol*, 1:63-69, 1984.

107. N. Butters, P. Miliotis, M.S. Albert, and D. Sax: "Memory Assessment: Evidence of the Heterogeneity of Amnesic Symptoms," *Advances in Clinical Neuropsychology*, edited by G. Goldstein, pp. 127-159. New York: Plenum Press, 1984.

108. C. Gebhardt, M. Naeser, and N. Butters: "Computerized Measures of CT Scans of Alcoholics: Thalamic Region Related to Memory," *Alcohol*, 1:133-140, 1984.

109. N. Butters: "Alcoholic Korsakoff's Syndrome: An Update," *Seminars in Neurology*, 4:226-244, 1984.

110. M. Martone, N. Butters, M. Payne, J. Becker, and D. Sax: "Dissociations Between Skill Learning and Verbal Recognition in Amnesia and Dementia," *Archives of Neurology*, 41:965-970. 1984.

111. N. Butters and J. Brandt: "The Continuity Hypothesis: The Relationship of Long-Term Alcoholism to the Wernicke-Korsakoff Syndrome," *Recent Developments in Alcoholism, Volume 3*, edited by M. Galanter, pp. 207-226, New York: Plenum Press, 1985.

112. N. Butters and P. Miliotis: "Amnesic Disorders," *Clinical Neuropsychology, 2nd Edition*, edited by K. Heilman and E. Valenstein, pp. 403-451. New York: Oxford University Press, 1985.

113. N. Butters: "Alcoholic Korsakoff's Syndrome: Some Unresolved Issues Concerning Etiology, Neuropathology, and Cognitive Deficits," *Journal of Clinical and Experimental Neuropsychology*, 7:181-210, 1985.

114. N. Butters, J. Wolfe, M. Martone, E. Granholm, and L.S. Cermak: "Memory Disorders Associated with Huntington's Disease: Verbal Recall, Verbal Recognition and Procedural Memory," *Neuropsychologia*, 6:729-744, 1985.

115. A.L. Glass and N. Butters: "The Effect of Associations and Expectations on Lexical Decision Making in Normals, Alcoholics and Alcoholic Korsakoff Patients," *Brain and Cognition*, 4:465-476, 1985.

116. E. Granholm, J. Wolfe, and N. Butters: "Affective-Arousal Factors in the Recall of Thematic Stories by Amnesic and Demented Patients," *Developmental Neuropsychology*, 1:317-333, 1985.

117. M. Martone, N. Butters, and D. Trauner: "Some Analyses of Forgetting of Pictorial Material in Amnesic and Demented Patients," *Journal of Clinical and Experimental Neuropsychology*, 8:161-178, 1986.

118. N. Butters, J. Wolfe, E. Granholm, and M. Martone: "An Assessment of Verbal Recall, Recognition, and Fluency Abilities in Patients with Huntington's Disease," *Cortex*, 22:11-32, 1986.

119. N. Butters: "The Clinical Aspects of Memory Disorders: Contributions from Experimental Studies of Amnesia and Dementia," *Clinical Application of Neuropsychological Test Batteries*, edited by T. Incagnoli, G. Goldstein, and C. Golden, pp. 361-382. New York: Plenum Press, 1986.

120. C. Ryan and N. Butters: "The Neuropsychology of Alcoholism," *The Neuropsychology Handbook: Behavioral and Clinical Perspectives*, edited by D. Wedding, A.M. Horton and J. Webster, pp. 376-409. New York: Springer Publishing Co., 1986.

121. J. Brandt and N. Butters: "The Alcoholic Wernicke-Korsakoff Syndrome and its Relationship to Long-Term Alcohol Abuse," *Neuropsychological Assessment of Neuropsychiatric Disorders*, edited by I. Grant and K. Adams, pp. 441-477. New York: Oxford University Press, 1986.

122. N. Butters and L.S. Cermak: "A Case Study of the Forgetting of Autobiographical Knowledge: Implications for the Study of Retrograde Amnesia," *Autobiographical Memory*, edited by D. Rubin, pp. 253-272. New York: Cambridge University Press, 1986.

123. J. Brandt and N. Butters: "The Neuropsychology of Huntington's Disease," *Trends in Neuroscience*, 9, No. 3, 9:3:118-120, 1986.

124. W. Beatty and N. Butters: "Further Analysis of Encoding in Patients with Huntington's Disease," *Brain and Cognition*, 5:387-398, 1986.

125. W. Beatty, N. Butters, and D. Janowsky: "Patterns of Memory Failure After Scopolamine Treatment: Implications for the Cholinergic Hypothesis of Dementia," *Behavioral and Neural Biology*, 45:192-211, 1986.

126. M. Moss, M.S. Albert, N. Butters, and M. Payne: "Differential Patterns of Memory Loss Among Patients with Alzheimer's Disease, Huntington's Disease and Alcoholic Korsakoff's Syndrome," *Archives of Neurology*, 43:239-246, 1986.

127. M. Grossman and N. Butters: "The Appreciation of Affect in Alcoholic Korsakoff Patients," *International Journal of Neuroscience*, 30:1-9, 1986.

128. N. Butters and D. Salmon: "Etiology and Neuropathology of Alcoholic Korsakoff's Syndrome: New Findings and Speculation," *Neuropsychiatric Correlates of Alcoholism*, edited by I. Grant, pp. 61-108. Washington, D.C.: American Psychiatric Press, 1986.

129. D. Salmon, N. Butters, and M. Schuckit: "Memory for Temporal Order and Frequency of Occurrence in Detoxified

130. N. Butters, M. Martone, B. White, E. Granholm and J. Wolfe: "Clinical Validators: Comparisons of Demented and Amnesic Patients," *Handbook of Clinical Memory Assessment of the Older Adult*, edited by L. Poon, pp. 337-352. Washington, D.C.: American Psychological Association, 1986.

131. J. Becker, N. Butters, P. Rivoira and P. Miliotis: "Asking the Right Questions: Problem-Solving in Alcoholics and Alcoholics with Korsakoff's Syndrome," *Alcoholism: Clinical and Experimental Research*, 10:641-646, 1986.

132. D. Salmon and N. Butters: "Recent Developments in Learning and Memory: Implications for the Rehabilitation of the Amnesic Patient," *Neuropsychological Rehabilitation*, edited by M. Meier, L. Diller, and A. Benton. pp. 280-293. London: Churchill Livingstone, 1987.

133. O. Parsons, N. Butters, and P. Nathan, editors: *Neuropsychology of Alcoholism: Implications for Diagnosis and Treatment*, New York: Guilford Press, 1987.

134. D. Salmon and N. Butters: "The Etiology and Neuropathology of Alcoholic Korsakoff's Syndrome: Some Evidence for the Role of the Basal Forebrain," *Recent Developments in Alcoholism*, Volume 5, edited by M. Galanter, pp. 27-58. New York: Plenum Press, 1987.

135. N. Butters, O. Parsons and P. Nathan: "Research Directions: The Next Decade," *Neuropsychology of Alcoholism: Implications for Diagnosis and Treatment*, edited by O. Parsons, N. Butters, and P. Nathan, pp. 392-403. New York: Guilford Press, 1987.

136. N. Butters and E. Granholm: "The Continuity Hypothesis: Some Conclusions and Their Implications for the Etiology and Neuropathology of the Alcoholic Korsakoff's Syndrome,"*Neuropsychology of Alcoholism: Implications for Diagnosis and Treatment*, edited by O. Parsons, N. Butters and P. Nathan, pp. 176-206. New York: Guilford Press, 1987.

137. W. Beatty, D. Salmon, N. Bernstein, M. Martone, L. Lyon and N. Butters: "Procedural Learning in a Patient with Amnesia due to Hypoxia," *Brain and Cognition*, 6:386-402, 1987.

138. N. Butters, E. Granholm, D. Salmon, I. Grant, and J. Wolfe: "Episodic and Semantic Memory: A Comparison of Amnesic and Demented Patients," *Journal of Clinical and Experimental Neuropsychology*, 9:479-497, 1987.

139. L. Judd, L. Squire, N. Butters, D. Salmon, and K. Paller: "Effects of Psychotropic Drugs on Cognition and Memory in Normal Humans and Animals," *Psychopharmacology: The Third Generation of Progress*, edited by H. Meltzer, pp. 1467-1475. New York: Raven Press, 1987.

140. N. Butters, D. Salmon, E. Granholm, W. Heindel, and L. Lyon: "Neuropsychological Differentiation of Amnesic and Dementing States," *Cognitive Neurochemistry*, edited by S. Stahl, S. Iversen, and E.C. Goodman, pp. 3-20. London: Oxford University Press, 1987.

141. A. Shimamura, D. Salmon, L. Squire, and N. Butters: "Memory Dysfunction and Word Priming in Dementia and Amnesia," *Behavioral Neuroscience*, 101:347-351, 1987.

142. M.A. Schuckit, N. Butters, L. Lyn, and M. Irwin: "Neuropsychologic Deficits and the Risk for Alcoholism," *Neuropsychopharmacology*, 1:1:45-53, 1987.

143. J. Wolfe, E. Granholm, N. Butters, E. Saunders, and D. Janowsky: "Verbal Memory Deficits Associated with Major Affective Disorders: A Comparison of Unipolar and Bipolar Patients," *Journal of Affective Disorders*, 13:83-92, 1987.

144. W. Beatty, D. Salmon, N. Bernstein, and N. Butters: "Remote Memory in a Patient with Amnesia Due to Hypoxia," *Psychological Medicine*, 17:657-665, 1987.

145. S. Smith, R. White, L. Lyon, E. Granholm, and N. Butters: "Priming Semantic Relations in Patients with Huntington's Disease," *Brain and Language*, 33:27-40, 1988.

146. S. Smith, N. Butters, and E. Granholm: "Activation of Semantic Relations in Alzheimer's and Huntington's Disease." *Neuropsychological Studies of Non-Focal Brain Damage: Dementia and Trauma*, edited by H. Whitaker, pp. 265-285. New York: Springer Verlag, 1988.

147. W. Heindel, N. Butters, and D. Salmon: "Impaired Learning of a Motor Skill in Patients with Huntington's Disease," *Behavioral Neuroscience*, 102:1:141-147, 1988.

148. N. Butters, D. Salmon, W. Heindel, and E. Granholm: "Episodic, Semantic and Procedural Memory: Some Comparisons of Alzheimer's and Huntington's Disease Patients," *Aging and the Brain*, edited by R. Terry, pp. 63-87. New York: Raven Press, 1988.

149. D. Salmon, B. Lasker, W. Beatty, and N. Butters: "Remote Memory in a Patient with Circumscribed Amnesia," *Brain and Cognition*, 7:201-211, 1988.

150. W. Beatty, D. Salmon, N. Butters, W. Heindel, and E. Granholm: "Retrograde Amnesia in Patients with Alzheimer's and Huntington's Disease," *Neurobiology of Aging*, 9:181-186, 1988.

151. N. Butters, D. Salmon, C.M. Cullum, P. Cairns, A. Tröster, D. Jacobs, M. Moss, and L.S. Cermak: "Differentiation of Amnesic and Demented Patients with the Wechsler Memory Scale Revised," *The Clinical Neuropsychologist*, 2:133-148, 1988.

152. D. Delis, C.M. Cullum, N. Butters, P. Cairns, and A. Prifitera: "The Wechsler Memory Scale-Revised and California Verbal Learning Test: Convergence and Divergence," *The Clinical Neuropsychologist*, 2:188-196, 1988.

153. H. Goodglass and N. Butters: "Psychobiology of Cognitive Processes," *Steven's Handbook of Experimental Psychology*, 2nd edition, edited by R. Atkinson, R. Herrnstein, G. Lindzey, and R. Luce, pp. 863-952. New York: Wiley Interscience, 1988.

154. E. Granholm and N. Butters: "Associative Encoding and Retrieval in Alzheimer's and Huntington's Disease," *Brain and Cognition*, 7:335-347, 1988.

155. D. Salmon, A. Shimamura, N. Butters, and S. Smith: "Lexical and Semantic Priming Deficits in Patients with Alzheimer's Disease," *Journal of Clinical and Experimental Neuropsychology*, 10:477-494, 1988.

156. L. Cermak and N. Butters: "Information Processing Deficits in Amnesia and Dementia," *Aphasiology*, 2:265-270, 1988.

157. D. Salmon, E. Granholm, D. McCullough, N. Butters, and I. Grant: "Recognition Memory Span in Mild and Moderately Demented Patients with Alzheimer's Disease," *Journal of Clinical and Experimental Neuropsychology*, 11:429-443, 1989.

158. W. Heindel, D. Salmon, and N. Butters: "Neuropsychological Differentiation of Memory Impairments in Dementia," *Memory, Aging and Dementia* edited by G. Gilmore, P. Whitehouse, and M. Wykle, pp. 112-139. New York: Springer Publishing Company, 1989.

159. N. Butters, D. Salmon, and W. Heindel: "Processes Underlying the Memory Impairments of Demented Patients," *Contemporary Neuropsychology and the Legacy of Luria* edited by E. Goldberg, pp. 99-126. New York: L. Erlbaum, 1990.

160. R. Katzman, T. Brown, L. Thal, P. Fuld, M. Aronson, N. Butters, M. Klauber, W. Wiederholt, M. Pay, X. Renbing, W. Ooi, R. Hofstetter, and R. Terry: "Comparison of Rate of Annual Change of Mental Status Score in Four Independent Studies of Patients with Alzheimer's Disease," *Annals of Neurology*, 24:384-389, 1988.

161. D. Salmon, W. Heindel, and N. Butters: "Neuropsychological Deficits in Early Alzheimer's Disease," *Bulletin of Clinical Neurosciences*, 53:25-31, 1988.

162. M. Irwin, N. Butters, T. Smith, S. Brown, S. Baird, and and M. Schuckit: "Graded Neuropsychological Impairment and Elevated Gamma Glutamyl Transferase in Chronic Alcoholic Men," *Alcoholism: Clinical and Experimental Research*, 13:99-103, 1989.

163. W. Heindel, D. Salmon, C. Shults, P. Walicke and N. Butters: "Neuropsychological Evidence for Multiple Implicit Memory Systems: A Comparison of Alzheimer's, Huntington's and Parkinson's Disease Patients," *Journal of Neuroscience*, 9:582-587, 1989.

164. A. Troster, D. Jacobs, N. Butters, C.M. Cullum, and D. Salmon: "Differentiating Alzheimer's from Huntington's disease with the Wechsler Memory Scale-Revised," *Clinics in Geriatric Medicine*, 5:611-632, 1989.

165. N. Butters and D. Stuss: "Diencephalic Amnesia," *Handbook of Neuropsychology*, Volume 3, edited by F. Boller and J. Grafman, pp. 107-148. The Netherlands: Elsevier, 1989.

166. D. Salmon, P. Kwo-on-Yuen, W. Heindel, N. Butters, and L. Thal: "Differentiation of Alzheimer's Disease and Huntington's Disease with the Dementia Rating Scale," *Archives of Neurology*, 46:1204-1209, 1989.

167. A. Troster, D. Salmon, D. McCullough, and N. Butters: "A Comparison of the Category Fluency Deficits Associated with Alzheimer's and Huntington's Disease," *Brain and Language*, 37:500-513, 1989.

168. T. Jernigan and N. Butters: "Neuropsychological and Neuroradiological Distinctions Between Alzheimer's and Huntington's Diseases," *Neuropsychology*, 3:283-290, 1989.

169. R. Dupont, T. Jernigan, N. Butters, D. Delis, J. Hesselink, W. Heindel, and J. Gillin: "Subcortical Abnormalities Detected in Bipolar Affective Disorder Using Magnetic Resonance Imaging: Clinical and Neuropsychological Significance," *Archives of General Psychiatry*, 47:55-59, 1990.

170. L. Hansen, D. Salmon, D. Galasko, E. Masliah, R. Katzman, R. De Teresa, L. Thal, M. Pay, R. Hofstetter, M. Klauber, V. Rice, N. Butters, and M. Alford: "The Lewy Body Variant of Alzheimer's Disease: A Clinical and Pathological Entity," *Neurology*, 40:1-8, 1990.

171. D. Jacobs, D. Salmon, A. Troster, and N. Butters: "Intrusion Errors in the Figural Memory of Patients with Alzheimer's and Huntington's Disease," *Archives of Clinical Neuropsychology*, 5:49-57, 1990.

172. C.M. Cullum, N. Butters, A. Toster, and D. Salmon: "Normal Aging and Forgetting Rates on the Wechsler Memory Scale- Revised," *Archives of Clinical Neuropsychology*, 5:23-30, 1990.

173. N. Butters, W. Heindel, and D. Salmon: "Dissociation of Implicit Memory in Dementia: Neurological Implications," *Bulletin of the Psychonomic Society*, 28:4:359-366, 1990.

174. D. Jacobs, A. Troster, N. Butters, D. Salmon and L. Cermak: "Intrusion Errors on the Visual Reproduction Test of the Wechsler Memory Scale and the Wechsler Memory Scale-Revised: An Analysis of Demented and Amnesic Patients," *The Clinical Neuropsychologist*, 4:177-191, 1990.

175. D. Salmon, L. Thal, N. Butters, and W. Heindel: "Longitudinal Evaluation of Dementia of the Alzheimer type: A comparison of Three Standardized Mental Status Examinations," *Neurology*, 40:1225-1230, 1990.

176. W. Heindel, D. Salmon, and N. Butters: "Pictoral Priming and Cued Recall in Alzheimer's and Huntington's Disease," *Brain and Cognition*, 13:282-295. 1990.

177. P. Massman, D. Delis, N. Butters, B. Levin, and D. Salmon: "Are all Subcortical Dementias Alike?: Verbal Learning and memory in Parkinson's and Huntington's Disease Patients," *Journal of Clinical and Experimental Neuropsychology*, 12:729-744, 1990.

178. N. Butters, I. Grant, J. Haxby, and L. Judd et al.: "Assessment of AIDS-Related Cognitive Changes: Recommendations of the NIMH Work Group on Neuropsychological Assessment Approaches," *Journal of Clinical and Experimental Neuropsychology,* 12:963-978, 1990.

179. J. Hodges, D. Salmon, and N. Butters: "Differential Impairment of Semantic and Episodic Memory in Alzheimer's and Huntington's Disease: A Controlled and Prospective Study," *Journal of Neurology, Neurosurgery and Psychiatry,* 53:1089-1095, 1990.

180. T. Jernigan, D. Salmon, N. Butters, and J. Hesselink: "Cerebral Structure on MRI, Part II: Specific Changes in Alzheimer's and Huntington's Diseases," *Biological Psychiatry,* 29:68-8,. 1991.

181. D. Delis, P. Massman, N. Butters, D. Salmon, L.S. Cermak, and J. Kramer: "Profiles of Demented and Amnesic Patients on the California Verbal Learning Test: Implications for the Assessment of Memory Disorders," *Psychological Assessment: A Journal of Consulting and Clinical Psychology,* 3:19-26, 1991.

182. K. Welsh, N. Butters, J Hughes, R. Mohs, and A Heyman: "Detection of Abnormal Memory Decline in Mild Cases of Alzheimer's Disease Using CERAD Neuropsychological Measures," *Archives of Neurology,* 48:278-281, 1991.

183. W. Heindel, D. Salmon, and N. Butters: "Alcoholic Korsakoff's Syndrome," *Memory Disorders: Research and Clinical Practice,* edited by T. Yangihara and R. Peterson, pp. 227-253. New York: Marcel Dekker, Inc., 1991.

184. G. DiTraglia, D. Press, N. Butters, T. Jernigan, L.S. Cermak, et al.: "Assessment of Olfactory Deficits in Detoxified Alcoholics," *Alcohol,* 8:109-115, 1991.

185. S. Ancoli-Israel, M. Klauber, N. Butters, L. Park and D. Kripke: "Dementia in Institutionalized Elderly: Relation to Sleep Apnea," *Journal of the American Geriatrics Society,* 39:258-263, 1991.

186. W. Heindel, D. Salmon, and N. Butters: "The Biasing of Weight Judgments in Alzheimer's and Huntington's Disease: A Priming or Programming Phenomenon?," *Journal of Clinical and Experimental Neuropsychology,* 13:189-203, 1991.

187. T. Jernigan, K. Schafer, N. Butters, and L.S. Cermak: "Magnetic Resonance Imaging of Alcoholic Korsakoff Patients," *Neuropsychopharmacology*, 4:175-186, 1991.

188. T. Jernigan, N. Butters, G. DiTraglia, K. Schafer, T. Smith, M. Irwin, I. Grant, M Schuckit, and L.S. Cermak: "Reduced Cerebral Grey Matter Observed in Alcoholics Using Magnetic Resonance Imaging," *Alcoholism: Clinical and Experimental Research*, 15:418-427, 1991.

189. B. Jones and N. Butters: "Neuropsychological Assessment," *The Clinical Psychology Handbook*, 2nd Edition, edited by M. Hersen, A. Kazdin, and A. Bellack, pp. 406-429. New York: Pergamon Press, 1991.

190. J. Hodges, D. Salmon, N. Butters: "The Nature of the Naming Deficit in Alzheimer's and Huntington's Disease," *Brain* , 114:1547-1558, 1991.

191. K. Schafer, N. Butters, T. Smith, M. Irwin, et al.: "Cognitive Performance of Alcoholics: A Longitudinal Evaluation of the Role of Drinking History, Depression, Liver Function, Nutrition and Family History," *Alcoholism: Clinical and Experimental Research*, 15:4:653-660, 1991.

192. R. Terry, E. Masliah, D. Salmon, R. DeTeresa, R. Hill, N. Butters, L. Hansen, R. Katzman: "Physical Basis of Cognitive Alterations in Alzheimer's Disease: Synapse Loss is the Major Correlate of Cognitive Impairment," *Annals of Neurology*. 30: 572-580, 1991.

193. M. O'Connor, N. Butters, R. Miliotis, P. Eslinger, and L.S. Cermak: "The Dissociation of Anterograde and Retrograde Amnesia in a Patient with Herpes Encephalitis," *Journal of Clinical and Experimental Neuropsychology*, 2: 159-178, 1992.

194. D. Delis, P. Massman, N. Butters, D. Salmon, P. Shear, T. Demadura and J. Filoteo: "Spatial Cognition in Alzheimer's Disease: Subtypes of Global-Local Impairment," *Journal of Clinical and Experimental Neuropsychology*, 14:463-477, 1992.

195. I. Rouleau, D. Salmon, N. Butters, C. Kennedy and K. McGuire: "Quantitative and Qualitative Analyses of Clock Drawings in Alzheimer's and Huntington's Disease," *Brain and Cognition*, 18:70-87, 1992.

196. K. Welsh, N. Butters, J. Hughes, R. Mohs and A. Heyman: "Detection and Staging of Dementia in Alzheimer's Disease. "*Archives of Neurology*, 49:448-452, 1992.

197. N. Butters: "Memory Remembered: 1970-1991," *Archives of Clinical Neuropsychology*, 7:285-295, 1992.

198. J. Hodges, D. Salmon and N. Butters: "Semantic Memory Impairment in Alzheimer's Disease: Failure of Access or Degraded Knowledge?", *Neuropsychologia*, 30:301-314, 1992.

199. P. Massman, D. Delis, N. Butters, R. Dupont and J.C. Gillin: "The Subcortical Dysfunction Hypothesis of Memory Deficits in Depression: Neuropsychological Validation in a Subgroup of Patients," *Journal of Clinical and Experimental Neuropsychology*, 14:687-706, 1992.

200. D. Salmon, W. Heindel and N. Butters: "Semantic Memory, Priming and Skill Learning in Alzheimer's Disease, " *Memory Functioning in Dementia*, pp. 99-118. Edited by L. Backman, Amsterdam: Elsevier Science Publishers, 1992.

201. N. Butters: "Explicit and Implicit Memory Disorders Associated with Dementia," in *Neuropsychology: The Neuronal Basis of Cognitive Function*, pp. 67-79, Thieme Medical Publishers: New York, 1992.

202. P. Sutker, A. Allain, J. Johnson and N. Butters: "Memory and Learning Performances in POW Survivors with History of Malnutrition and Combat Veteran Controls", *Archives of Clinical Neuropsychology*, 7:431-444, 1992.

203. P. Shear, N. Butters, T. Jernigan, G. DiTraglia, M. Irwin, M. Schuckit and L.S. Cermak: "Olfactory Loss in Alcoholics: Correlations with Cortical and Subcortical MRI Indices," *Alcohol*, 9:247-255, 1992.

204. L. Squire and N. Butters (Editors): *Neuropsychology of Memory*, 2nd Edition, New York: Guilford Press, 1992.

205. D. Salmon and N. Butters: "Neuropsychological Assessment of Dementia in the Elderly," in *Principles of Geriatric Neurology*, R. Katzman and J. Rowe (Editors), pp. 144-164. Philadelphia: F.A. Davis, 1992.

206. J.V Filoteo, D. Delis, P. Massman, T. Demadura, N. Butters and David Salmon: "Directed and Divided Attention in Alzheimer's Disease: Impairment in Shifting of Attention to Global and Local Stimuli," *Journal of Clinical and Experimimental Neuropsychology*, 14: 871-883, 1992.

207. T. Diamond, R. White, R. Myers, C. Mastromauro, W. Koroshetz, N. Butters, D. Rothstein, M. Moss and J. Vasterling: "Evidence of Presymptomatic Cognitive Decline in Huntington's Disease," *Journal of Clinical and Experimental Neuropsychology*, 14: 961-975, 1992.

208. A.U. Monsch, M.W. Bondi, N. Butters, D.P. Salmon, R. Katzman and L.J. Thal: "Comparisons of Verbal Fluency Tasks in the Detection of Dementia of the Alzheimer Type, *Archives of Neurology*, 49: 1253-1258, 1992.

209. T. Jernigan, N. Butters and L.S. Cermak: "Studies of Brain Structure in Chronic Alcoholism Using Magnetic Resonance Imaging," in *Research Monograph 21: Imaging in Alcohol Research*, S. Zakhari and E. Witt (editors), pp. 121-134, National Institute on Alcohol Abuse and Alcoholism: Rockville, MD., 1992.

210 J. Paulsen, N. Butters, D. Salmon, W. Heindel and M. Swenson: "Prism Adaptation in Alzheimer's and Huntington's Disease," *Neuropsychology*, 7:73-81, 1993.

211. W.C. Heindel, D.P. Salmon and N. Butters: "Cognitive Approaches to the Memory Disorders of Demented Patients," in *Comprehensive Handbook of Psychopathology* (2nd edition), P.B. Sutker and H.E. Adams (editors), pp. 735-761, Plenum Press: NY, 1993.

212. P.J. Massman, D.C. Delis and N. Butters: "Does Impaired Primacy Recall Equal Impaired Long-Term Storage?: Serial Position Effects in Huntington's and Alzheimer's Disease," *Developmental Neuropsychology*, 9:1-15, 1993.

213. P.J. Eslinger, H. Damasio, A.R. Damasio and N. Butters: "Nonverbal Amnesia and Asymmetric Cerebral Lesions Following Encephalitis," *Brain and Cognition*, 21:140-152, 1993.

214. A. Chan, N. Butters, J. Paulsen, D. Salmon, M. Swenson and L. Maloney: "An Assessment of the Semantic Network in Patients with Alzheimer's Disease", *Journal of Cognitive Neuroscience*, 5:254-261, 1993.

215. P. Massman, D. Delis, V. Filoteo, N. Butters, D. Salmon, nd T. Demadura: "Mechanisms of Spatial Impairment in Alzheimer's Disease Subgroups: Differential Breakdown of Directed Attention to Global-Local Stimuli", *Neuropsychology*, 7:172-181, 1993.

216. M. Bondi, A. Monsch, N. Butters, D. Salmon and J. Paulsen: "Utility of a Modified Version of the Wisconsin Card Sorting Test in the dectection of Dementia of the Alzheimer's Type", *The Clinical Neuropsychologist*, 7:161-170, 1992.

217. W.C. Widerholt, D. Cahn, N. Butters, D. Salmon, D. Kritz-Silverstein, E. Barrett-Connor: "Effects of Age, Gender and Education on the Selected Tests in an Elderly Community Cohort", *JAGS*, 41:639-647, 1993.

218. J.R. Hodges, D.P Salmon, N. Butters: "Recognition and Naming of Famous Faces in Alzheimer's Disease: A Cognitive Analysis", *Neuropsychologia*, 31:775-788, 1993.

219. D. P. Salmon, N. Butters, W.C. Heindel: "Alcohol Dementia and Related Disorders," *Neuropsychology of Alzheimer's Disease and Other Dementias*, edited by R.W. Parks, R.F. Zec, R.S. Wilson, pp. 186-209, New York: Oxford University Press, 1993.

220. A. Troster, N. Butters, D. Salmon, C.M. Cullum, D. Jacobs, J. Brandt and R. White: "The Diagnostic Utility of Saving Scores: Differentiating Alzheimer's and Huntington's Disease with the Logical Memory and Visual Reproduction Tests", *Journal of Clinical and Experimental Neuropsychology*, 15:773-788, 1993.

221. N. Butters, A Chan, D.P. Salmon and K. McGuire: "Dimensionality and Clustering in the Semantic Network of Patients with Alzheimer's Disease", *Psychology and Aging*, 8:411-419. 1993.

222. M.A. Butters, D.P. Salmon and N. Butters: Neuropsychological Assessment of Dementia". In M. Storandt and G. VandenBos (Eds) *Neuropsychological assessment of older adults: Dementia and Depression.* American Psychological Association, Washington, DC (In Press)

223. N. Butters, D.P. Salmon and W.C. Heindel: Specificity of the Memory Deficits Associated with Basil Ganglia Dysfunction", *Revue Neurologique* (Paris). (In Press)

224. A.U. Monch, M.W. Bondi, N. butters, J.S. Paulsen, D. Salmon P. Brugger, and M.R. Swensen: "A Comparison of Category and Letter Fluency in Alzheimer's Disease and Huntington's Disease", *Neuropsychology,* 8:25-30, 1994.

225. P.K. Shear, T.L. Jernigan and N. Butters: "Volumetric Magnetic Resonance Imaging Quantification of Logitudinal Brain Changes in Abstinent Alcoholics", *Alcohol, Clinical and Experimental Research*, 18:172-176, 1994.

226. J.C. Gillin, T.L. Smith, M. Irwin, N. Butters, A. Demodena and M. Schuckit. "Increased Pressure for Rapid Eye Movement Sleep at Time of Hospital Admission Predicts Relapse in Nondepressed Patients with Primary Alcoholism at 3-Month Follow-up. *Archives of General Psychiatry* 51:189-197, 1994.

227. K.A. Welsh, N. Butters, R.C. Mohs, D. Keekley, S. Edland G. Fillenbaum, and A. Heyman. "The Consortium to Establish a Registry of Alzheimer's Disease (CER^A^D, Part V: A normative study of the neuropsychological battery. *Neurology*, 44:609-614, 1994.

228. P.J. Massman, N. Butters and D.C. Delis: Some Comparisons of the Verbal Learning Deficits Alzheimer's Dementia, Huntington's and Depression". In V.O. Emery and T. E. Oxman (Eds.), *DEMENTIA: Presentations, Differential Diagnosis, and Nosology.* The Johns Hopkins University Press, Pgs. 232-248, 1994.

229. M. Bondi, D. Salmon and N. Butters. Neuropsychological features of memory disorders in Alzheimer's Disease. In R.D. Terry, R. Katzman and K. Bick (Eds.), *Alzheimer Disease*, Raven Press: Pgs. 41-63, 1994.

230. J.V. Filoteo, D.C. Delis, P.J. Massman and N. Butters. Visuospatial dysfunction in dementia and normal aging. In F.A. Huppert, C. Brayne, and D. W. O'Connor (Eds.), *Dementia and normal aging.* New York: Cambridge University Press, Pgs. 366-381, 1994.

231. N. Butters, M. O'Connor and M. Verfaellie. Investigations of the Explicit and Implicit Memory Abilities of a Patient with Nonverbal Memory Problems, Retrograde Amnesia, and a Visual Imaging Deficit. In R. Campbell and M. Conway (Eds.), *Broken Memories.* Blackwell Publishers, Oxford, England. (In Press)

232. W. Samuel, R. Terry, R. De Teresa, N. Butters, and E. Masliah. Clinical correlates of cortical and nucleus basalis pathology in Alzheimer's Disease. *Archives of Neurology.* (In Press)

Index

ISBN 0-306-44983-8
90000

9 780306 449833